PET and PET/CT Stud

Andrzej Moniuszko • Adam Sciuk

PET and PET/CT Study Guide

A Review for Passing the PET Specialty Exam

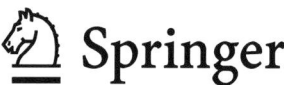

Andrzej Moniuszko
Department of Nuclear Medicine
Resurrection Medical Center
Chicago, IL, USA

Adam Sciuk
Department of Radiology
Resurrection Medical Center
Chicago, IL, USA

ISBN 978-1-4614-2286-0   ISBN 978-1-4614-2287-7 (Ebook)
DOI 10.1007/978-1-4614-2287-7
Springer New York Heidelberg Dordrecht London

Library of Congress Control Number: 2012947031

© Springer Science+Business Media, LLC 2013
This work is subject to copyright. All rights are reserved by the Publisher, whether the whole or part of the material is concerned, specifically the rights of translation, reprinting, reuse of illustrations, recitation, broadcasting, reproduction on microfilms or in any other physical way, and transmission or information storage and retrieval, electronic adaptation, computer software, or by similar or dissimilar methodology now known or hereafter developed. Exempted from this legal reservation are brief excerpts in connection with reviews or scholarly analysis or material supplied specifically for the purpose of being entered and executed on a computer system, for exclusive use by the purchaser of the work. Duplication of this publication or parts thereof is permitted only under the provisions of the Copyright Law of the Publisher's location, in its current version, and permission for use must always be obtained from Springer. Permissions for use may be obtained through RightsLink at the Copyright Clearance Center. Violations are liable to prosecution under the respective Copyright Law.
The use of general descriptive names, registered names, trademarks, service marks, etc. in this publication does not imply, even in the absence of a specific statement, that such names are exempt from the relevant protective laws and regulations and therefore free for general use.
While the advice and information in this book are believed to be true and accurate at the date of publication, neither the authors nor the editors nor the publisher can accept any legal responsibility for any errors or omissions that may be made. The publisher makes no warranty, express or implied, with respect to the material contained herein.

Springer is part of Springer Science+Business Media (www.springer.com)

I would like to dedicate this work to my brother Jerzy, my sister-in-law Teresa, and my dear nieces Jola, Violetka, and Margie for all their help and indefatigable support at the beginning of my new medical journey.

Andrzej Moniuszko

To my lovely wife Kasia, son Jakub, and daughter Ola for their love, support, and inspiration.

Adam Sciuk

Preface

The *PET and PET/CT Study Guide* is designed for technologists, practitioners, and trainees in medical imaging to serve as a practical tool to study multiple aspects of PET and PET/CT. The book was written and reviewed by individuals from a wide spectrum of nuclear medicine expertise: an experienced nuclear medicine technologist, a new graduate of nuclear medicine technology program, a practicing nuclear medicine physician, and a nuclear medicine college teacher. A broad assembly of authors and contributors, with different nuclear medicine experiences, provides an array of problems that technologists, practitioners, and trainees can, and will, encounter in everyday practice. Some of the questions are easy, and some of them are not. In either case, the book is not designed to test the reader's knowledge. Rather, it should be viewed as tool to learn and build the skills necessary in utilizing this compelling modality in daily practice. It is said that a picture is worth a thousand words. Our book includes more than 75 images, graphics, and diagrams. It is our goal for these illustrations to help readers get to the bottom of the problem and to come up with the right solution quickly.

The book is divided into five chapters and an appendix. We kick things off with a chapter on test taking strategies, which is designed to equip readers with practical tools and methods to successfully navigate through the multiple-choice exam. It was written by a recent graduate and the hands-on experience provides readers with valuable insider tips.

Chapters 2–5 contain the test problems. Each test includes multiple-choice questions with a total number of 650 problems; chapters are organized into levels of complexity, from the easiest to the most difficult.

Generally, tagging questions as easy or difficult is a tricky matter, and highly subjective. Nevertheless, for learning purposes, the proposed classification will be beneficial to readers. Each chapter is a separate entity with answers and optional short explanations included. This will work like building blocks, where the completion of the first test will prepare the reader to progress to the second test, and so on.

Appendix A consists of the critical formulas, numbers, and normal range values for some of the quantitative nuclear medicine procedures. It is suggested, for those preparing for the licensee examination, to commit these to memory; for others, it is for reference purposes only.

Appendix B offers a list of commonly used abbreviations that are encountered in everyday nuclear medicine practice, and beyond. The list can appear as too short or simply too long. Some readers will find the included terms as "unnecessary"; some readers will not find the abbreviation they are looking for. One size never fits all, and thus the subjective choices, as is our selection, are not perfect. Use it to your advantage. There is enough space between the lines, and in the margins, to modify to your own preferences. Understanding the acronyms will pay off in the long run; simply being able to decode it, will be short-lived. Therefore, a thorough review of the abbreviations before the examinations can be very helpful, and highly suggested.

Appendix C presents a glossary of frequently used terms in nuclear medicine, and again, we strongly advise a thorough review of the terms.

Appendix D is comprised of web site addresses that offer priceless and free information on many topics related to the nuclear medicine field.

The present collection of problems mirrors the exam content as provided by NMTCB. The questions cover radiation safety, radionuclides, and instrumentation to name a few. The reader should never be discouraged when the type of "never heard of" or "it is over my head" problem is encountered. We advise students to go through these questions carefully, and answer diligently—you will be surprised how much you already know and how much you can still learn. Both factors serve as great motivators. Learning should be fun, entertaining, and contagious. Positron emission tomography is a powerful, challenging, and rapidly evolving field of medicine and the only way to keep pace with its development is through continuous learning. Make it fun, and make it a habit—this is the kind of addiction that you can afford. The benefits are overwhelming. You can receive the 24 continuing education credit hours and keep your professional license. You can read, you can study, you can investigate, and you can challenge yourself and others. Best of all you can exceed…your own expectations. The choice is yours.

We want to thank Prof. Joanne Metler, Coordinator of Nuclear Medicine Technology Program, College of DuPage, IL, for her patience in reviewing our manuscript. Her dedication, helpful criticism, and detailed oriented effort deserve nothing but our sincere appreciation. It is beyond the scope of words to express our appreciation for the opportunity of knowledge and her enthusiasm, suggestions, inspiration, and encouragement to write this book. Thank you for being with us through every chapter of our book.

We would also like to thank Mrs. Sabina Moniuszko for devotion and intractable eagerness when preparing diagrams and drawings we used in this book, to Dharmesh Patel for authoring math questions, and to Mr. George Chang, PACS coordinator, Resurrection Medical Center, for his priceless help in preparing clinical images.

About the Authors

Andrzej Moniuszko received an MD degree in 1977 from Medical University in Bialystok, Poland. In 1995 he moved to the US and two years later passed all exams required by the United States Medical Licensing Examination (USMLE). He completed a Nuclear Medicine Technology Program in College of DuPage, Glen Ellyn, IL and now works as a Nuclear Medicine Technologist in Resurrection Medical Center, Chicago, IL and holds CNMT, ARRT (N), PET and NCT certifications.

The dualistic nature of nuclear medicine, which combines interdisciplinary, state-of-the-art diagnostic imaging with the softer side of taking care of patients and helping people, perfectly fits Andrzej's (Andy's) personality. During the many years of his medical experience he has viewed revolutions of treatment regimens and transformations of imaging protocols. Through these changes he has learned that the only things that have not changed over time are the patients' fears, worries, and concerns, all of which he calls a lesson in humbleness.

Adam Sciuk is a polish-born physician who received his initial medical training at the Military Medical Academy in Poland. After finishing his internship he emigrated to United States and completed Diagnostic Radiology residency program at the Louisiana State University in Shreveport. Throughout his residency he participated in several clinical research projects, some of which resulted in presentations on the national level. For his achievements he was awarded with the Roentgen Resident/Fellow Research Award. Dr. Sciuk has also completed fellowships in Nuclear Medicine and Diagnostic Magnetic Resonance Imaging at the University of Wisconsin in Madison, where he focused on Positron Emission Tomography, its applications in oncology imaging, and correlation with whole body diffusion imaging. Dr. Sciuk is currently an attending radiologist at Resurrection Medical Center in Chicago where he combines clinical work with his research passion.

Contents

1	**Tackling the Multiple-Choice Test**	1
	Tackling the Test Anxiety	3
	Suggested Readings	4
2	**Practice Test # 1: Difficulty Level-Easy**	5
	Questions	5
	Answers	45
	References and Suggested Readings	73
3	**Practice Test # 2: Difficulty Level-Moderate**	77
	Questions	77
	Answers	120
	References and Suggested Readings	148
4	**Practice Test # 3: Difficulty Level-Hard**	153
	Questions	153
	Answers	191
	References and Suggested Readings	222
5	**Practice Test # 4: Bonus Questions**	227
	Questions	227
	Answers	240
	References and Suggested Readings	247
Appendix A:	**Numbers and Formulas**	249
Appendix B:	**Commonly Used Abbreviations and Symbols in Nuclear Medicine**	259
Appendix C:	**Glossary**	273
Appendix D:	**Useful Websites**	287
Author Index		291
Subject Index		295

Contributors

Andrzej Moniuszko, MD Nuclear Medicine Technologist, Department of Nuclear Medicine, CNMT, ARRT(N), NCT, PET, Resurrection Medical Center, Chicago, IL, USA

Marta L. Moniuszko, MBA, BS Lead System Analyst, HRO Outsourcing, Aon Hewitt, Lincolnshire, IL, USA

Sabina Moniuszko Student, Physical Therapy. Oakton Community College, Des Plaines, IL, USA

Dharmesh Patel Associate, Nuclear Medicine Technologist, Department of Nuclear Medicine, Resurrection Medical Center, Chicago, IL, USA

Adam Sciuk, MD Staff Radiologist, Department of Radiology, Resurrection Medical Center, Chicago, IL, USA

Chapter 1
Tackling the Multiple-Choice Test

The Positron Emission Tomography specialty exam is administered by Nuclear Medicine Technology Certification Board (NMTCB). Once you decide to take the exam, the first step you should take is to visit its web site and familiarize yourself with the test information provided. Make the effort to know the intimate details of NMTCB's exams. The PET exam is now available "on demand." This means that once you are notified that your application has been approved, you may choose when you'd like to take it, as opposed to a designated one-time examination date.

Multiple choice is the most common test format for standardized tests. It helps to understand the basic setup of this type of a test before tackling it.

A multiple-choice test is composed of three elements: stem, options, and distractors. The stem is the basic problem, and it may be either a question or an incomplete statement. Options are the list of responses available. The list contains one correct answer, and the remaining ones act as the distractors. The distractors are designed to appear as a plausible answer. You, as the test taker, must choose the best answers from the list of alternatives. Now, multiple-choice questions are, in fact, objective questions; they are based on information without the ambiguity of test taker's opinion or interpretation. This, coupled with the known and structured test format, allows the candidate to actually approach the test strategically.

Let us lay down the different methods and strategies for taking the multiple-choice test.

- Cover the list of responses with your hand, read the stem carefully, and actually try to answer the question before looking at the possible choices. By doing so, you will not be negatively influenced or confused by the available choices. Pick the response which best matches your initial answer.
- Read the stem thoroughly (you can write down the important words), determine what is being asked, and then read all the answers carefully. Compare each choice to what you think is the correct answer, eliminate the obviously incorrect answers, and choose your answer from the remaining options.

- Another useful approach is to read the stem together with each of the options, one by one. Treat each combination as if it was a True/False question. If the combined statement is false, you can eliminate that option; if it appears to be correct, mark it as a possible answer. Repeat this for all alternatives.
- For questions that are more complicated or difficult, try to simplify the stem, and summarize or rephrase the answers. In this way, both the stem and the options will be clearer, and make more sense to you, making the question more manageable.
- If none of the choices available to you match your predetermined answer, you can use one of the following techniques to narrow down to the probable answer:
  - Usually the positive answer or the longer/st response with most information is more likely to be the correct.
  - Responses containing phrases such as "All of the Above" or "None of the Above" are also more likely to be true. However, you must be careful. Do read all of the preceding responses, and ensure all of them apply.
  - Be cautious of trap words such as "never," "every," "always," "only," and "completely." Read the alternatives containing these words very thoroughly. Keep in mind that options with absolute phrases suggest that the statement is always true, which is rarely correct.
  - On the other hand, words such as "may," "generally," "some," "usually," and "often" are clues that the answer might be correct.
  - Eliminate answers that are otherwise true but do not apply to the stem. In other words, if the option is only partially true or incorrect as it relates to the stem, reject it.
  - If two answers have similar one or two words or words that sound or look similar, choose one of the two.
- It is a good and advised practice to first answer the questions you are comfortable with, and not to get distracted if you cannot answer a question. Instead, tag each appropriately, and then go back and reattempt to find the answers. Remember, the entire test is full of hints, and information contained in one part may help you in another.
- Keep in mind, usually your first choice is the correct one. Unless you determine based on information further along in the test or you are certain you misread the stem or the alternatives, you should not change your answer.
- If all of the above fail, guess, but do not guess until you have eliminated all of the definitely incorrect options. There is no penalty for incorrect answers.

In general, as it applies, you are not able to skip a question (leave it unanswered), but you may mark it, and come back to it later. You might also be allowed to review your choices, and change any answer before submitting the test. Each test administrator offers a brief test tutorial before the examination with sample questions. These are designed to help you familiarize yourself with the test process, and format of the questions.

Reading this section should arm you with a good selection of strategies to help you make your way through the multiple-choice test. Simultaneously, you are probably beginning to feel a slight hint of anxiety. The nervousness is likely to increase as you near your test exam date, and will peak during the actual examination. It is just as equally important, therefore, to look into the arsenal of anxiety-fighting tools.

Tackling the Test Anxiety

Preparation, both mental and physical, is said to be the number one killer of text anxiety. We will first explore this weapon.

There is a myriad of literature on the subject of studying methods. Having gotten as far as you have in your life, I trust you must have had developed a good study technique that carried you this far. But for those that have been out of the study realm, let us review some of the basics of good study habits.

First of all, you must develop a study strategy. Depending on numerous factors, like available time, time length before the exam, mental agility, and subject familiarity, the study plan will be different. Be realistic; you know what works for you, and with your schedule, build the strategy accordingly. But also remember, as Dwight D. Eisenhower once said about preparing for the battle, "Plans are worthless, but planning is indispensable." Make plans, and adjust them as your personal circumstances change. The most important thing is to continuously manage your study time, and not to procrastinate. The study guide you hold in your hand is designed to help you navigate through the preparation. In a situation when you will find yourself lost in the piles of supplemental books, index cards, post-it notes, or tape recorders, here are a few study tips to get you back on track.

- Approach studying with positive attitude, and at the same time, eliminate any negative thoughts related to yourself or the actual studying.
- Arrange, or rearrange, your schedule to minimize any outside distractions. You should have a designated study area, preferably in a secluded, quite, and well-lighted place.
- Determine the part of the material you are going to study, and for how long. Have everything ready and within reach, and remove everything that is not related to the particular section. Stick to the plan.
- If you catch yourself day dreaming, or losing concentration, switch to a different study area or subject.
- Take breaks. You can stretch, take a brisk walk, or eat a snack. Stop when you are feeling tired or are simply no longer productive.

This will take care of preparing mentally for the exam, and reducing some of the anxiety that is uprooted from simply not being prepared. Just as importantly, you have to be physically ready. In general, the stronger the body is, the stronger the mind. Exercise throughout the entire study phase, but especially days before the examination. It will significantly reduce your stress level, and improve brain function. Get a good night's sleep the night before the exam, and eat a nourishing breakfast. Your brain cannot operate without glucose, and you will run out of energy without sufficient food in your body. Dress comfortably, preferably in layers, so you are able to adjust your attire to the temperature inside the testing center. Prepare everything you need for the test the day ahead, and leave yourself ample time to arrive at the destination. Being mentally and physically prepared is bound to eliminate the majority of the test-related anxiety. There is, however, always a small percentage of anxiety that will always be present in a high stakes environment. Accept it, it will actually help you stay alert, and sharpen your mental reflexes.

On the day of the examination it is critical to remain relaxed, and release any mental or physical anxiety. To do so, arrive early to the test site, and do not study or review the material after your arrival. Rather, take a moment to yourself to perform couple of slow-breathing exercises, and simultaneously visualize yourself at a peaceful place. This will allow you to stay calm and relaxed. During the examination, the outmost important thing is for you to concentrate on the question directly before. Do not fall into the trap of thinking about the question you just answered or the questions that follow. Your goal is to answer that question correctly. That is all that matters. The best tennis players win because they never let the ball out of their eyesight. Follow their winning practices. After the examination is completed, reflect back on your accomplishment, and reward yourself!

Thomas A. Edison once said: "Many of life's failures are people who did not realize how close they were to success when they gave up." If he did give up, we might still be sitting in the dark. Don't. Good luck!

Suggested Readings

Blackey R. So many choices, so little time: strategies for understanding and taking multiple-choice exams in history. Hist Teach. 2009;43(1):53–66.
Gloe D. Study habits and test-taking tips. Dermatol Nurs. 1999;11:493–9.
Kubistant T. Test performance: the neglected skill. Education. 2001;102(1):53–5.
Learning Express. Test taking power strategies. New York, NY: Learning Express; 2007.
Study Guides and Strategies. Overcoming test anxiety. http://www.studygs.net/tstprp8.htm. Accessed 12 Sep 2010.
Taking Multiple Choice Exams. http://www.uwec.edu/geography/Ivogeler/multiple.htm. Accessed 20 Sep 2010.

Chapter 2
Practice Test # 1: Difficulty Level-Easy

Questions

1. The exposure rate of an activity of 1 millicurie (mCi) measured at 1 centimeter (cm) is called:
   (A) Roentgen man equivalent (REM)
   (B) The exposure rate constant (ERC)
   (C) Total effective dose equivalent (TEDE)
   (D) Kilobecquerel (kBq)

2. Quantitative bias that refers to the underestimation of counts density which differs from what they should be is called:
   (A) Motion artifact
   (B) Partial-volume effect
   (C) Recovery coefficient
   (D) Truncation artifact

3. Truncation artifacts in PET/CT imaging are produced by:
   (A) Contrast medium
   (B) Difference in size of FOV between PET and the CT
   (C) Difference in scanning time between PET and the CT
   (D) Beds overlapping

Answers to Test #1 begin on page 45

4. Dental fillings, hip prosthetics, or chemotherapy port are examples of PET/CT imaging artifacts described as:
   (A) Truncation artifacts
   (B) Motion artifacts
   (C) Contrast medium artifacts
   (D) Metallic implants artifacts

5. Property of PET detectors that allows them faster timing signals for coincidence detection and to work at high count rates is called:
   (A) The stopping power
   (B) Energy resolution
   (C) The decay constant
   (D) The light output

6. The picturing, description, and measurement of biological processes at the particle and cellular level is known as:
   (A) Dynamic imaging
   (B) Molecular imaging
   (C) Static imaging
   (D) Dual point imaging

7. A PET system capacity to distinguish between two points after image reconstruction is called:
   (A) Contrast
   (B) Resolution
   (C) Attenuation
   (D) Emission

8. Allergic reaction that begins within seconds/minutes of contrast media administration and rapidly progresses to cause airway constriction, skin and intestinal irritation, and altered heart rhythms is called:
   (A) Urticaria
   (B) Anaphylaxis
   (C) Sepsis
   (D) Infarction

9. The first PET radiopharmaceutical to receive the U.S. Food and Drug Administration approval in 1989 was:
   (A) Rb-82
   (B) F-18 Fluoride
   (C) F-18 FDG
   (D) N-13 ammonia

10. Choose from the following responses to interpret this ECG:
    (A) Normal sinus rhythm
    (B) Electronic ventricular pacemaker
    (C) Atrial fibrillation
    (D) Ventricular bigeminy (Fig. 2.1)

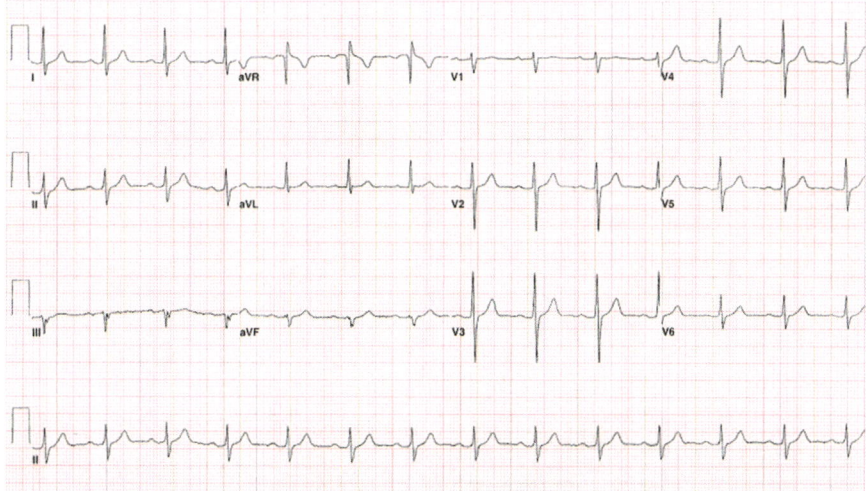

Fig. 2.1 ECG Sample Case: A 51-year-old man with atypical chest pain

11. The dose calibrator quality control procedure performed to assess the device's ability to measure accurately a range of a low to high activities is called:
    (A) Geometry
    (B) Accuracy
    (C) Linearity
    (D) Constancy

12. The following positron-emitting radionuclides are isotopes of natural elements present in most biochemical processes EXCEPT:
    (A) O-15
    (B) F-18
    (C) C-11
    (D) N-13

13. Two photons arising from the same annihilation event and detected by two detectors within the coincidence time-window are:
    (A) True coincidences
    (B) Random events
    (C) Scatter coincidences
    (D) Single events

14. Which of the following serve as the building blocks for proteins synthesis?
    (A) Amino acids
    (B) Phospholipids
    (C) Enzymes
    (D) Hormones

15. Positronium (Ps) is an arrangement of:
    (A) Two positrons
    (B) Two electrons
    (C) An electron and a positron
    (D) A positron and a neutrino

16. Which of the following regions is the most common site of brown fat localization?
    (A) Neck
    (B) Mediastinum
    (C) Paravertebral
    (D) Perinephric

17. Which of the following scintillators commonly used in PET imaging has the highest stopping power?
    (A) LSO (lutetium oxyorthosilicate)
    (B) BaF2 (barium fluoride)
    (C) BGO (bismuth germinate)
    (D) GSO (gadolinium orthosilicate)

18. A malignant neoplasm of the skin linked with approximately 75% of skin cancer–related mortality is called:
    (A) Basal cell carcinoma
    (B) Sarcoma
    (C) Melanoma
    (D) Squamous cell carcinoma

19. PET tracers have demonstrated significant potential utility and application in the following clinical areas EXCEPT:
    (A) Oncology
    (B) Cardiology
    (C) Pulmonology
    (D) Neurology

20. A dose of F-18 FDG is calibrated to have 14 mCi at 12:00 P.M. How many milicuries of F-18 FDG will be remaining at 12:40 P.M.?
    (A) 2.6 mCi
    (B) 11 mCi
    (C) 18 mCi
    (D) 19.6 mCi

21. The sum of the weighted equivalent doses in all the tissues and organs of the body is called:
    (A) Whole-body dose
    (B) Effective dose
    (C) Committed dose equivalent
    (D) Shallow dose equivalent

22. The combined whole-body effective dose for a clinically diagnostic PET/CT is typically in the range:
    (A) <10 mSv
    (B) 10–20 mSv
    (C) 20–30 mSv
    (D) >30 mSv

23. The positron has the same mass as an electron and an electric charge of:
    (A) –2
    (B) –1
    (C) 0
    (D) +1

24. The initial diagnosis of melanoma is established by:
    (A) PET examination
    (B) CT examination
    (C) Histologic evaluation
    (D) Dermatologist evaluation

25. In PET scanning process raw data acquired and identified as coincidence events along their LOR are stored in the raw data format called:
    (A) Histograms
    (B) Sinograms
    (C) Dextrograms
    (D) Pictograms

26. Which of the following is cyclotron produced positron-emitting radionuclide?
    (A) Copper-62
    (B) Nitrogen-13
    (C) Gallium-68
    (D) Rubidium-82

27. A piece of equipment that sorts out photons of different radionuclides with different photon energies and to separate scattered photons from the useful ones is called:
    (A) Photomultiplier tube
    (B) Pulse height analyzer
    (C) ADC converter
    (D) Optical window

28. DNA synthesis is a measure of cellular:
    (A) Apoptosis
    (B) Mutation
    (C) Proliferation
    (D) Metabolism

29. The F-18 fluoride bone uptake mechanism is similar to that of:
    (A) F-18 fluorodeoxyglucose (FDG)
    (B) Ga-68
    (C) Tc-99 m methylenediphosphonate (MDP)
    (D) In-111

30. The process by which new blood vessels are formed is called:
    (A) Angiogenesis
    (B) Embryogenesis
    (C) Morphogenesis
    (D) Organogenesis

31. Which of the following quality control procedures are required for proper functioning of the survey meter?
    (A) Calibration and linearity
    (B) Geometry and constancy
    (C) Calibration and constancy
    (D) Linearity and geometry

32. The Circle of Willis is a circle of arteries that supply blood to:
    (A) The heart
    (B) The lungs
    (C) The brain
    (D) The liver

33. The CT X-ray tube:
    (A) Detects the X-ray
    (B) Produces the X-ray
    (C) Shields from the X-ray
    (D) Measures the X-ray

34. The radiodensity of distilled water at standard pressure and temperature (STP) on the Hounsfield unit (HU) scale is equal to:
    (A) −1 HU
    (B) 0 HU
    (C) 1 HU
    (D) 10 HU

35. The dose calibrator quality control procedure testing a long-lived standard at each of the frequently used radionuclides settings is called:
   (A) Geometry
   (B) Accuracy
   (C) Linearity
   (D) Constancy

36. Which of the following radionuclides commonly used in PET imaging has the highest energy?
   (A) Carbon-11
   (B) Nitrogen-13
   (C) Oxygen-15
   (D) Fluorine-18

37. The PET scanner quality control procedure in which data are used with the transmission data in the computation of attenuation correction factors is called:
   (A) Normalization
   (B) Calibration
   (C) Blank scan
   (D) Attenuation correction

38. The property of the scintillation detector described as the number of scintillations produced by each incident photon is called:
   (A) The stopping power
   (B) Energy resolution
   (C) The decay constant
   (D) The light output

39. Which of the following compounds serves as a precursor for the synthesis of phospholipids?
   (A) Thymidine
   (B) Acetate
   (C) Choline
   (D) Tyrosine

40. What is the percent error of the dose calibrator reading if a 4 ml reference volume (expected) of geometry test reads 2.8 mCi, and the actual reading obtained in 10 ml volume is 2.5 mCi?
   (A) 12%
   (B) 10.7%
   (C) −10.7%
   (D) −12 %

41. The presented images labeled A, B, C, and D were obtained during a routine PET/CT scan. The image labeled "A" is described as:
    (A) Topogram
    (B) Fused coronal
    (C) Non-attenuation corrected
    (D) Maximum-intensity projection (Fig. 2.2)

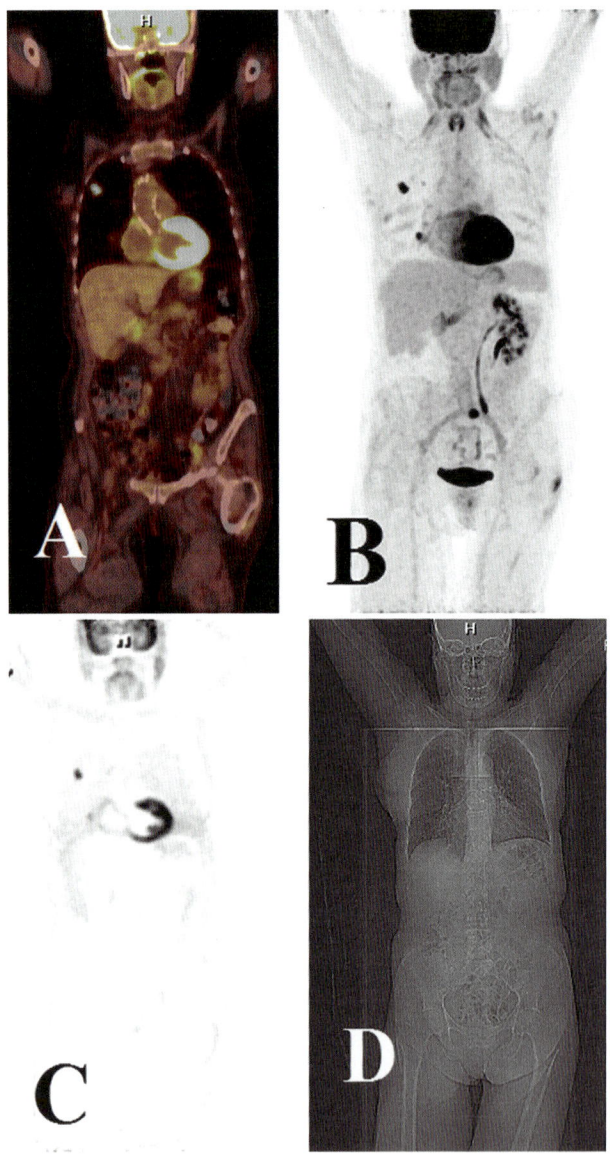

Fig. 2.2 PET/CT images

42. Which of the following is the correct order of scanning when a typical PET/CT protocol is applied?
    (A) Transmission CT, emission PET, topogram
    (B) Transmission CT, topogram, emission PET
    (C) Topogram, transmission CT, emission PET
    (D) Emission PET, transmission CT, topogram

43. Presence of the non-collinearity of the annihilation photons and the finite positron range are inherent properties of positron emission tomography resulting in:
    (A) Attenuation artifacts
    (B) Positional inaccuracy
    (C) Scatter
    (D) Truncation

44. Which of the following positron-emitting nuclides has the shortest half-life?
    (A) Rubidium-82
    (B) Oxygen-15
    (C) Nitrogen-13
    (D) Carbon-11

45. The cathode filament of the X-ray tube:
    (A) Emits electrons
    (B) Emits X-ray
    (C) Attracts electrons
    (D) Detects X-ray

46. An oncology patient referred for a positron emission tomography scan should fast prior to his/her appointment for at least:
    (A) 12 h
    (B) 8 h
    (C) 4 h
    (D) 2 h

47. Daily quality control checks on the PET scanner should be performed:
    (A) After the last procedure
    (B) During the uptake phase
    (C) At the end of the day
    (D) Before the patient is injected

48. Patients with malignant melanoma should be scanned with their arms:
    (A) Down
    (B) Crossed over the chest
    (C) Up
    (D) Beneath the patient

49. The presence of asbestos-related plaques, benign inflammatory pleuritis, tuberculous pleuritis, and pleural effusion can result in:
    (A) False-positive uptake in FDG-PET images of patients with malignant mesothelioma
    (B) True-positive uptake in FDG-PET images of patients with malignant mesothelioma
    (C) FDG-PET attenuation artifacts
    (D) FDG-PET motion artifacts

50. A 13 mCi dose of F-18 FDG is calibrated for 12:00 P.M. If the patient comes an hour early, how many millicuries will there be in the dose?
    (A) 3.6 mCi
    (B) 9 mCi
    (C) 19 mCi
    (D) 46 mCi

51. The earliest disposal of the decay-in-storage waste material is permitted if it was held for a minimum 10 half-lives and has decayed to less than:
    (A) Background level
    (B) Two times background levels
    (C) 0.05 mR/h
    (D) 0.5 mR/h

52. Organizing, problem solving, attention, and planning are controlled by the:
    (A) Frontal lobe of the brain
    (B) Occipital lobe of the brain
    (C) Parietal lobe of the brain
    (D) Temporal lobe of the brain

53. The recommended time interval for PET imaging after biopsy is:
    (A) 1 week
    (B) 2–4 weeks
    (C) 2–6 months
    (D) >6 months

54. The example of the anatomic diagnostic modality employed in the work-up of the patient with seizures is:
    (A) Electroencephalography (EEG)
    (B) Positron emission tomography (PET)
    (C) Magnetic resonance imaging (MRI)
    (D) Single-photon emission computed tomography (SPECT)

55. In the PET/CT acquisition, the CT component is performed for:
    (A) Scatter correction
    (B) Attenuation correction
    (C) Motion correction
    (D) Random correction

56. A series of organized, involuntary, smooth waves of muscular contractions of the alimentary canal is called:
    (A) Diverticulosis
    (B) Peristalsis
    (C) Cramps
    (D) Paralysis

57. Standardized uptake value (SUV) measurements are performed on:
    (A) Non-attenuation-corrected (NAC) images only
    (B) Attenuation-corrected (AC) images only
    (C) Non-attenuation-corrected (NAC) and attenuation-corrected (AC) images
    (D) Attenuation-corrected (AC) or non-attenuation-corrected (NAC) images

58. Which of the following positron-emitting nuclides has the longest half-life?
    (A) Fluorine-18
    (B) Oxygen-15
    (C) Nitrogen-13
    (D) Carbon-11

59. False-negative PET scans in lung cancer imaging occur predominantly because of:
    (A) Lesions that are too big to be evaluated by PET
    (B) Lesions that are too superficial to be evaluated by PET
    (C) Lesions that are too small to be evaluated by PET
    (D) Lesions that are too deep to be evaluated by PET

60. The presented CT image Fig. 2.3 is an example of an artifact described as a:
    (A) Beam hardening artifact
    (B) Contrast media artifact
    (C) Motion artifact
    (D) Streak artifact

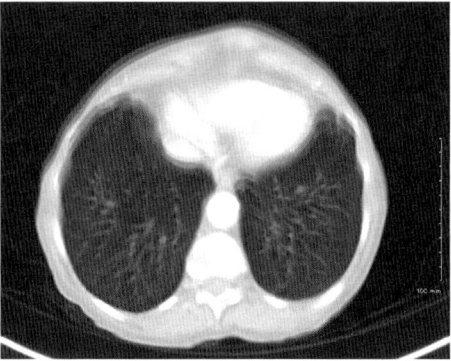

Fig. 2.3 CT axial slice

61. The principal measure of reducing radiation exposure to patients during PET/CT examination is reduce the:
    (A) Peak kilovoltage
    (B) Product of beam current and exposure time
    (C) Beam current
    (D) Product of beam current and peak kilovoltage

62. A minimally invasive surgical procedure used to detect the presence or absence of occult regional nodal metastases in patients without clinically noticeable nodal disease is called:
    (A) Lymphoscintigraphy
    (B) Sentinel node scintigraphy
    (C) Sentinel node biopsy
    (D) Lymph nodes mapping

63. According to minimal performance standards, the FDG uptake period that is required to minimize variability in SUV quantification should be at least:
    (A) 30 min
    (B) 45 min
    (C) 60 min
    (D) 75 min

64. Lung activity observed on F-18 FDG-PET/CT imaging:
    (A) Is more prominent on attenuation-corrected images
    (B) Increases from the posterior to the anterior segments
    (C) Increases from the inferior to the superior segments
    (D) Is more prominent on non-attenuation-corrected images

65. Which of the following methods, in clinical practice, is the most commonly applied to determine SUV?
    (A) Isocontour ROIs
    (B) Manual ROIs
    (C) SUV max
    (D) SUV peak

66. CT and PET scans demonstrate different aspects of disease indicating regions with:
    (A) Altered metabolism (PET) and areas of structural change (CT)
    (B) Altered metabolism (CT) and areas of structural change (PET)
    (C) Altered metabolism (PET) and areas of structural change (PET)
    (D) Altered metabolism (CT) and areas of structural change (CT)

67. If the pretest probability of disease is high and then a negative PET is more likely to be:
    (A) False negative
    (B) False positive
    (C) True negative
    (D) True positive

68. Multiple focal cortical and subcortical defects on FDG study indicate diagnosis of:
    (A) Vascular dementia
    (B) Alzheimer's disease
    (C) Parkinson's disease
    (D) Radiation necrosis

69. The process of aligning images so that corresponding features can easily be related is called:
    (A) Image smoothing
    (B) Image filtering
    (C) Image registration
    (D) Image processing

70. The NRC requires that all wipe tests be recorded in disintegrations per minute (dpm). If 230 net counts per minute (cpm) were acquired with 86% well counter efficiency, what is the result of the wipe test in disintegrations per minute (dpm)?
    (A) 37 dpm
    (B) 198 dpm
    (C) 267 dpm
    (D) 344 dpm

71. The concept of clinical SPECT/CT system can be described as:
    (A) A single-head scintillation camera positioned in front of a CT scanner
    (B) A dual-head scintillation camera positioned in front of a CT scanner
    (C) A CT scanner positioned in front of a dual-head scintillation camera
    (D) A CT scanner positioned in front of a single-head scintillation camera

72. A normal, physiological uptake of F-18 FDG in the stomach can be described as:
    (A) Distal stomach uptake is higher than proximal stomach uptake
    (B) Anterior stomach uptake is higher than posterior stomach uptake
    (C) Proximal stomach uptake is higher than distal stomach uptake
    (D) Posterior stomach uptake is higher than anterior stomach uptake

73. The recommended time interval for PET-FDG imaging after chemotherapy is:
    (A) 1 week
    (B) > 10 days
    (C) 2–6 months
    (D) > 6 months

74. An area of focal FDG uptake in the lungs, without corresponding finding on CT scan, most likely represents:
    (A) Pulmonary nodule
    (B) Radiation necrosis
    (C) An injected blood clot
    (D) Rib fracture

75. The display shown in Fig. 2.4 presents attenuation-corrected and reconstructed positron emission tomography (PET-FDG) viability study. The reoriented tomographic slices are:
    (A) Short-axis slices
    (B) Vertical long-axis slices
    (C) Oblique short-axis slices
    (D) Horizontal long axis

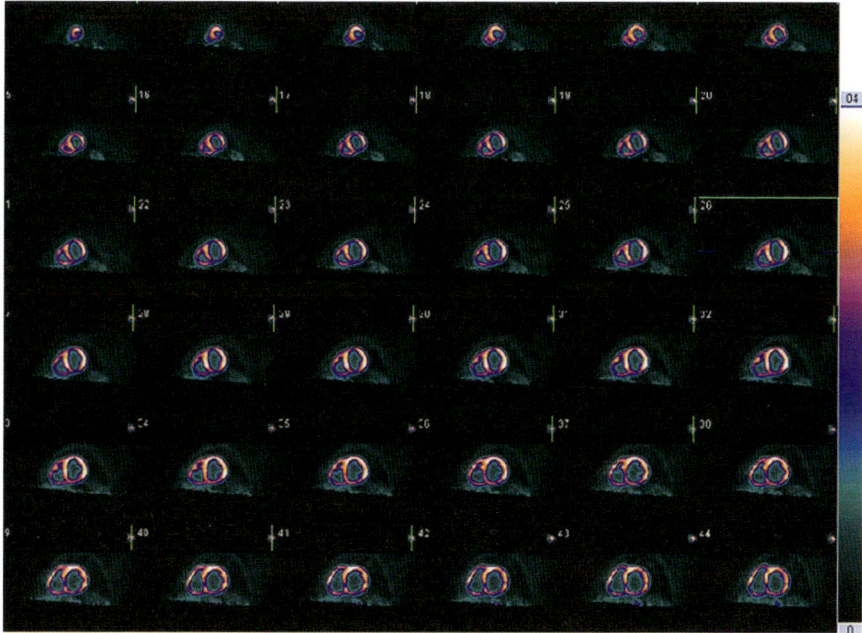

Fig. 2.4 PET/CT-FDG viability study

76. A hyperinsulinemic state affects the diagnostic quality of FDG-PET imaging and it is typically associated with:
    (A) Diffuse liver and splenic uptake
    (B) Diffuse muscular and myocardial uptake
    (C) Diffuse stomach and pancreatic uptake
    (D) Diffuse brown fat and brain uptake

77. Malignant tumors of the chest wall include all of the following EXCEPT:
    (A) Lipoma
    (B) Chondrosarcoma
    (C) Osteosarcoma
    (D) Ewing sarcoma

78. A group of lung diseases characterized by chronic obstruction of lung airflow that interferes with normal breathing and is not fully reversible is called:
    (A) Chronic bronchitis
    (B) Emphysema
    (C) Chronic obstructive pulmonary disease
    (D) Hospital acquired pneumonias

79. The beta-amyloid uptake can be assessed through positron emission tomography (PET) using the radiopharmaceutical:
    (A) Carbon-11-labeled Pittsburgh Compound B (C-11 PiB)
    (B) Fluor-18 fluoromisonidazole (F-18 MISO)
    (C) Fluor-18-3-fluorothymidine (F-18FLT)
    (D) Carbon-11-labeled methionine (C-11 Met)

80. Calculate the effective half-life of a radiopharmaceutical using the following information:
    Physical half-life is 110 min
    Biological half-life is 360 min
    (A) 470 min
    (B) 235 min
    (C) 84.3 min
    (D) 3.2 min

81. Which of the following scintillators has the highest light output?
    (A) LSO (lutetium oxyorthosilicate)
    (B) NaI (Tl) (thallium-doped sodium iodide)
    (C) BGO (bismuth germinate)
    (D) GSO (gadolinium orthosilicate)

82. The main organs of the digestive system include:
    (A) Teeth
    (B) Liver
    (C) Pancreas
    (D) Pharynx

83. F-18 FDG-PET is considered as a superior modality, compared with CT, for evaluating posttreatment response in lymphoma patients because of:
    (A) The ability to provide anatomical information
    (B) The ability to differentiate viable tumor from fibrosis
    (C) Higher resolution
    (D) Shorter imaging

84. Which of the following types of non-Hodgkin lymphomas is most common?
    (A) Burkitt's lymphoma
    (B) Lymphoblastic lymphoma
    (C) Diffuse large B-cell lymphoma
    (D) Anaplastic large T-cell/null cell lymphoma

85. The major limitation of PET in the head and neck imaging is its:
    (A) Poor sensitivity
    (B) Poor spatial resolution
    (C) Prolonged scanning time
    (D) Radiation exposure

86. The most common cell type found in lymphoid tissue is:
    (A) Lymphocyte
    (B) Stem cell
    (C) Erythrocyte
    (D) Monocyte

87. In order to achieve precise attenuation correction data for transmission scan they should be obtained using:
    (A) Low-dose CT
    (B) High-dose CT
    (C) Germanium-68
    (D) Cobalt-56

88. Hiatal hernias can cause large foci of increased F-18 FDG uptake in/at:
    (A) The hilar region
    (B) The gastroesophageal junction
    (C) The pyloric sphincter
    (D) The stomach fundus

89. The lymphoma that has come back after it has been treated is called:
    (A) Aggressive
    (B) Intermittent
    (C) Indolent
    (D) Recurrent

90. The diagram for the process of positron–electron annihilation is shown in Fig. 2.5. Which of the following labels identifies the annihilation photon(s)?
    (A) D
    (B) C
    (C) B
    (D) A

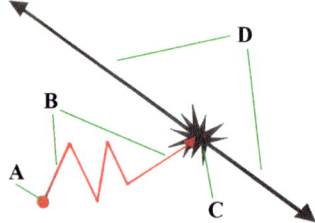

Fig. 2.5 Positron–electron annihilation diagram. *Illustration by Sabina Moniuszko*

91. The use of a low-dose CT scan in place of a conventional PET transmission scan:
    (A) Increases the scan duration
    (B) Reduces confidence of the scan interpretation
    (C) Decreases throughput
    (D) Improves accuracy of the scan interpretation

92. The one of disadvantages of nuclear medicine study over PET-FDG study in infection and inflammation imaging lies in its:
    (A) Low resolution
    (B) Faster time to results
    (C) Quantitation abilities
    (D) High sensitivity

93. Dual time point FDG-PET imaging is reflecting:
    (A) The dynamics of lesion glucose metabolism
    (B) The dynamics of lesion growth
    (C) The dynamics of blood pool glucose clearance
    (D) The dynamics of blood pool activity

94. Clinical stress perfusion studies with Rb-82 are usually limited to pharmacologic stress because of Rb-82's:
    (A) High kinetic energy
    (B) Short half-life
    (C) Positron range
    (D) High cost

95. Image-guided transthoracic needle aspiration or biopsy can be achieved with all of the following EXCEPT:
    (A) Computed tomography (CT)
    (B) Positron emission tomography (PET)
    (C) Fluoroscopy
    (D) Ultrasonography (USG)

96. Stomach reflux disease can result in increased FDG uptake in/at:
    (A) The hilar region
    (B) The gastroesophageal junction
    (C) The pyloric sphincter
    (D) The stomach fundus

97. The use of PET gating for specific applications in PET/CT scanning:
    (A) Reduces motion artifacts
    (B) Increases scanning time
    (C) Increases spatial resolution
    (D) Decreases sensitivity

98. The lymphatic system is not a separate system of the body, but it is considered a part of the:
    (A) Digestive system
    (B) Hematopoietic system
    (C) Circulatory system
    (D) Respiratory system

99. All of the following positron emission tomography myocardial perfusion tracers are cyclotron produced EXCEPT:
    (A) Water O-15
    (B) Rubidium Rb-82
    (C) Acetate C-11
    (D) Ammonia N-13

100. The presented images labeled A, B, C, and D were obtained during a routine PET/CT scan. The image labeled "B" is described as:
    (A) Topogram
    (B) Fused coronal
    (C) Non-attenuation corrected
    (D) Maximum-intensity projection (Fig. 2.6)

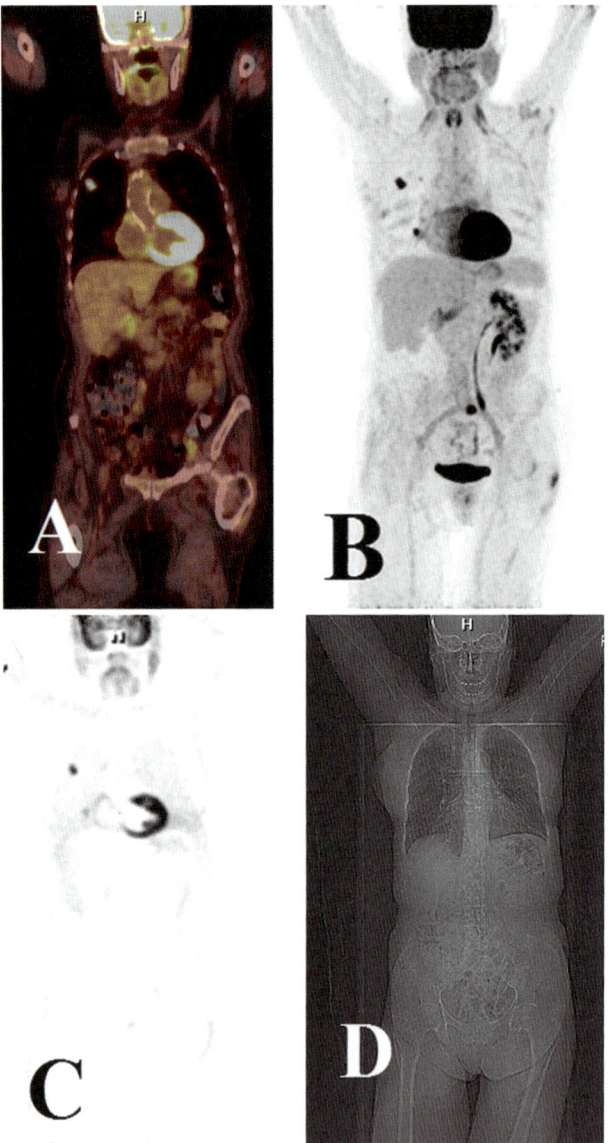

Fig. 2.6 PET/CT images

101. All of the following are examples of conventional diagnostic imaging procedures that evaluate normal anatomy via radiologic images EXCEPT:
    (A) X-ray
    (B) Ultrasonography
    (C) Magnetic resonance imaging
    (D) Positron emission tomography

102. The cerebellum is located posteriorly just below the cerebrum and is responsible for the proper control of:
    (A) Body temperature
    (B) Skeletal muscles
    (C) Emotions
    (D) Vision

103. A topographic image of the body used to confirm proper patient positioning is called:
    (A) The blank scan
    (B) The scout scan
    (C) The delayed scan
    (D) The rescan

104. The TNM (tumor, node, metastasis) staging system that is generally used for solid tumors is not applicable to lymphoma, since:
    (A) Lymphoma spreads in a predictable pattern
    (B) Lymphoma is a rapidly progressing disease
    (C) Lymphoma begins in multiple sites simultaneously
    (D) Lymphoma spreads in an unpredictable pattern

105. Rb-82 is a monovalent cationic analog of potassium and has a biologic activity similar to:
    (A) Gallium Ga-67
    (B) Thallium Tl-201
    (C) Technetium Tc-99 m
    (D) Fluorine F-18

106. A pulmonary nodule (PN) is defined as a separate opacity that is entirely surrounded by lung parenchyma and has a diameter of:
    (A) 4 cm or less
    (B) 3 cm or less
    (C) 2 cm or less
    (D) 1 cm or less

107. Which of the following positron emission tomography myocardial perfusion tracers is described as a model tracer for flow quantitation?
    (A) Water O-15
    (B) Rubidium Rb-82
    (C) Acetate C-11
    (D) Ammonia N-13

108. All of the following diagnostic procedures can be utilized to evaluate patients with lymphoma EXCEPT:
    (A) Ga-67 scintigraphy
    (B) Bone marrow biopsy
    (C) Lymphangiogram
    (D) Sentinel node localization

109. All of the following quantitative methods have been used to explore the prognostic value of FDG uptake in malignant tumors EXCEPT:
    (A) Standard uptake value max (SUV max)
    (B) Tumor's glycolytic volume (TGV)
    (C) Metabolic tumor volume (MTV)
    (D) Standard uptake value min (SUV min)

110. The presented images labeled A, B, C, and D were obtained during a routine CT of the brain. The image described as D represents:
    (A) Lateral brain localizer image
    (B) Coronal slice of the brain
    (C) Saggital slice of the brain
    (D) Tranverse slice of the brain (Fig. 2.7)

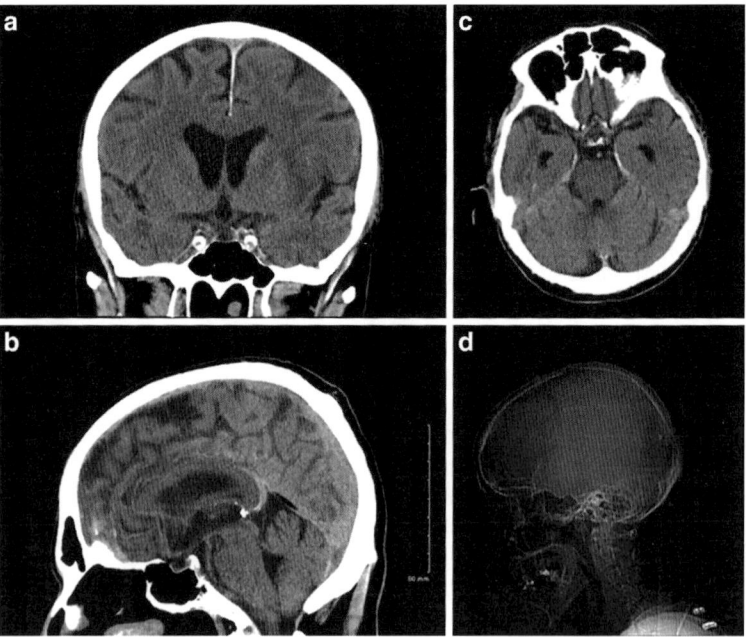

Fig. 2.7 Brain CT scans

111. Which of the following components of the PET/CT protocol delivers the highest radiation dose to the patient?
    (A) Topogram
    (B) Low-dose CT
    (C) Diagnostic CT
    (D) Dose of 370 MBq of F-18FDG

112. Computed tomography (CT) assessment of pulmonary nodules includes all of the following EXCEPT:
    (A) Lobar and segmental localization
    (B) Growth rate evaluation
    (C) Metabolic lesion characteristics
    (D) Size and/or volume measurement

113. Which of the following substrates, under normal conditions, are the major sources of myocardial energy?
    (A) Ketone bodies and amino acids
    (B) Lactate and pyruvate
    (C) Free fatty acids and glucose
    (D) Insulin and proteins

114. All of the following organs belong to the lymphatic system EXCEPT:
    (A) Thymus
    (B) Thyroid
    (C) Tonsils
    (D) Spleen

115. Colorectal cancer imaging, when PET utilizes F-18FDG as a tracer, is covered by Medicare in all of the following settings EXCEPT:
    (A) Screening
    (B) Diagnosis
    (C) Staging
    (D) Restaging

116. The principal division of the lungs is called:
    (A) Segment
    (B) Lobe
    (C) Acinus
    (D) Lobule

117. Which of the following PET cardiac tracers is a FDA-approved indicator of myocardial viability?
    (A) Water O-15
    (B) Rubidium Rb-82
    (C) Ammonia N-13
    (D) F-18 fluorodeoxyglucose

118. The pattern of F-18 FDG uptake in the bowel most likely associated with a neoplastic process can be described as:
    (A) Segmental
    (B) Diffuse
    (C) Focal
    (D) Absent

119. The fundamental limit of restricted spatial resolution of PET scanners is due to:
    (A) The distance positrons travel before they annihilate with an electron
    (B) The non-collinearity of the pair of annihilation photons
    (C) The scanner geometry
    (D) The crystals light output

120. A heterogeneous group of hematologic malignancies arising from lymphocytes is called:
    (A) Anemia
    (B) Leukemia
    (C) Lymphoma
    (D) Thrombocytopenia

121. A breast-feeding patient referred for PET imaging should:
    (A) Discontinue breast-feeding 12 h before injection of radiotracer
    (B) Discontinue breast-feeding 6 h before injection of radiotracer
    (C) Discontinue breast-feeding for at least 6 h after injection of radiotracer
    (D) Discontinue breast-feeding for at least 12 h after injection of radiotracer

122. Differentiated thyroid cancer (DTC) is divided into:
    (A) Papillary and follicular
    (B) Medullary and insular
    (C) Anaplastic and papillary
    (D) Medullary and follicular

123. Dose extravasation at the antecubital injection site can cause:
    (A) Ipsilateral inguinal node uptake
    (B) Contralateral axillary node uptake
    (C) Ipsilateral axillary node uptake
    (D) Contralateral inguinal node uptake

124. The portion of the large intestine that runs across the abdomen from the hepatic flexure to the splenic flexure is called the:
    (A) Sigmoid colon
    (B) Transverse colon
    (C) Ascending colon
    (D) Descending colon

125. A much higher sensitivity of positron emission tomography (PET) imaging over single-photon emission computed tomography (SPECT) results in all of the following EXCEPT:
    (A) Improved noise-to-signal ratios
    (B) Improved temporal resolution
    (C) Shorter scanning time
    (D) Improved image quality

126. The most common primary symptom of dementia is/are:
    (A) Personality changes
    (B) Diminished thinking ability
    (C) Changes in memory
    (D) Depression

127. Noninvasive, accepted methods for improving the diagnostic accuracy of FDG-PET include all of the following EXCEPT:
    (A) Furosemide administration in kidney tumor
    (B) Stomach distention in gastric carcinoma
    (C) Beta blockers in suspected brown adipose tissue uptake
    (D) Valium administration in dementia imaging

128. According to the Centers for the Medicare & Medicaid Services (CMS), an inconclusive test is a test(s) whose results are NOT:
    (A) Equivocal
    (B) Reproducible
    (C) Technically uninterpretable
    (D) Discordant with a patient's other clinical data

129. Stunned or hibernating myocardium is:
    (A) Nonviable
    (B) Dysfunctional but viable
    (C) Dysfunctional and nonviable
    (D) Functional

130. In the image in Fig. 2.8, what structure is depicted by line "b"?
    (A) Right ventricle
    (B) Liver
    (C) Left ventricle
    (D) Aorta

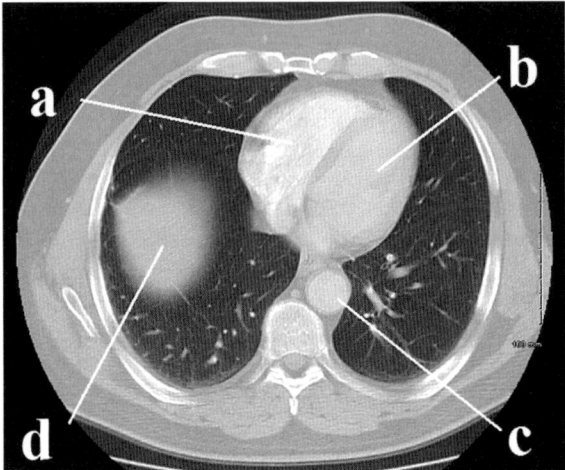

Fig. 2.8 Chest CT scan

131. After completion of the F-18 FDG study, the patient's fluid intake:
    (A) Should be stopped
    (B) Should be continued
    (C) Is not relevant
    (D) Is contraindicated

132. The duodenum, jejunum, and ileum make up:
    (A) The small intestine
    (B) The stomach
    (C) The large intestine
    (D) The rectum

133. A PET quantifier, calculated as the tracer activity concentration within a volume of interest, divided by the injected dose per unit body weight is called:
    (A) Fractional uptake value
    (B) Standardized upload value
    (C) Standardized uptake value
    (D) Fractional upload value

134. For optimal patient care and interpretation of FDG-PET images, the following information from the patient referred for PET scanning should be obtained EXCEPT:
    (A) Breast-feeding info
    (B) Recent surgery info
    (C) Use of medication info
    (D) Housing info

135. In the image in Fig. 2.9, which of the following arrows is pointing to the gallbladder?
    (A) d
    (B) c
    (C) b
    (D) a

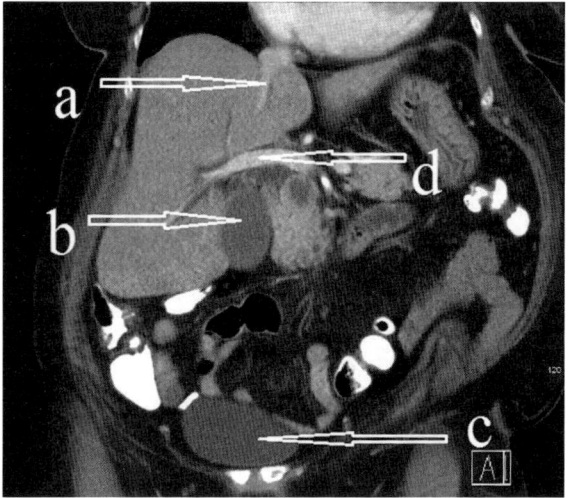

Fig. 2.9 Abdomen CT scan

136. The patient should remain relaxed and avoid talking, chewing, or hyperventilating during the uptake phase after F-18 FDG injection in order to:
    (A) Minimize physiologic lung uptake
    (B) Minimize physiologic muscular uptake
    (C) Maximize physiologic muscular uptake
    (D) Maximize physiologic liver uptake

137. A condition of an abnormally low number of neutrophils is called:
    (A) Neutrophilia
    (B) Leukocytosis
    (C) Neutropenia
    (D) Leucopenia

138. The temporal lobe is located on either side of the brain around the level of the ears and controls:
    (A) Auditory information
    (B) Visual information
    (C) Smell sensation
    (D) Tactile sensation

139. PET-FDG provides beneficial information in all of the following areas of lymphoma evaluation EXCEPT:
    (A) Diagnosis
    (B) Response to therapy
    (C) Recurrence detection
    (D) Staging

140. It is permitted by a facility to combine two unit doses of F-18 FDG, as long as they originated from the same lot number. There are two 14 mCi/2 ml contingency doses possessing the same lot number of F-18 FDG calibrated for 13:00 h. If a patient needs to be injected at 14:00 h for a PET/CT scan with a 14 mCi of dose, how much volume must be drawn from one unit dose to make another unit dose of 14 mCi?
    (A) 0.3 ml
    (B) 0.6 ml
    (C) 0.9 ml
    (D) 1.2 ml

141. The main source of potential radiation hazard to a breast-feeding infant of the postpartum woman undergoing PET scanning is from:
    (A) Ingested milk
    (B) Proximity to the breast
    (C) Background radiation
    (D) Scanning device

142. All of the following are well-established indications for PET functional imaging in patients with suspected recurrent colorectal carcinoma EXCEPT:
    (A) Falling CEA levels in the absence of a known source
    (B) Staging recurrent colorectal carcinoma
    (C) Preoperative staging
    (D) Equivocal lesion on conventional imaging

143. Which of the following kinds of treatment/therapy has the promoting effect on the spleen and bone marrow?
    (A) Antibiotic treatment
    (B) Bone pain therapy with Sm –153-lexidronam
    (C) Granulocyte colony-stimulating factor (G-CSF) therapy
    (D) Brachytherapy for prostate carcinoma

144. Anxiolytic medication given before a PET scanning:
    (A) Induces hyperglycemia
    (B) Relaxes patient
    (C) Prevents hyperinsulinemia
    (D) Forces diuresis

145. Administration of highly concentrated intravenous agent and/or high-density barium-based oral agents during routine CT scanning will yield:
    (A) Overestimated standardized uptake value (SUV)
    (B) Unchanged standardized uptake value (SUV)
    (C) Underestimated standardized uptake value (SUV)
    (D) Standardized uptake value (SUV) equal to 1

146. The pattern of F-18 FDG in the normal palatine and lingual tonsils is described as:
    (A) Absent
    (B) Asymmetrical and increased
    (C) Symmetrical and increased
    (D) Asymmetrical

147. In quantitative PET imaging, e.g., SUV calculation, the following scanner related parameters need to be corrected EXCEPT:
    (A) Correction for random coincidences
    (B) Correction for scatter coincidences
    (C) Correction for effects of attenuation
    (D) Correction for table speed

148. The section of the image assessed for count content reflecting either the flow of radionuclide or concentration of radionuclide in that area is called:
    (A) Polar map
    (B) Region of interest
    (C) Background region
    (D) Activity curve

149. Positrons are subatomic particles that have all of the characteristics of electrons EXCEPT:
    (A) Mass
    (B) Magnitude of charge
    (C) Size
    (D) Polarity of charge

150. The diagram for the process of positron–electron annihilation is shown in Fig. 2.10. Which of the following labels identifies the positron–electron annihilation event?
    (A) D
    (B) C
    (C) B
    (D) A

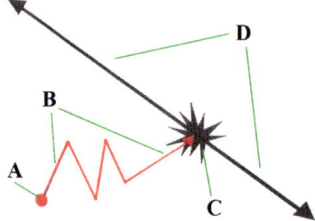

Fig. 2.10 Positron–electron annihilation diagram. *Illustration by Sabina Moniuszko*

151. Wipe testing to detect removable contamination in each area of use must be performed:
    (A) Daily
    (B) Weekly
    (C) Biweekly
    (D) Monthly

152. The parameters as perfusion, permeability, and transit time offer an insight into the functional status of the:
    (A) Respiratory system
    (B) Gastrointestinal system
    (C) Vascular system
    (D) Reproductive system

153. An event assigned to a line of response (LOR) joining the two relevant detectors is called:
    (A) An annihilation event
    (B) A random event
    (C) A coincidence event
    (D) A Scatter event

154. A hormone vital to regulating carbohydrate and fat metabolism in the body by causing cells in the liver, muscle, and fat tissue to take up glucose from the blood is called:
    (A) Inulin
    (B) Parathormone
    (C) Insulin
    (D) Estrogen

155. Which of the following routes of F-18 FDG administration is acceptable if intravenous access is not available?
    (A) Subcutaneous
    (B) Intramuscular
    (C) Oral
    (D) Rectal

156. The medication given to relieve myocardial ischemia that works by causing both venous and arterial dilation is called:
    (A) Propranolol
    (B) Aminophylline
    (C) Nitroglycerine
    (D) Digoxin

157. All of the following interventions can be used to reduce urinary tract F-18 FDG activity EXCEPT:
    (A) Furosemide administration
    (B) Foley catheter placement
    (C) Patient hydration
    (D) Valium administration

158. The infiltrated dose can result in all of the following EXCEPT:
    (A) Masked myocardial ischemia
    (B) Lowered counting statistics
    (C) Altered distribution of the radiopharmaceutical
    (D) Decreased biological half-life of the radiopharmaceutical

159. Advantages of positron emission tomography myocardial perfusion imaging versus single-photon emission computed tomography include all of the following EXCEPT:
    (A) Shorter acquisition time
    (B) Higher extraction fraction of tracers
    (C) More equivocal reports
    (D) Higher spatial, temporal, and contrast resolution

160. Convert 14 mCi to megabecquerels (MBq).
    (A) 518 MBq
    (B) 378 MBq
    (C) 0.518 MBq
    (D) 0.378 MBq

161. The radiation sensitivity of a tissue is inversely proportional to the:
    (A) Degree of cell differentiation
    (B) Distance from the source of radiation
    (C) Time of radiation exposure
    (D) Rate of cell proliferation

162. All of the following conditions can lead to false-positive results in PET/CT scanning EXCEPT:
    (A) Mastitis
    (B) Tuberculosis
    (C) Necrosis
    (D) Sarcoidosis

163. After F-18FDG administration, a 20- to 30-mL saline flush is recommended in order to:
    (A) Prevent the dose infiltration
    (B) Reduce the dose venous retention
    (C) Hydrate the patient
    (D) Reduce radiation exposure

164. The Y-axis of the data plotted on PET sinogram represents:
    (A) The angle of orientation of the LOR
    (B) The shift of the LOR from the center of gantry
    (C) The window of coincidence of the LOR
    (D) Displacement of the LOR from center of FOV

165. Diffuse, symmetric uptake of F-18 FDG observed in the thyroid gland:
    (A) Indicates hypothyroidism
    (B) Indicates malignancy
    (C) Is a normal variant
    (D) Is always abnormal

166. The type of study defined as flow either per unit volume or per unit mass of tissue is called:
    (A) Perfusion study
    (B) Bolus study
    (C) Wash-in study
    (D) Wash-out study

167. When septa separate each crystal ring and coincidences are only recorded between detectors within the same ring and/or in closely neighboring rings the data are acquired:
    (A) In hybrid mode
    (B) In 2D mode
    (C) In 3 D mode
    (D) In 4D mode

168. Spatial information is converted to frequency information by the mathematical process known as:
    (A) Fourier transform
    (B) Convolution
    (C) Filtering
    (D) Fourier rebinning

169. A graph that records the electrical activity of the heart is called:
    (A) The echocardiogram
    (B) The encephalogram
    (C) The electrocardiogram
    (D) The elastogram

170. The presented images labeled A, B, C, and D were obtained during a routine PET/CT scan. The image labeled "C" is described as:
    (A) Topogram
    (B) Fused coronal
    (C) Non-attenuation corrected
    (D) Maximum-intensity projection (Fig. 2.11)

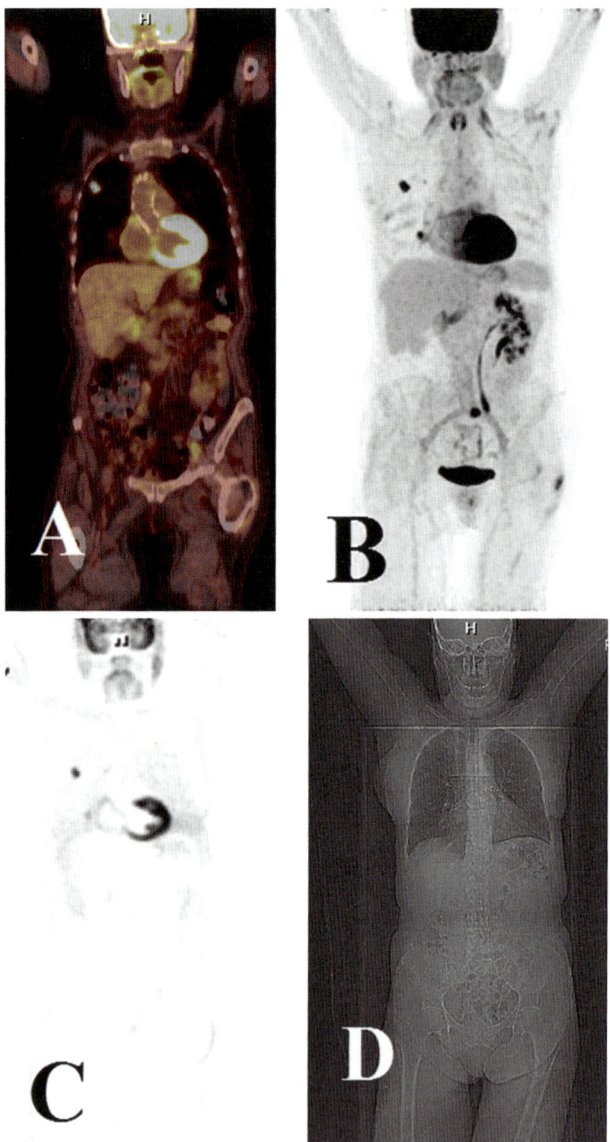

Fig. 2.11 PET/CT images

171. The whole-body dosimeter should be issued to personnel who might exceed minimum whole-body doses of:
    (A) 100 mrem/year (1 mSv/year)
    (B) 200 mrem/year (2 mSv/year)
    (C) 300 mrem/year (3 mSv/year)
    (D) 500 mrem/year (5 mSv/year)

172. Advantages of FDG-PET over conventional scintigraphy in the demonstration of infectious and inflammatory processes include all of the following EXCEPT:
    (A) Rapid reporting
    (B) High radiation burden
    (C) Superior resolution
    (D) Higher lesion-to-background ratios at early time points

173. An organ, attaining its largest size at the time of puberty, gradually shrinks and almost disappears. This organ, which serves as the site of T-cell differentiation, is called:
    (A) Thyroid
    (B) Thrombus
    (C) Thymus
    (D) Thalamus

174. The pharmacological effect of dipyridamole and adenosine, used as pharmacological stress agents in patients who cannot exercise, depends on:
    (A) Vasoconstriction
    (B) Tachycardia
    (C) Vasodilation
    (D) Hypertension

175. When monitoring response to treatment with PET-FDG imaging is essential to obtain:
    (A) Baseline PET-FDG scan
    (B) Interim PET-FDG scan
    (C) PET-FDG scan on the last day of therapy
    (D) PET-FDG scan two days after therapy

176. A low blood glucose level, accompanied by the signs and symptoms of increased activity of the autonomic nervous system and depressed activity of the central nervous system, is called:
    (A) Hypoxemia
    (B) Hypothermia
    (C) Hypoglycemia
    (D) Hypoinsulinemia

177. Which of the following patient/lesion characteristics suggests lung malignancy?
    (A) Lesion has a smooth margin on CT
    (B) Patient is nonsmoker
    (C) Lesion is 3 mm in size
    (D) Patient has hemoptysis

178. The 2010 Guidelines for Cardiopulmonary resuscitation (CPR) and Emergency Cardiovascular Care (ECC) of American Heart Association (AHA) recommend in adults a compression rate of at LEAST:
    (A) 120/min
    (B) 100/min
    (C) 80/min
    (D) 60/min

179. Medicare coverage specific for FDG-PET non-small cell lung cancer (NSLC) imaging includes all of the following EXCEPT:
    (A) Screening
    (B) Diagnosis
    (C) Staging
    (D) Restaging

180. A 15-year-old child needs to have a PET/CT scan prior to chemotherapy. The child's weight is 142 pounds and an adult dose for a PET/CT scan in this facility is 13 mCi. Using Clark's formula, calculate the pediatric F-18 FDG dose.
    (A) 6.5 mCi
    (B) 7.3 mCi
    (C) 8.0 mci
    (D) 12.3 mCi

181. The computed tomography X-ray tube:
    (A) Shields the patient from X-ray
    (B) Moves the patient table
    (C) Rotates the scanner detectors
    (D) Produces the beam of X-ray

182. In the process of interpretation and analysis of PET/CT images, a normal study with further investigations or clinical follow-up excluding focal inflammation or malignancy is called:
    (A) False positive
    (B) False negative
    (C) True negative
    (D) True positive

183. The relative variations in count densities between adjacent areas in the image of an object are called:
    (A) Contrast
    (B) Background
    (C) Noise
    (D) Shadow

184. FDG uptake by cancer cells tends to decline as:
    (A) Blood glucose and insulin levels decrease
    (B) Blood glucose level decreases and insulin levels increase
    (C) Blood glucose and insulin levels increase
    (D) Blood glucose increases and insulin levels decreases

185. Which of the following positron emission tomography myocardial perfusion tracers has the highest kinetic energy?
    (A) Water O-15
    (B) Rubidium Rb-82
    (C) FDG F-18
    (D) Ammonia N-13

186. The pattern of FDG uptake/glucose metabolism in patients with multi-infarct dementia is characterized by the presence of:
    (A) Frontal hypometabolism
    (B) Scattered foci of hypometabolism
    (C) Occipital hypometabolism
    (D) Parietotemporal hypometabolism

187. All of the following are the U.S. Food and Drug Administration (FDA)-approved cardiac PET tracers EXCEPT:
    (A) Water O-15
    (B) Rubidium Rb-82
    (C) Ammonia N-13
    (D) F-18 fluorodeoxyglucose

188. Fatigue, anemia, altered bowel function, and weight loss are frequently presenting symptoms of the:
    (A) Lung cancer
    (B) Brain cancer
    (C) Prostate cancer
    (D) Colorectal cancer

189. The sensitivity and specificity of PET-FDG for detecting and characterizing malignant lung nodules greater than 1 cm are correspondingly:
    (A) 96% and 57%
    (B) 96% and 77%
    (C) 56% and 57%
    (D) 56% and 77%

190. What is seen in this ECG?
    (A) Normal sinus rhythm
    (B) Electronic ventricular pacemaker

(C) Atrial fibrillation
(D) Ventricular bigeminy (Fig. 2.12)

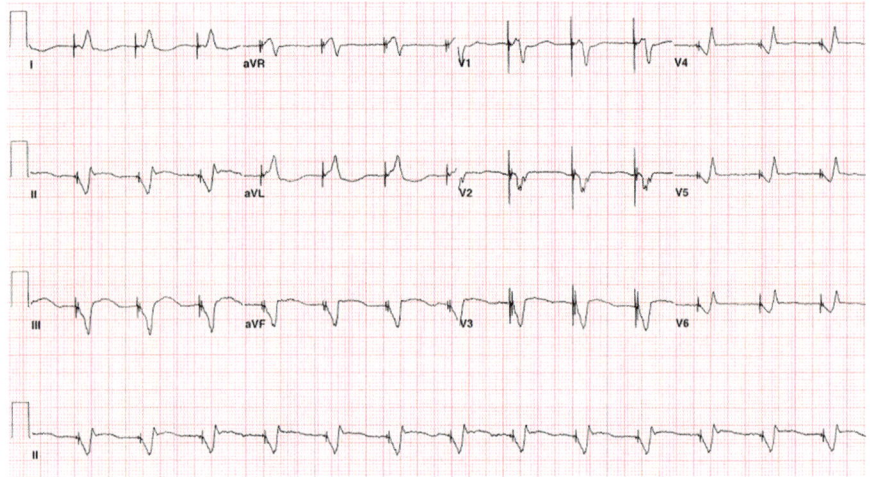

Fig. 2.12 ECG Sample Case: A 65-year-old man with dyspnea

191. If an approximate dose received from a PET scan is 25 millisieverts (mSv), what is the dose received in Roentgen equivalent man (rems)?
    (A) 2.5 rems
    (B) 250 rems
    (C) 2,500 rems
    (D) 25,000 rems

192. Common causes of needle-stick injuries include all of the following EXCEPT:
    (A) Recapping needles
    (B) Disposing sharps
    (C) Using Luer-activated devices
    (D) Accessing IV tubing with needles

193. Pulmonary mass is defined as having any pulmonary, pleural, or mediastinal lesion seen on chest radiographs and having a diameter:
    (A) >1 cm
    (B) >2 cm
    (C) >3 cm
    (D) >4 cm

194. The following data are necessary for calculating standardized uptake value (SUV) EXCEPT:
    (A) Patient height
    (B) Patient weight
    (C) Injected dose
    (D) Patient age

195. A package of F-18 FDG is producing an exposure rate of 2 mR/h at a distance of 3.3 ft. How many meters away should one stand to secure a background level of 0.03 mR/h? (1 m = 3.3 ft)
    (A) 7.6 ft.
    (B) 8.2 m
    (C) 26.94 m
    (D) 76 ft.

196. A substance used to enhance the visibility of a structure or fluid in the body for medical imaging is called:
    (A) Contrast media
    (B) Radiotracer
    (C) Filter
    (D) Buffer agent

197. A PET scanner parameter defined as the coincident count rate in a measurement that does not include scattered or random coincidences is called:
    (A) Noise equivalent count rate (NECR)
    (B) Contrast
    (C) Signal-to-noise ratio (SNR)
    (D) Sensitivity

198. A group of age-related symptoms involving progressive impairment of brain function resulting in diminished thinking ability, loss of memory, and personality changes is called:
    (A) Parkinson's disease
    (B) Dementia
    (C) Schizophrenia
    (D) Huntington's disease

199. The following types of therapy can be employed in the treatment of patients with lymphomas EXCEPT:
    (A) Chemotherapy
    (B) Radiotherapy
    (C) Radioimmunotherapy
    (D) Magnotherapy

200. The exposure rate from a radioactive source is 100 millirem per hour (mR/h) at 3 m. What is the new exposure rate if the distance from the radiation source is increased to 6 m?
    (A) 75 mR/h
    (B) 55 mR/h
    (C) 25 mR/h
    (D) 15 mR/h

Answers

1. B – The exposure rate constant (ERC)

   For positron emitters, the exposure rate constant (ERC) is about 6 R/h per millicurie at 1 cm. The exposure rate of a 10 mCi dose of F-18 is approximately six times greater than that of a 10 mCi dose of Tc-99 m at a distance of approximately 8 inches.
   (PET Radiation Safety. Duke 2011))

2. B – Partial-volume effect

   PVE is caused by the finite spatial resolution of the imaging system which reveals how far the signal "spills out" around its actual location. The signal spreading falsely increases the object size and volume. Image sampling, where voxels in ROI include the signal from underlying tissues, also contributes to the phenomenon known as partial-volume effect.
   (Soret et al. 2007)

3. B – Difference in size of FOV between PET and the CT

   Discrepancy between fields of view (FOVs) in a PET/CT scanner—70 cm causes a truncation artifact when imaging extends beyond the CT FOV-50 cm; as a result no attenuation correction values for the truncated anatomy are being applied.
   (Sureshbabu and Mawlawi 2005)

4. D – Metallic implants artifacts

   Metallic implants create streaking artifacts on CT images because of their high photon absorption. Higher Hounsfield numbers consequently produce high PET attenuation coefficients and an overestimation of PET findings.
   (Sureshbabu and Mawlawi 2005)

5. C – The decay constant

   The decay constant decides how long the scintillation flashes in the crystal; a short decay time reduces detector dead time and as a result higher annihilation rates can be accepted.
   (Saha 2005)

6. B – Molecular imaging

   Radionuclide originated molecular imaging techniques such as positron emission tomography
      (PET) and single-photon emission computed tomography (SPECT) capture functional or phenotypic changes associated with pathology and unfold the molecular abnormalities responsible to form basis of many diseases.
   (Vallabhajosula 2007)

7. B – Resolution

   A PET system resolution, according to NEMA guidelines, is assessed by imaging a point source in the air and reconstructing the images with no smoothing or transformation of images. The resolution of the system is affected by the annihilation ambiguities, the detector ring diameter and the size of the scintillation crystal.
   (Nuclear Medicine/PET GE 2011)

8. B – Anaphylaxis

   Like the majority of other allergic reactions, anaphylaxis is caused by the release of histamine and other chemicals from mast cells (type of white blood cell found in vast numbers in the airways, digestive system, and skin).
   (Robbins and Cotran 2010)

9. A – Rb-82

   Sr 82- Rb 82 generator (Cardiogen-82; Bracco Diagnostics, Inc, Princeton, NJ) for myocardial perfusion imaging studies.
   (Vallabhajosula et al. 2011)

10. A – Normal sinus rhythm

    Normal sinus rhythm is the reference physiologic rhythm of the heart. By convention, normal sinus rhythm is usually defined as sinus rhythm with a heart rate between 60 and 100 beats/min.
    (Goldberger 2006)

11. C – Linearity

    Linearity is performed at installation and quarterly. The DC must function linearly between the lowest and highest activities used in the NM department.
    (Early and Sodee 1995)

12. B – F-18

    The PET radiopharmaceuticals O-15, C-11, and N-13 are biochemically indistinguishable from their natural counterparts. On the other hand, the half-lives of these three PET radionuclides are not perfect for routine clinical use.
    (Vallabhajosula et al. 2011)

13. A – True coincidences

    A true coincidence (event) is registered each time contained by the coincidence time-window when neither photon is undergoing any form of interaction prior to discovery. Singles are coincidence events which are lost due to, e.g., dead time, tissue attenuation.
    (Nuclear Medicine/PET GE 2011)

14. A – Amino acids

    The tumor growth and development are described by an increase in the rate of protein synthesis. Because amino acids (AAs) are the building blocks for protein synthesis, transport of AAs into cells is one of the most important and essential steps in protein synthesis.
    (Vallabhajosula et al. 2011)

15. C – An electron and a positron

    Being unstable, the two particles annihilate each other converting all its mass into energy and in that way emitting two photons of 511 keV each (which is resting energy of the electron or positron) in opposite direction.
    (Shukla and Kumar 2006)

16. A – Neck

    Brown adipose tissue is especially abundant in newborns and in hibernating mammals. Studies using PET scanning of adult humans have shown that brown fat is related not to white fat, but to skeletal muscle and it is still present in adults (females > males, children > adults) in the upper chest and neck (neck (2.3%) > paravertebral (1.4%) > mediastinum (0.9%) > perinephric (0.8%), overall up to 4%).
    (Cannon and Nedegaard 2004)

17. C – BGO (bismuth germinate)

    The stopping power of the scintillators governs the mean distance the photon travels before it stops, and depends on the density and effective Z of the detector material.
    (Lin and Alavi 2009)

18. C – Melanoma

    Although melanoma mainly is found in the skin, it can also arise in mucosal surfaces (anus, vaginal surfaces), ocular locations, or meningeal surfaces.
    (Karakousis 2011)

19. C – Pulmonology

    Because of the complication associated with cancer biology, the PET radiopharmaceutical use in oncology accounts for most applications. The recent advancement in tracers' development in neurology and cardiology, a PET/CT application in these areas, might even top the current PET/CT utility in oncology.
    (Vallabhajosula et al. 2011)

20. B 11 mCi
    (Formula 16A)

21. B – Effective dose

    It is given by the expression: $E = \text{SUM}(\text{WT} \times \text{CDE})$
    where:
    E = the effective whole-body dose, WT = the tissue weighting factor, CDE = committed dose equivalent.
    (Lombardi 1999)

22. C – 20–30 mSv

    The combined whole-body effective dose can be reduced to 5–15 mSv if a low-dose CT is used.
    (Patton et al. 2009)

23. D – +1

    The positron or antielectron is the antiparticle or the antimatter counterpart of the electron.
    (Early and Sodee 1995)

24. C – Histologic evaluation

    The diagnosis of a melanoma is made by pathologic analysis of the excisional biopsied specimen.
    (Karakousis and Czerniecki 2011)

25. B – Sinograms

    PET data are acquired directly into sinograms in a manner similar to matrix mode in planar imaging and all necessary corrections are often applied at the time of sinograms formation.
    (Wahl 2009)

26. B – Nitrogen-13

    Cu-62 (parent radionuclide Zinc-62), Ga-68 (parent Germanium-68), and Rb-82 (parent Strontium-82) are generator produced radionuclides.
    (Wahl 2009)

27. B – Pulse height analyzer

    The signal from the photomultiplier tube goes into a PHA in order to do this energy distinction. Only signals of a certain size (height) will pass the analyzer and become registered. This pulse height is preset by defining a voltage window (ΔE) between a lower level (LL) and an upper level (UL). In the PET systems the window of PHA is centered on 511 keV with LL of 350 keV and UL of 650 keV.
    (Saha 2005)

Answers 49

28. C – Proliferation

Cell proliferation, increased mitotic rate, and lack of differentiation are considered as the focal reasons accountable for accelerated malignant growth.
(Vallabhajosula et al. 2011)

29. C – Tc-99 m methylenediphosphonate (MDP)

Fluoride ions diffuse through capillaries into the bone extracellular fluid and chemisorb onto the bone surface by exchanging with hydroxyl (OH) groups in hydroxyapatite crystal of bone to form fluoroapatite. The uptake of Tc-99 m MDP and F-18 fluoride in malignant bone lesions reflects the increased regional blood flow and bone turnover.
(Blake et al. 2001)

30. A – Angiogenesis

Angiogenesis is required in various physiological as well as pathological processes, including physical development, wound repair, reproduction, response to ischemia, solid tumor growth, and metastatic tumor spread.
(Wahl 2009)

31. C – Calibration and constancy

Calibration or accuracy is performed before the first use of the instrument, annually, and after repair. Constancy QC of the survey meter is performed daily with a long half-life reference source.
(Christian et al. 2004)

32. C – The brain

The Circle of Willis is formed by the merging of the anterior, middle, and posterior cerebral arteries and the anterior and posterior communicating arteries (connect the left and right sides of an artery).
(Christian et al. 2004)

33. B – Produces the X-ray

X-ray photons are produced by bombarding the target in the vacuum tube with a stream of fast-moving electrons; X-rays are produced when the electrons are suddenly decelerated upon collision with the metal target. ("Bremsstrahlung" or "braking radiation")
(Wahl 2009)

34. B – 0 HU

The radiodensity of distilled water at standard pressure and temperature (STP) is defined as zero Hounsfield units (HU), while the radiodensity of air at STP is defined as −1,000 HU.
(Prokop and Galanski 2003)

35. D – Constancy

    Daily readings of the standard, e.g., Cs-137 should fall within the tolerance limits +/− 10% for NRC regulated states.
    (Christian et al. 2004)

36. C – Oxygen-15

    Oxygen-15: half-life of 2 min, mean energy 735 8.2 keV, and positron range in water of 8.2 mm.
    (Wahl 2009)

37. C – Blank scan

    The blank scan is acquired daily using transmission rod sources and can be used to monitor system (crystals, blocks, and modules) stability. It represents the sensitivity response to the transmission source without attenuating material or patient in the gantry (blank).
    (Christian et al. 2004)

38. D – The light output

    The scintillation process means the conversion of high-energy photons into visible light via interaction with a scintillating material. A scintillation detector or scintillation counter is obtained when a scintillator is coupled to an electronic light sensor such as a photomultiplier tube (PM). Among the properties listed above, the light output is the most important, as it affects both the efficiency and the resolution of the detector.
    (Early and Sodee 1995)

39. C – Choline

    All cells use choline for the biosynthesis of phospholipids, which are fundamental components of all cellular walls.
    (Roivainen et al. 2000)

40. B – 10.7%

    The given volume is additional information and must be disregarded, since the percent error formula does not utilize it.
    (Formula 8A)

41. B – Fused coronal
    (Wahl 2009)

42. C – Topogram, transmission CT, emission PET

    In general, PET/CT is performed using a protocol comprising a topogram followed by a low-dose CT for attenuation correction (CT-AC) and anatomical correlation and by PET scan.
    (Wahl 2009)

Answers

43. B – Positional inaccuracy

    Other characteristics of PET offset this disadvantage. "Native" or "built in" positional inaccuracy is not present in, e.g., conventional single-photon emission techniques (SPECT).
    (Wahl 2009)

44. A – Rubidium-82

    Rubidium Rb-82 decays by positron emission and associated gamma emission with a physical half-life of 75 s and necessitates on-site generator use. CardioGen-82 is a closed system used to produce rubidium Rb-82 chloride injection for intravenous administration.
    (Wahl 2009)

45. A – Emits electrons

    The electrons are discharged from the cathode only when the filament is heated to the right temperature. Temperature is controlled by the tube current (mA).
    (Wahl 2009)

46. C – 4 h

    A delay time of 90 min postinjection is recommended for lesions where FDG uptake is relatively low, e.g., in breast cancer, and for suspected liver lesions in patients with colorectal cancer.
    (Lin and Alavi 2009)

47. D – Before the patient is injected

    It is important that QC be performed for PET and for CT machines by established protocols in accordance with predetermined daily, weekly, and quarterly schedules.
    (Christian et al. 2004)

48. A – Down

    Patients with melanoma need the whole body captured.
    (Lin and Alavi 2009)

49. A – False-positive uptake in FDG-PET images of patients with malignant mesothelioma

    Most benign pleural processes have an SUV < 2.2, although epithelioid tumors might not be FDG avid, and consequently, may be a source of false-negative results.
    (Lin and Alavi 2009)

50. C – 19 mCi

    $13\text{mCi} = I_o \times e^{-(0.693)(60\,\text{min}/110\,\text{min})} = 19\text{mCi}$ (Formula 16B)

51. B – Two times background levels

    Before disposing of the waste, all radiation symbols and signs should be removed or defaced.
    (Christian et al. 2004)

52. A – Frontal lobe of the brain

    The frontal lobe is the anterior portion of the brain. It is responsible for "higher cognitive functions" including emotions, creativity, and behavior (abstract thinking, creative thought, intellect, initiative, judgment). The frontal lobe is also involved in motor skills.
    (Christian et al. 2004)

53. A – 1 week

    To avoid false-positive/false-negative results in PET imaging, the time interval of 2–6 months is recommended for postradiation therapy scans.
    (Lin and Alavi 2009)

54. C – Magnetic resonance imaging (MRI)

    Magnetic resonance imaging (MRI) remains the imaging modality of choice when structural or anatomic abnormalities are suspected.
    (Placantonakis and Schwartz 2009)

55. B – Attenuation correction

    Attenuation correction and anatomical correlation enhance PET/CT specificity compared with PET alone.
    (Lin and Alavi 2009)

56. B – Peristalsis

    Once broken up, the food bolus is forced into the pharynx and beyond to the esophagus and stomach through peristalsis and gravity.
    (Frohlich 2001)

57. B – Attenuation-corrected (AC) images only

    AC must be completed before SUV is calculated — if not, the amounts would depend upon the extent of attenuation.
    (Lin and Alavi 2009)

58. A – Fluorine-18

    Fluorine-18 has a physical half-life of 110 min and carbon-11, nitrogen-13, or oxygen-15 with physical half-lives of 20, 10, and 2 min, respectively. Mnemonic: ONC -2,10,20.
    (Wahl 2009)

Answers

59. C – lesions that are too small to be evaluated by PET

    Also, bronchioloalveolar carcinoma, differentiated adenocarcinoma, carcinoid, and mucoepidermoid carcinoma seem to have poor FDG avidity, and can be a source of false negatives.
    (Lin and Alavi 2009)

60. C – Motion artifact

    Motion can be voluntary, e.g., patient movement or involuntary, e.g, respiration. The most efficient way to reduce motion artifacts is to reduce the scanning time. Methods to reduce patient motion artifacts also include patient immobilization, ECG-gated CT, and some correction algorithms.
    (Lin and Alavi 2009)

61. B – Product of beam current and exposure time

    Modifying kVp will also reduce radiation exposure, but to a lesser extent.
    (Patton et al. 2009)

62. C – sentinel node biopsy

    Best identification of the sentinel node (SN) is currently achieved by using preoperative SN localization lymphoscintigraphy and dual-modality intraoperative detection, using the γ probe and a blue dye.
    (Karakousis and Czerniecki 2011)

63. C – 60 min

    At least 60 min time interval allows sufficient uptake in the tumor and contrast with the background. According to the minimal performance standards, the use of longer uptake time intervals is allowed.
    (Boellaard 2011)

64. D – Is more prominent on non-attenuation-corrected images

    Normal FDG uptake in the lungs is faint and homogeneous on AC images.
    (Lin and Alavi 2009)

65. C – SUV max

    Although SUV max is easily measured, it is highly dependent on the statistical quality of the images, and the size of the maximal pixel.
    (Wahl 2009)

66. A – Altered metabolism (PET) and areas of structural change (CT)

    Both the CT and PET CT fusion images are used to localize PET uptake abnormalities.
    (Lin and Alavi 2009)

67. A – False negative

    A positive PET scan in this circumstance is more likely to be true positive. Pretest probability is the probability that a person suffers from a disease before the test is executed.
    (Lin and Alavi 2009)

68. A – Vascular dementia

    Lower metabolism differentiating vascular dementia from Alzheimer's disease (AD) is mainly observed in the deep gray nuclei, cerebellum, primary cortices, middle temporal gyrus, and anterior cingulate gyrus.
    (Lin and Alavi 2009)

69. C – Image registration

    Registration aligns images by applying transformations to one of the images so that it matches the other; image registration aids in many critical tasks such as diagnosis, performing image guided surgery, planning radiotherapy, and/or surgery etc.
    Hajnal et al. 2001

70. C – 267 dpm

    The background counts are subtracted from the given gross counts to obtain the net counts. If the net counts are given, there is no need for background counts subtractions.
    (Formula 11)

71. B – A dual-head scintillation camera positioned in front of a CT scanner

    Equipment manufacturers are using dual-head scintillation cameras positioned in front of a CT scanner and sharing a common imaging table.
    (Patton et al. 2009)

72. C – Proximal stomach uptake is higher than distal stomach uptake

    Moderate diffuse stomach uptake is also considered as a normal, physiologic variation.
    (Lin and Alavi 2009)

73. B – >10 days

    This time allows avoidance of the chemotherapeutic effect, and of transient fluctuations in F-18 -FDG uptake due to stunning or flare of tumor uptake.
    (Wahl 2009)

Answers

74. C – An injected blood clot

    The injury to the venous endothelium during injection causes formation of blood clots at the site of injury, which consecutively detach from the vein, settle in the pulmonary vasculature, and are noted as hot spots in the lung.
    (Lin and Alavi 2009)

75. A – Short-axis slices

    The short-axis tomograms is displayed with the apical slices always shown first, then progressing serially toward the cardiac base. The orientation is as if the viewer were observing the heart from the cardiac apex, with the left ventricle to the viewer's right and the right ventricle to the viewer's left.
    ACC/AHA/SNM 1992

76. B – Diffuse muscular and myocardial uptake

    A hyperinsulinemic state is caused by increased serum insulin levels from either exogenous administration or endogenous secretion of insulin associated with insufficient fasting.
    (Lin and Alavi 2009)

77. A – Lipoma

    On FDG-PET imaging, malignant tumors generally appear as hypermetabolic lesions with uptake correlating well with the tumor histologic grade. A lipoma, the most common form of soft tissue tumor, is a benign tumor composed of adipose tissue.
    (Hickeson and Abikhzer 2011)

78. C – Chronic obstructive pulmonary disease

    "Chronic bronchitis" and "emphysema" are included within the chronic obstructive pulmonary disease (COPD) diagnosis.
    (Kumar and Abbas 2010)

79. A – Carbon-11-labeled Pittsburgh Compound B (C-11 PiB)

    The beta-amyloid protein, by forming a major part of the amyloid plaque, is implicated in Alzheimer's development and increased C-11 PiB uptake is observed in patients with AD.
    (Wahl 2009)

80. C – 84.3 min
    (Formula 14)

81. B – NaI (Tl)

    The property of the scintillation detector described as the number of scintillations produced by each incident photon is called the light output. Sodium iodide doped with thallium-NaI (Tl) scintillator has the highest light output, it is hygroscopic, has low stopping power-low linear attenuation coefficient for 511 keV, long decay time, and is no longer used in PET imaging.
    (Lin and Alavi 2009)

82. D – Pharynx

    The main organs of the digestive system also comprise: mouth, esophagus, stomach, and small and large intestines.
    (Christian and Bernier 2004)

83. B – The ability to differentiate viable tumor from fibrosis

    Up to 64% of patients with Hodgkin Lymphoma (HL) will present with a residual mass on CT following treatment, but only 18% will actually relapse.
    (Iagaru et al. 2008)

84. C – Diffuse large B-cell lymphoma

    Diffuse large B cell can occur at any age, and it is slightly more common in men than women, making up approximately 40% of all cases. Diffuse large B-Cell lymphoma is considered a high-grade lymphoma and therefore requires prompt treatment.
    (Jhanwar and Straus 2006)

85. B – Poor spatial resolution

    PET/CT scanners use the high spatial resolution of CT and as a result PET/CT is superior to either PET or CT alone for the evaluation of head malignancy.
    (Wahl 2009)

86. A – Lymphocyte

    The two most common lymphocytes are the B cell and the T cell that protect the body against germs by producing antibodies (B cells) against fungi, viruses, and bacteria (T cells).
    (Kumar 2010)

87. C – Germanium-68

    Attenuation correction factors measured by CT are only scaled up for 511 keV and PET-CT enables only segmental attenuation correction. Typical transmission scans with a rotating rod add about 3–6 min to the single-bed imaging time. This is acceptable for cardiac imaging, but a significant drawback for multi-bed position oncology scans.
    (Wahl 2009)

Answers

88. B – The gastroesophageal junction

    Increased FDG uptake at the gastroesophageal junction can result in a false-positive study imitating a distal esophageal neoplasm or node.
    (Lin and Alavi 2009)

89. D – Recurrent

    A recurrent lymphoma does not have to return to the same site of the body or be the exact same subtype in order to be considered a recurrent lymphoma. Indolent Non-Hodgkin's lymphoma (NHL), represents a group of incurable slow growing lymphomas, e.g., follicular lymphoma, a small lymphocytic lymphoma that is highly responsive to initial therapy, but relapses with less responsive disease.
    (Andreoli et al. 2001)

90. A – D

    Electron–positron annihilation occurs when an electron (e−) and a positron (e+, the electron's antiparticle) collide. The result of the collision is the annihilation of the electron and positron, and the creation of two gamma ray photons.
    (Wahl 2009)

91. D – Improves accuracy of the scan interpretation

    The coregistered, high-resolution anatomy accurately aligned with PET data localizes functional abnormalities and clarifies equivocal situations.
    (Patton et al. 2009)

92. A – Low resolution

    Increased FDG activity in infection and inflammation depends on its uptake in activated granulocytes and macrophages with increased rates of glucose metabolism.
    (Wahl 2009)

93. A – The dynamics of lesion glucose metabolism

    Result of the percentage change in SUV of a lesion from early to delayed imaging is reflecting the dynamics of lesion glucose metabolism. The auxiliary value of the dual time point FDG-PET is problematic, mainly because of the substantial overlap of benign and malignant nodule FDG-PET characteristics.
    (Barger and Nandular 2012)

94. B – Short half-life

    Exercise stress is somewhat difficult with Rb-82 due to its short half-life, breathing motion from immediate postexercise imaging, and close patient contact that may significantly increase the radiation exposure to the staff.
    (Zaret and Beller 2005)

95. B – Positron emission tomography (PET)

    Pneumothorax and hemorrhage are the most common complications of transthoracic needle biopsy.
    (Houseni et al. 2011)

96. B – The gastroesophageal junction

    In patients without a specific history of esophagogastric disease, a gastroesophageal maximum SUV of less than 4 is usually not associated with gastroesophageal neoplasia.
    (Lin and Alavi 2009)

97. A – Reduces motion artifacts

    Gated acquisitions improved quantification over nongated acquisitions by 8% and 10% for 2D and 3D modes accordingly.
    (Vines et al. 2007)

98. C – Circulatory system

    The lymphatic system is comprised of a network of conduits called lymphatic vessels that transport excess fluids away from interstitial spaces in body tissue and return the fluids to the bloodstream.
    (Kumar and Abbas 2010)

99. B – Rubidium Rb-82

    Rb-82 is produced from a strontium-82 (Sr-82)/Rb-82 generator, which can be eluted every 10 min. The half-life (T1/2) of Sr-82 is 25.5 days, which results in a generator life of 4–8 weeks.
    (Zaret and Beller 2005)

100. D – Maximum-intensity projection

    Maximum-Intensity Projection (MIP) is a simple image-order rendering technique. MIP involves visualizing the regions/structures with the highest intensity values.
    (Lin and Alavi 2009)

101. D – Positron emission tomography

    PET images describe function, in that they represent metabolic or biochemical processes (physiology), while the other imaging modalities, such as CT and MRI, visualize structure and shape (anatomy).
    (Christian et al. 2004)

102. B – Skeletal muscles

   The cerebellum coordinates voluntary movements such as posture, balance, coordination, and speech, resulting in smooth, balanced muscular activity.
   (Christian et al. 2004)

103. B – The scout scan

   A scout scan can be obtained with a transmission scan using a Ge-68 source on a dedicated PET unit, with a low-dose CT on PET/CT scanners, or with an emission image after injection of a small activity in labs using Rb-82.
   (Di Carli and Lipton 2007)

104. A – Lymphoma spreads in a predictable pattern

   The staging system used for lymphomas is an anatomical classification, which is created upon the model that lymphoma spreads in a foreseeable pattern of neighboring disease. Lymphoma starts at a single lymph node and then advances to neighboring lymph nodes via the lymphatic system, before disseminating to distant sites and organs.
   (Kumar and Abbas 2010)

105. B – Thallium Tl-201

   During one capillary pass, Rb-82 is incompletely extracted by the myocardial cells via the Na+/K+ adenosine triphosphatase pump, and extraction is inversely and nonlinearly proportional to perfusion. Furthermore, extraction and retention, at a given perfusion level, may be affected by drugs, severe acidosis, hypoxia, and ischemia.
   (Zaret and Beller 2005)

106. B – 3 cm or less

   By definition PN is not associated with the hilum or mediastinum and is not linked to atelectasis, pleural effusion, or lymphadenopathy.
   (Houseni et al. 2011)

107. A – Water O-15

   Water O-15 uptake is linearly correlated to flow and a single compartment model is used for flow quantitation.
   Al-Mallah et al. 2010

108. D – Sentinel node localization

   The route of the initial lymph drainage and extent of tumor spread can be determined by locating the sentinel lymph node—the first node that filters lymph fluid draining from the melanoma or breast carcinoma.
   (Wahl 2009)

109. D – Standard uptake value min (SUV min)

    Metabolic bulk-based parameters, metabolic tumor volume (MTV), tumor's glycolytic volume (TGV), and total lesion glycolysis (TLG=MTV x SUV mean), seem to be better indicators of primary tumor aggressiveness and, as a result, more sensitive than the single-pixel-derived SUV max.
    (Gerbaudo et al. 2011)

110. A – Lateral brain localizer image

    A localizer ("scout" or "scanogram" or "topogram" depending on vendor) is usually a specific image that is not really a cross-section but a projection image.
    (Brant et al. 2007)

111. C – Diagnostic CT

    An average effective dose from diagnostic CT is 2–3 times higher than that from F-18 FDG.
    (Brix et al. 2005)

112. C – Metabolic lesion characteristics

    CT is in general used to further differentiate nodules that are detected on other imaging tests such as chest radiography.
    (Prokop and Galanski 2003)

113. C – Free fatty acids and glucose

    The heart metabolizes a comprehensive variety of substrates such as free fatty acids, glucose, lactate, pyruvate, ketone bodies, and amino acids, but under normal conditions, free fatty acids and glucose are the most important sources of energy.
    (Bengel et al. 2009)

114. B – Thyroid

    The bone marrow, lymph nodes, lymph vessels, and the appendix are also parts of the lymphatic system. The spleen is the only lymphatic organ responsible for filtering blood.
    (Kumar and Abbas 2010)

115. A – Screening

    Determining location of tumors if rising CEA level suggests recurrence was the earliest indication approved for Medicare reimbursement. Whole-body PET scans for assessment of recurrence of colorectal cancer cannot be ordered more frequently than once every 12 months, unless medical necessity documentation supports a separate reevaluation settings of a rising CEA within this period.
    (CMS 2011)

Answers

116. B – Lobe

    The right lung is divided into three lobes, superior, middle, and inferior, by two interlobular fissures and the left lung is divided into two lobes, an upper and a lower, by an interlobular fissure.
    (Hansell et al. 2008)

117. D – F-18 fluorodeoxyglucose

    Medicare covers FDG-PET for the determination of myocardial viability as a primary or initial diagnostic study prior to revascularization, or following an inconclusive SPECT.
    (NCD 2012)

118. C – Focal

    The focal uptake associated with GI pathology is observed in ~70% of cases. The incidence of false-positive results, e.g., normal, focal uptake in the ascending colon, is lower with PET/CT imaging.
    (Lin and Alavi 2009)

119. B – The non-collinearity of the pair of annihilation photons

    PET scanners have insufficient spatial resolution, due to instrumentation and physical factors when compared with other imaging modalities, such as CT and MR. The key limiting factor is attributable to the distance that positrons, once released from the parent nucleus, must travel before they lose energy and annihilate with an electron in tissue.
    (Zaidi and Thompson 2009)

120. C – Lymphoma

    The malignant lymphocytes accumulate in lymph nodes, causing enlargement and appearance of solid masses. The lymphocytes can also infiltrate extranodal tissues eg. bone marrow and various organs (gastrointestinal tract, lung, skin, central nervous system).
    (Kumar and Abbas 2010)

121. D – discontinue breast-feeding for at least 12 h after injection of radiotracer

    The short physical half-life of 18 F and the low excretion of FDG into breast milk support the use of PET as the preferred oncologic imaging procedure in nursing mothers if imaging cannot otherwise be avoided. Some authors concluded that cessation of breast-feeding is unnecessary after PET studies but close contact should be avoided.
    (SNM 2011)

122. A – Papillary and follicular

    DTC is divided into papillary cancer (classic type and encapsulated, follicular variant, and aggressive variants such as sclerosing, columnar, or tall cell variants) and follicular cancer (classic, Hurthle, and clear cell types).
    (Kumar and Abbas 2010)

123. C – Ipsilateral axillary node uptake

    Node uptake at the draining lymph node is due to particle formation and subsequent phagocytosis.
    (Lin and Alavi 2009)

124. B – Transverse colon

    The ascending colon is located on the right side of abdomen up to the hepatic flexure and the descending colon is located on the left side of the abdomen from the splenic flexure to the iliac crest.
    (Moore et al. 2010)

125. A – Improved noise-to-signal ratios

    Increases in sensitivity enhance signal-to-noise ratios (SNRs) in the data, which also corresponds to advances in image SNR.
    (Rahmim and Zaidi 2008)

126. C – change in memory

    The word dementia comes from the Latin de meaning "apart" and mens from the genitive mentis meaning "mind".
    (Symptoms of Dementia 2011)

127. D – Valium administration in dementia imaging

    Sedatives, antipsychotic medications, drugs such as amphetamines, and narcotics modify cerebral metabolism and it should not be used in the brain metabolism imaging.
    (Wahl 2009)

128. B – Reproducible

    The above definition is applied when the PET scan, whether at rest alone or rest with stress, is used following a SPECT that was found to be inconclusive.
    (CMS 2011)

129. B – Dysfunctional but viable

    Stunned or hibernating myocardium has the capacity to return to normal or display substantial improvement in contractile function with revascularization.
    (Takalkar et al. 2011)

Answers

130. C – left ventricle

    Cardiac imaging with CT and MR imaging always relies on technical developments because high temporal and spatial resolution is necessary for the satisfactory evaluation of heart vascular systems.
    (Madden 2007)

131. B – Should be continued

    After completion of the study, the patient should be instructed to continue with fluid intake and voiding to minimize radiation exposure.
    (Hamblen and Lowe 2003)

132. A – The small intestine

    The small intestine is suspended from the body wall by an extension of the peritoneum called the mesentery. It is the major site of chemical digestion and absorption of nutrients by the body.
    (Moore et al. 2010)

133. C – Standardized uptake value

    Standarized uptake value (SUV) — sometimes known as the dose uptake ratio (DUR), or dose absorption ratio (DAR) — is a method for normalizing whole-body PET images relative to volume of distribution in the patient and injected dose.
    (Hallett 2004)

134. D – Housing info

    Information on recent chemotherapy and/or radiation therapy, presence of inflammatory conditions, and other relevant features (e.g., claustrophobia, difficulty with lying flat) is also necessary for optimal patient care and interpretation of FDG-PET images.
    (Wahl 2009)

135. C – b

    The gallbladder is a small pouch that sits just under the liver. In adults, the gallbladder measures approximately 8 cm (3.1 in) in length and 4 cm (1.6 in) in diameter when fully distended. It is divided into three sections: fundus, body, and neck.
    (Madden 2007)

136. B – Minimize physiologic muscular uptake

    This is particularly important in patients with head and neck cancer to minimize uptake in local laryngeal and masticatory muscles.
    (Wahl 2009)

137. C – Neutropenia

Neutrophils in normal conditions make up 50–70% of circulating white blood cells and serve as the primary defense against infections by fighting bacteria in the blood.
(Frohlich 2001)

138. A – Auditory information

The temporal lobes are responsible for hearing, speech recognition, and music. They are also responsible for short-term memory and for help in sorting out new information.
(Christian et al. 2004)

139. A – Diagnosis

FDG-PET is rarely used in the diagnosis of lymphoma because most suspicious lesions usually proceed directly to biopsy for tissue diagnosis. A bone marrow biopsy may also be done to determine if the bone marrow has been affected.
(Andreoli et al. 2001)

140. C – 0.9 ml

To solve this problem, first decay 14 mCi for 1 h to 14:00 h, which equals 9.6 mCi. Subtract 9.6 mCi from 14 mCi, which equals 4.4 mCi. 4.4 mCi is the amount you need to obtain from the other unit dose; however, the answer is needed in volume. To obtain the needed volume, first calculate the concentration; therefore, divide 9.6 mCi by 2 ml's, (since the original concentration was 14 mCi/2 ml at 13:00 h), which equals 4.8 mCi/ml at 14:00 h. Since the needed activity to obtain 14 mCi at 14:00 h is 4.4 mCi, the 4.4 mCi dose needs to be divided by the concentration of 4.8 mCi/ml (what you want/what you have) to obtain the volume needed, which is 0.9 ml.
(Formula 16A and 18)

141. B – Proximity to the breast

High uptake of FDG in the lactating breast appears to be related to suckling. There is, however, little secretion of activity into breast milk. The normal lactation schedule can be maintained with a breast pump during the 24-h period.
(Hicks et al. 2001)

142. A – Falling CEA levels in the absence of a known source

CEA (carcinoembryonic antigen) is a type of protein molecule that is typically associated with certain tumors—most frequently in cancer of the colon and rectum—a rising CEA level indicates progression or recurrence of the cancer.
(Kumar and Abbas 2010)

143. C – Granulocyte colony-stimulating factor (G-CSF) therapy

    The stimulating effect that G-CSF therapy has on the spleen and bone marrow must be taken into account when performing a FDG-PET scan, as it can be an important source of false-positive results.
    (Lin and Alavi 2009)

144. B – Relaxes patient

    The most common anxiolytics—anti-anxiety medications—can be grouped in categories:
    Antidepressants (Prozac, Paxil, Zoloft), antihistamines (Atarax, Benadryl), and benzodiazepines (Ativan, Valium, Xanax). Diazepam (Valium) is commonly used orally for the short-term management of anxiety disorders and acute alcohol withdrawal.
    (Mycek and Harvey 2008)

145. A – Overestimated standardized uptake value (SUV)

    The presence of contrast agent produces an erroneous increase in the Hounsfield units, and as a result, an overestimation of the attenuation in these areas. The increase is linear with increasing contrast agent concentration.
    (Visvikis et al. 2004)

146. C – Symmetrical and increased

    Increased FDG uptake is a result of physiologic activity associated with the lymphatic tissue in Waldeyer's ring (a ring of lymphatic tissue formed by the two palatine tonsils, the pharyngeal tonsil, the lingual tonsil, and intervening lymphoid tissue). Symmetry is helpful in evaluating FDG uptake in the head and neck.
    (Lin and Alavi 2009)

147. D – Correction for table speed

    Differences in detector efficiencies, detection geometry, and dead-time effects also need to be taken into account to ensure the accuracy of performed quantifications.
    (Visvikis et al. 2004)

148. B – Region of interest

    For quantitative assessment, computer-derived regions, or regions of interest (ROI), drawn by the software users', e.g., nuclear medicine physician or technologist, are commonly applied. Manual definitions, maximum pixel value, three-dimensional isocontour at a percentage of maximum pixel value or fixed-size ROI centered on maximum pixel value methods of ROI placement are used to measure SUV.
    (Lin and Alavi 2009)

149. D – Polarity of charge

Positively charged positrons (e+), which are produced when radioactive substances decay, are the antimatter equivalents of electrons (e−).
(Christian et al. 2004)

150. B – C

The image illustrates the principles of a positron emission tomographY (PET). It shows how during the annihilation process two photons are emitted in ~1,800 opposing directions.
(Lin and Alavi 2009)

151. B – Weekly

An area 10 cm x 10 cm should be wiped with cotton swab or a filter paper disk; wipes should be then counted in well counter and data should be recorded in disintegrations per min. The survey frequency may be increased if the RSO deems that contamination has increased to levels that could pose an exposure problem or cause regulatory concern.
(Christian et al. 2004)

152. C – Vascular system

The vascular system plays an ultimate role in the pathogenesis of the cardiovascular disease and cancer and is a crucial element in inflammatory processes.
(Miles et al. 2007)

153. C – A coincidence event

Each PET detector records an incident photon and generates a timed pulse. Consequently these pulses are then combined in coincidence circuitry, and if the pulses fall within a narrow time-window, they are considered to be coincident.
(Wahl 2009)

154. C – Insulin

Insulin is produced within the body in a proportion to remove excess glucose from the blood. When blood glucose levels fall below a certain level, the glycogen stored in the liver and muscles is broken down and can then be utilized as an energy source (glucogenolysis).
(Mycek and Harvey 2008)

155. C – Oral

The same delay time used with iv administration before imaging can be applied after oral dosing. However, because of the considerable amount of F-18 FDG preserved in the gut, cautious interpretation will be needed when disease of the GI tract is being evaluated.
(Nair et al. 2007)

156. C – nitroglycerine

    The combination of pharmacological action of nitroglycerine is very effective in reducing myocardial ischemia: venodilation causes the amount of blood returning to the heart to decrease myocardial oxygen demand, while arterial dilation produces an increase to the amount of blood flowing to the myocardium.
    (Mycek and Harvey 2008)

157. D – Valium administration

    Elimination of artifactual collection of FDG in the colon and urinary system is essential if primary cancer, associated adenopathy, or faint recurrences are to be evaluated in FDG-PET imaging of the abdomen and pelvis.
    (Lin and Alavi 2009)

158. D – Decreased biological half-life of the radiopharmaceutical

    Lowered counting statistics results in a poor quality study and changed distribution can cause uptake in lymph nodes.
    (Burrell and MacDonald 2006)

159. C – More equivocal reports

    Improved image quality leads to more assurance in reporting, and less frequent equivocal reports.
    (Zaret and Beller 2005)

160. A – 518 MBq

    Since 1 Ci = 37 GBq, it is easy to convert 14 mCi to 0.014 Ci and multiply it by 37 which will give you 0.518 GBq, which then multiply by 1,000 to obtain 518 MBq.
    Another easier conversion is as follows, 1 mCi = 37 MBq, so all you have to do is multiply 14 mCi × 37 MBq/mCi = 518 MBq.
    (Formula 7A and B)

161. A – Degree of cell differentiation

    Blood forming organs and reproductive organs are more sensitive to radiation than highly specialized (differentiated) tissues of the nervous system.
    (Lombardi 1999)

162. C – Necrosis

    Non-metabolically active constituents, that is, necrotic tissue, fibrotic scar, or mucin, may reduce FDG uptake in tumors and lead to false negative in PET/CT scanning.
    (Kumar et al. 2009)

163. B – Reduce the dose venous retention

    The glucose measurement, F-18FDG administration with 20- to 30-mL saline flush, and postinjection activities should be performed with minimal interruption.
    (Hamblen and Lowe 2003)

164. A – The angle of orientation of the LOR

    The values along a particular horizontal row in the sinogram represent counts acquired along matching LORs at the angle that relates to that row. Angular location of the given point can be determined from the phase of the sine wave (y-axis).
    (Fahey 2002)

165. C – Is a normal variant

    Diffuse symmetric uptake can be seen in the normal thyroid gland in about 2% of scans. Diffuse thyroid uptake can occur in association with thyroiditis (particularly Hashimoto thyroiditis) or Graves' disease.
    (Lin and Alavi 2009)

166. A – Perfusion study

    Perfusion study is the most important single index that can be measured. In wash-out studies the time–concentration curve for an agent during its passage out of a tissue bed is analyzed.
    (Miles et al. 2007)

167. B – In 2D mode

    Septa are thin rings (~1 mm thick) of lead or tungsten. The outer diameter of the septal rings is equal to the ring diameter of the scanner, with the difference between the inner and outer diameters of the septa varying from 7 to 10 cm, depending on the manufacturer.
    (Wahl 2009)

168. A – Fourier transform

    This approach is comparable to an equalizer in a sound system. An equalizer exchanges the incoming sound signal into its constituent frequency bands creating a frequency spectrum from the low, or bass, frequencies to the high, or treble, frequencies.
    (Groch and Erwin 2000)

169. C – The electrocardiogram

    The electrocardiogram (ECG or EKG) registers cardiac electrical currents (voltages, potentials) by measures of metal electrodes placed on the surface of the body.
    (Goldberger 2006)

Answers

170. C – Non-attenuation corrected

171. D – 500 mrem/year (5 mSv/year)

    The whole-body dosimeter, worn at workers' chest or waist, is required by any worker who is likely to receive 10% of the occupational dose limit.
    (Lombardi 1999)

172. B – High radiation burden

    PET-FDG scanning can be completed in approximately 2 h from the injection with high quality of images (resolution of 4–8 mm for PET vs. 10–15 mm for SPECT) and does not require handling of potentially infected blood products (WBC).
    (Balink and Collins 2009)

173. C – Thymus

    The thymus is a specific organ of the immune system. The thymus produces and "instructs" T-lymphocytes (T cells) — each T cell targets a foreign substance which it identifies with its receptor.
    (Kumar and Abbas 2010)

174. C – Vasodilation

    Adenosine acts by inducing vasodilatation (A2 receptors) of precapillary sphincters in the arterioles and increasing in myocardial blood flow and oxygen supply.
    (Mycek and Harvey 2008)

175. A – Baseline PET-FDG scan

    To monitor response to therapy and to reduce the risk of false-negative and false-positive readings, it is recommended that a baseline scan be available for assessment.
    (Lin and Alavi 2009)

176. C – Hypoglycemia

    In general hypoglycemia is present at a fasting plasma glucose concentration of <60 ml/dl. The most common forms of hypoglycemia occur as a complication of treatment of diabetes mellitus with insulin or oral medications. Hypoglycemia is less common in nondiabetic persons and can occur at any age.
    (Andreoli et al. 2001)

177. D – Patient has hemoptysis

    Lesion's spiculated margin, smoking, and lesion diameter >3.0 cm are suggestive of malignancy.
    (Houseni et al. 2011)

178. B – 100/min

The number of chest compressions delivered per minute during CPR is an important determinant of return of spontaneous circulation (ROSC) and survival with good neurologic function.
(AHA 2011)

179. A – Screening

Medicare coverage for solitary pulmonary nodule imaging is approved, if the scan is performed for characterization of nodules indeterminate on CT.
(CMS 2012)

180. D – 12.3 mCi
(Formula 19A)

181. D – Produces the beam of X-ray

X-ray photons are produced by bombarding the target in the vacuum tube with the stream of fast moving electrons; a cathode emits electrons into the vacuum and an anode collects the electrons and consequently establishing a flow of electrical current.
(Prokop and Galanski 2003)

182. C – True negative

A study demonstrating a focal localized disease process, confirmed by additional investigations, as being the cause of fever of unknown origin (FUO) or malignancy is called true positive.
(Munro 2005)

183. A – Contrast

Image contrast to demarcate a lesion relies on its size relative to system resolution and its surrounding background. If a minimum size of a lesion does not grow bigger than system resolution, contrast may not be sufficient to appreciate the lesion, even at higher count density.
(Wahl 2009)

184. C – Blood glucose and insulin levels increase

FDG-PET imaging in uncontrolled diabetic patients may result in false-negative studies.
(Kumar et al. 2009)

185. B – Rubidium Rb-82

Rb-82 has the highest, 1.48 MeV, kinetic energy of the commonly used PET tracers, but the related long positron range of 2.6 mm reduces the spatial resolution with PET imaging.
(Zaret and Beller 2005)

Answers 71

186. B – Scattered foci of hypometabolism

 The scattered regions of hypometabolism are corresponding to the areas of prior infarct(s).
 (Mittra and Quon 2009)

187. A – Water O-15

 The absence of FDA approval has limited water O-15 to research applications in the USA
 (NCD 2012)

188. D – Colorectal cancer

 Hepatomegaly, ascites, and cachexia indicate presence of metastatic disease.
 (Abeloff and Armitage 2008)

189. B – 96% and 77%

 By incorporating the CT component into PET acquisition, the number of false-positive lesions is decreased, and overall specificity of PET/CT reaches 85% (sensitivity ~97%).
 (Kim et al. 2007)

190. B – Electronic ventricular pacemaker

 When a ventricular pacemaker fires, it produces a sharp vertical deflection (the pacemaker spike) followed by a QRS complex (representing depolarization of the ventricle).
 (Goldberger 2006)

191. A – 2.5 rems

 1 sievert = 100 rems, you have 25 millisieverts, which is 0.025 Sieverts; therefore, if 1 Sievert = 100 rems, then 0.025 Sieverts = 2.5 rems.
 (Formula 7D)

192. C – Using Luer-activated device

 Luer-activated device, prepierced septum/blunt catheter, and pressure activated safety valve devices are available needless systems.
 (Perry and Potter 2010)

193. C – >3 cm

 The term "mass" usually indicates a solid or partly solid opacity; its contour, border, or density characteristics can be evaluated with CT.
 (Hansell et al. 2008)

194. D – Patient age

In the most common approach, SUV is defined as the tracer activity concentration within a volume of interest, divided by the injected dose per unit body weight. The patient's weight and height are needed for the estimation of parameters such as the lean body mass and SUVLBM or body surface area and SUVBSA.
(Lucignani et al. 2004)

195. B – 8.2 m

The answer required is in meters; therefore, it is very important to convert to the appropriate units. You must read the question carefully and determine which units are requested. It is very easy to come up with a wrong answer that is presented as one of the multiple-choice answers; therefore, special attention must be paid to problems containing varying units.
(Formula 12)

196. A – Contrast media

Iodine and barium are the most common types of contrast agents for enhancing X-ray-based imaging methods (CT). Gadolinium is used in magnetic resonance imaging as a MRI contrast agent and microbubble contrast agents are used to aid the sonographic imaging, e.g., echocardiograms in the detection of a cardiac shunt.
(Prokop and Galanski 2003)

197. A – Noise equivalent count rate (NECR)

NECR or effective count rate is comparative to the signal-to-noise ratio in the ending reconstructed images and works as a good parameter to evaluate the performances of different PET machines. NECR is given by: $NECR = T2/T + S + R$ where T, R, and S are the true, random, and scatter coincidence count rates accordingly.
(Saha 2005)

198. B – Dementia

Alzheimer's disease is by far the most common cause of dementia and accounts for two-thirds of dementia cases.
(Newberg and Alavi 2010)

199. D – Magnotherapy

Radioimmunotherapy, with highly specific monoclonal antibodies directed at lymphoma cells, and high-dose chemotherapy, with bone marrow or stem cell transplantation, are new treatment options; they are being used in initial treatments and for select patients who relapse after standard treatment.
(Andreoli et al. 2001)

200. C – 25 mR/h

This problem is a representation of the Inverse Square Law — radiation exposure is reduced to three-quarters of the original intensity by doubling the distance from the radiation source. The exposure rate is 100mR/h at 3 m and 25mR/h at 6 m.
(Formula 12)

References and Suggested Readings

Abeloff DM, Armitage OJ. Abeloff's clinical oncology. 4 thth ed. Philadelphia, PA: Churchill Livingstone Elsevier; 2008.
AHA. Guidelines for CPR and ECC. http://www.heart.org/idc/groups/heart-public/@wcm/@ecc/documents/downloadable/ucm_317350.pdf
Al-Mallah HM, Sitek A, Moore CS, et al. Assessment of myocardial perfusion and function with PET and PET/CT. J Nucl Cardiol. 2010;17:498–513.
Andreoli TE, Bennett JC, et al. Cecil essentials of medicine. 5th ed. Philadelphia, PA: WB Saunders Company; 2001.
Balink H, Collins J. F-18 FDG PET/CT in the diagnosis of fever of unknown origin. Clin Nucl Med. 2009;34(12):862–8.
Barger RL, Nandular RK. Diagnostic performance of dual-time 18 F-FDG PET in the diagnosis of pulmonary nodules: a meta-analysis. Acad Radiol. 2012;19(2):153–8.
Bengel MF, Higuchi T, Javadi SM, et al. Cardiac positron emission tomography. J Am Coll Cardiol. 2009;54:1–15.
Blake GM, Park-Holohan SJ, Cook GJ, et al. Quantitative studies of bone with the use of 18 F-fluoride and 99mTc-methylene diphosphonate. Semin Nucl Med. 2001;31:28–49.
Boellaard R. Need for standardization of F-18 FDG PET/CT for treatment response assessments. J Nucl Med. 2011;52:93s.
Brant EW, Helms AC, Webb RW. Fundamentals of body CT. 3rd ed. Philadelphia, PA: Saunders Elsevier; 2007.
Brix G, Lechel U, Glatting G, et al. Radiation exposure of patients undergoing whole-body dual-modality 18 F-FDG PET/CT examinations. J Nucl Med. 2005;46:608–13.
Burrell S, MacDonald A. Artifacts and pitfalls in myocardial perfusion imaging. J Nucl Med Technol. 2006;34:193–211.
Cannon B, Nedegaard J. Brown adipose tissue: function and physiological significance. Physiol Rev. 2004;84(1):277–359.
Chen W, Li G, Parsons M, et al. Clinical significance of incidental focal versus diffuse thyroid uptake on FDG-PET imaging. PET Clin. 2007;2:321–9.
Christian PE, Bernier DR, Langan JK. Nuclear medicine and PET: technology and techniques. 5th ed. St. Louis, MO: Mosby; 2004.
CMS. National Coverage Determination.https://www.cms.gov/medicare-coverage-database/details/ncd. Accessed 25 Dec 2011.
Dementia. http://www.medicalnewstoday.com/articles/142214.php. Accessed june15, 2011.
Di Carli MF, Lipton MJ, editors. Cardiac PET and PET/CT imaging. New York, NY: Springer; 2007.
Early PJ, Sodee BD. Principles and practice of nuclear medicine. 2nd ed. St. Louis, MO: Mosby; 1995.
Fahey HF. Data acquisition in PET imaging. J Nucl Med Technol. 2002;30(2):39–49.
Frohlich ED. Rypin's basic sciences review. 18th ed. Philadelphia, PA: J.B. Lippincott Company; 2001.

Gerbaudo HV, Katz IS, Nowak KA, et al. Multimodality imaging review of malignant pleural mesothelioma diagnosis and staging. PET Clin. 2011;6:275–97.
Goldberger LA. Clinical electrocardiography: a simplified approach. 7th ed. St. Louis, MO: Mosby Elsevier; 2006.
Groch MW, Erwin WD. SPECT in the Year 2000. Basic principles. J Nucl Med Technol. 2000;2000(4):233–44.
Hajnal GV, Hill LGD, Hawkes JD. Medical image registration (Biomedical engineering). Boca Raton, FL: CRC Press; 2001.
Hallett WA. Quantification in clinical fluorodeoxyglucose positron emission tomography. Nucl Med Commun. 2004;25(7):647–50.
Hamblen MS, Lowe JV. Clinical F-18 FDG oncology patient preparation techniques. J Nucl Med Technol. 2003;31(1):3–7.
Hansell DM, Bankier AA, MacMahon H, et al. Fleischner Society: glossary of terms for thoracic imaging. Radiology. 2008;246(3):697–722.
Hicks JR, Binns D, Stabin GM. Pattern of uptake and excretion of F-18 FDG in the lactating breast. J Nucl Med. 2001;42(8):1238–42.
Hickeson M, Abikhzer G. Review of physiologic and pathophysiologic sources of fluorodeoxyglucose uptake in the chest wall on PET. PET Clin. 2011;6:339–64.
Houseni M, Chamroonrat W, Zhuang J, et al. Multimodality imaging assessment of pulmonary nodules. PET Clin. 2011;6:231–50.
Iagaru A, Goris LM, Gambhir SS. Perspectives of molecular imaging and radioimmunotherapy in Lymphoma. Radiol Clin N Am. 2008;46:243–52.
Jhanwar SY, Straus JD. The role of PET in Lymphoma. J Nucl Med. 2006;47:1326–34.
Karakousis CG, Czerniecki JB. Diagnosis of melanoma. PET Clin. 2011;6:1–8.
Kim SK, Allen-Auerbach M, Goldin J, et al. Accuracy of PET/CT in characterization of solitary pulmonary lesions. J Nucl Med. 2007;48(2):214–20.
Kumar V, Abbas KA, Faust N. Robbins and Cotran pathologic basis of disease. 7 th ed. Elsevier Saunders, 2005.
Kumar R, Rani N, et al. False-negative and false-positive results in FDG-PET and PET/CT in breast cancer. PET Clin. 2009;4:289–98.
Lin EC, Alavi A. PET and PET/CT. A clinical guide. 2nd ed. New York, NY: Thieme Medical Publishers; 2009.
Lombardi MH. Radiation safety in nuclear medicine. Boca Raton, FL: CRC Press; 1999.
Lucignani G, Paganelli G, Bombardieri E. The use of standardized uptake values for assessing FDG uptake with PET in oncology: a clinical perspective. Nucl Med Commun. 2004;25(7):651–6.
Madden EM. Introduction to sectional anatomy workbook and board review guide (Point). 2nd ed. Philadelphia, PA: Lippincott Williams & Wilkins; 2007.
Miles AK, Blomley JKM, et al. Functional and physiological imaging in Grainger & Allison´s diagnostic radiology. New York: Churchill Livingstone; 2007.
Mittra E, Quon A. Positron emission tomography/computed tomography: the current technology and applications. Radiol Clin N Am. 2009;47:147–60.
Moore LK, Dalley FA, Agur RMA. Clinically oriented anatomy. 6th ed. Philadelphia, PA: Lippincott Williams & Wilkins (a Walters Kluwer business); 2010.
Munro HB. Statistical methods for health care research. 5th ed. Philadelphia, PA: Lippincott Williams & Wilkins; 2005.
Mycek MJ, Harvey RA. Lippincott's illustrated reviews: pharmacology. 3rd ed. Philadelphia, PA: Lippincott; 2008.
Nair A, Agrawal A, Jaiswar R. Substitution of Oral F-18 FDG for Intravenous F-18 FDG in PET Scanning. J Nucl Med Technol. 2007;35(2):100–4.
Newberg BA, Alavi A. Normal patterns and variants in PET Brain Imaging. PET Clin. 2010;5: 1–13.
Nuclear Medicine/PET http://gecommunity.gehealthcare.com Accessed 21 July 2011.

References and Suggested Readings

Patton JA, Townsend WD, Brian F, Hutton FB. Hybrid imaging technology: from dreams and vision to clinical devices. Semin Nucl Med. 2009;39:247–63.

Perry AG, Potter PA. Clinical nursing skills and techniques. 7th ed. St. Louis, MO: Mosby Elsevier; 2010.

PET Radiation Safety. http://www.safety.duke.edu/radsafety/slides/pet_rad_safe.pps. Accessed 20 Dec 2011

Placantonakis GD, Schwartz HT. Localization in Epilepsy. Neurol Clin. 2009;27:1015–30.

Prokop M, Galanski M. Spiral and multislice computed tomography of the body. New York, NY: Thieme; 2003.

Rahmim A, Zaidi H. PET versus SPECT: strengths, limitations and challenges. Nucl Med Commun. 2008;29:193–7.

Robbins SL, Cotran RS. Pathologic basis of disease. 8th ed. Philadelphia, PA: Saunders Elsevier; 2010.

Roivainen A, Forsback S, Grönroos T, et al. Blood metabolism of [methyl-11 C]choline; implications for in vivo imaging with positron emission tomography. Eur J Nucl Med. 2000;27: 25–32.

Saha GB. Basics of PET imaging. New York, NY: Springer; 2005.

Shukla AK, Kumar U. Positron emission tomography: An overview. J Med Phys. 2006;31:1.

Soret M, Bacharach SL, Buvat I. Partial-volume effect in PET tumor imaging. J Nucl Med. 2007;48:932–45.

Sureshbabu W, Mawlawi O. PET/CT imaging artifacts. J Nucl Med Technol. 2005;33:156–61.

Takalkar A, Agarwal A, Adams S, et al. Cardiac assessment with PET. PET Clin. 2011;6:313–26.

The SNM Procedure Guideline for General Imaging 6.0. http://interactive.snm.org/docs/General_Imaging_Version_6.0.pdf. Accessed 22 Dec. 2011.

Vallabhajosula S. 18 F-labeled positron emission tomographic radiopharmaceuticals is oncology: an overview of radiochemistry and mechanisms of tumor localization. Semin Nucl Med. 2007;37:400–19.

Vallabhajosula S, Solnesn L, Vallabhajosula B. Broad overview of positron emission tomography radiopharmaceuticals and clinical applications: what is new? Semin Nucl Med. 2011;41: 246–64.

Vines CD, Keller H, et al. Quantitative PET comparing gated with nongated acquisitions using a NEMA phantom with respiratory-simulated motion. J Nucl Med Technol. 2007;35:246–51.

Visvikis D, Turzo A, et al. Technology related parameters affecting quantification in positron emission tomography imaging. Nucl Med Commun. 2004;25(7):637–341.

Wahl LR, Jacene H. From RECIST to PERCIST: evolving considerations for PET response criteria in solid tumors. J Nucl Med. 2009;50 Suppl 5:122s–50s.

Wahl RL. Principles and practice of PET and PET/CT. 2nd ed. Philadelphia, PA: Lippincott and Wilkins; 2009.

Zaidi H, Thompson C. Evolution and developments in instrumentation for positron emission mammography. PET Clin. 2009;4:317–27.

Zaret BL, Beller GA. Clinical nuclear cardiology: state of the art and future directions. 3rd ed. Philadelphia, PA: Mosby; 2005.

Chapter 3
Practice Test # 2: Difficulty Level-Moderate

Questions

1. Which of the following cardiac imaging studies deliver the highest estimated effective radiation dose?
   (A) Rb-82 rest and stress
   (B) Calcium scoring
   (C) N-13 ammonia rest and stress
   (D) O-15 water rest and stress

2. Quantitative bias that refers to the underestimation of counts density which differs from what they should be is called the partial-volume effect (PVE). Which of the following statements describing the PVE is TRUE?
   (A) PVE is more prominent in smaller tumor
   (B) PVE is more prominent in metastatic tumor
   (C) PVE is less prominent in tumor in situ
   (D) PVE is less prominent in bigger tumor

3. Truncation is the source of streaking artifacts at the edge of the CT image. The presence of streaking artifacts:
   (A) Overestimates the attenuation coefficients
   (B) Produces image misregistration
   (C) Underestimates the attenuation coefficients
   (D) Necessitates use of shielding

Answers to Test #2 begin on page 120

4. All of the following are the most commonly seen artifacts on PET/CT images EXCEPT:
   (A) Respiratory motion
   (B) Partial-volume effect
   (C) Truncation
   (D) Contrast medium

5. The inverse of the mean distance traveled by photons before they deposit energy in the crystal is called:
   (A) The stopping power
   (B) Energy resolution
   (C) The decay constant
   (D) The light output

6. Post-processing measures such as scaling, segmentation, or a combination of the two has been used in the PET/CT systems in order to:
   (A) Correct for scatter coincidences
   (B) Convert the CT attenuation coefficients to those corresponding to PET
   (C) Correct for random coincidences
   (D) Convert PET emission data to the CT attenuation coefficients

7. The reconstruction method in which the comparison is made between the numerical projection data and the measured projection data in a feedback loop is called:
   (A) Filtered Back Projection (FBP)
   (B) Iterative Reconstruction (IR)
   (C) Ordered-Subset Expectation Maximization (OS-EM)
   (D) Maximum Likelihood—Expectation Maximization (ML-EM)

8. Which of the following statements describing the role of PET in the diagnostic work-up of patients with melanoma is FALSE?
   (A) PET is a standard modality in evaluation of recurrent melanoma
   (B) Melanin content influences lesion detectability by PET
   (C) PET is most valuable in stage III disease
   (D) PET is more accurate for systemic staging than regional staging

9. According to the Practice of Medicine and Pharmacy laws, all the clinical FDG-PET imaging work is complete by prescription by a physician and dispensing by registered:
   (A) Nurse
   (B) Radiologist
   (C) Pharmacist
   (D) Nuclear medicine physician

10. If a radiopharmaceutical has a physical half-life of 110 min, and a biological half-life of 6 h, what is the effective half-life of the radiopharmaceutical in hours?
    (A) 5.7 h
    (B) 2 h
    (C) 1.83 h
    (D) 1.4 h

11. Choose the correct interpretation of this ECG (Fig. 3.1):
    (A) Normal sinus rhythm
    (B) Electronic ventricular pacemaker
    (C) Atrial fibrillation
    (D) Ventricular bigeminy

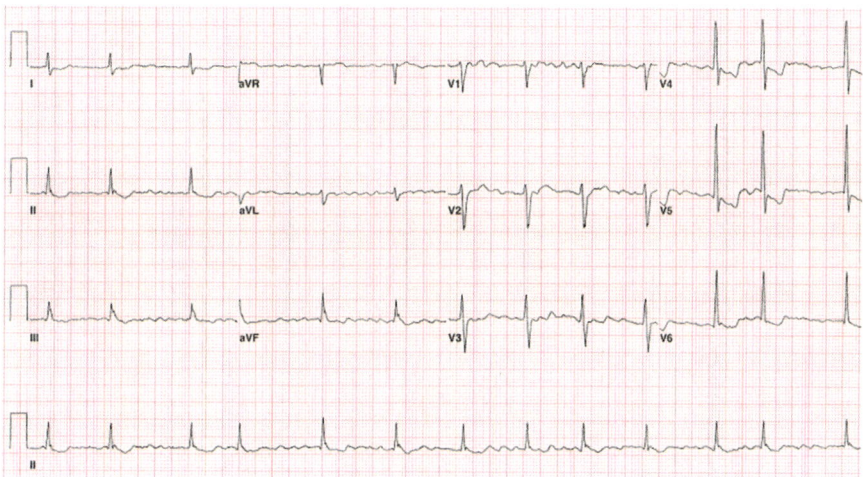

Fig. 3.1 ECG Sample Case: A 59-year-old woman with shortness of breath

12. The temporal improvement in contractile function of a dysfunctional myocardial region after restoration of blood flow describes:
    (A) Myocardial infarction
    (B) Myocardial viability
    (C) Diastolic dysfunction
    (D) Systolic dysfunction

13. Linear attenuation coefficient determines the scintillator:
    (A) Stopping power
    (B) Energy resolution
    (C) Decay constant
    (D) Light output

14. Administration/consumption of which of the following before F-18 FDG dosing will DECREASE uptake of the radiotracer by BAT (Brown Adipose Tissue)?
    (A) Ephedrine
    (B) Propranolol
    (C) Caffeine
    (D) Nicotine

15. The breathing protocols applied during PET/CT acquisition, e.g., respiratory gating, the breath-hold at inspiration protocol, and the shallow breathing protocol are utilized to eliminate:
    (A) Truncation artifacts
    (B) Misregistration artifacts
    (C) Contrast media artifacts
    (D) Streaking artifacts

16. In which of the following clinical circumstances is the application of standardized uptake value (SUV) most likely to be useless?
    (A) Prognosis of the disease
    (B) Diagnosis of the disease
    (C) Staging of the disease
    (D) Therapy monitoring of the disease

17. Which of the following scintillators is commercially available in a time-of-flight (TOF) PET imaging?
    (A) GSO
    (B) BaF2
    (C) BGO
    (D) LYSO

18. Administration of water-equivalent contrast agent when performing PET/CT imaging:
    (A) Underestimates SUV
    (B) Overestimates SUV
    (C) Does nOt affect SUV
    (D) Produces streaking artifacts

19. The presented PET MIP image in Fig. 3.2 was obtained in routine PET/CT examination. Which of the following expressions can be found in the body of the radiologist's report describing the exam's findings?
    (A) Hypermetabolic activity in the infracarinal region…increased activity in both adrenal glands…
    (B) Mass at the right lung base with rim of increased activity…increased activity in the left adrenal…
    (C) The chest demonstrates several punctate hypermetabolic foci….liver metastases
    (D) The chest demonstrates several punctate hypermetabolic foci…physiologic uptake in the abdomen and pelvis

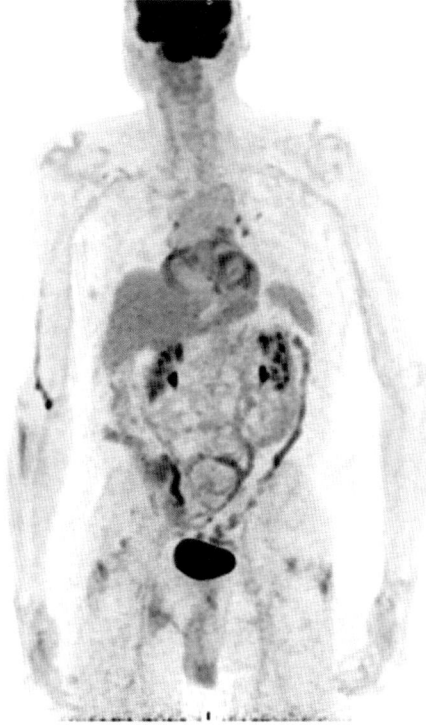

Fig. 3.2 PET/CT examination

20. Calculate a 14-year-old child's dose for a PET scan using Webster's formula with the following parameters:
    Adult dose—13 mCi
    Child's weight—149 lb
    Child's height—5' 6"
    (A) 5.7 mCi
    (B) 7.0 mCi
    (C) 9.2 mCi
    (D) 12.6 mCi

21. A state of chronically reduced contractility in viable myocardial tissue, caused by prolonged or repetitive reductions in myocardial flow, is called:
    (A) Scarred myocardium
    (B) Ischemic myocardium
    (C) Stunned myocardium
    (D) Hibernatic myocardium

22. The 2010 Guidelines for Cardiopulmonary resuscitation (CPR) and Emergency Cardiovascular Care (ECC) of American Heart Association (AHA) recommend in adults a compression depth of at LEAST:
    (A) 1 in.
    (B) 1.5 in.
    (C) 2 in.
    (D) 2.5 in.

23. If a truncated CT scan is used for the attenuation correction of a larger transaxial field of view PET scan, the activity estimates outside the measured CT field of view will be:
    (A) Underestimated
    (B) Overestimated
    (C) Unchanged
    (D) Equal to 0

24. A global reduction in the brain function assessed by F-18 FDG uptake is observed in:
    (A) Dementia
    (B) Parkinson's disease
    (C) Hypothyroidism
    (D) Hyperthyroidism

25. Medicare reimbursement for PET-FDG Myocardial Viability imaging is available in all of the following settings EXCEPT:
    (A) Primary diagnosis
    (B) Following an inconclusive SPECT
    (C) Initial diagnosis
    (D) Following an inconclusive CCTA

26. The histological presence of extracellular β-amyloid plaques (Aβ) and intraneuronal neurofibrillary tangles (NFTs) in the cerebral cortex defines:
    (A) Parkinson's disease
    (B) Alzheimer's disease
    (C) Dementia
    (D) Glioma

27. In the typical PET/CT acquisition, the CT component is performed as:
    (A) A non-contrast low radiation dose scan
    (B) A non-contrast high radiation dose scan
    (C) High radiation dose scan with a contrast
    (D) Low radiation dose scan with a contrast

28. Ovarian uptake of F-18 FDG in a postmenopausal patient indicates:
    (A) A normal finding
    (B) Malignancy
    (C) Pregnancy
    (D) Ovulating ovary

29. Which of the following radiopharmaceuticals has been developed as the PET tracer to measure a cell proliferation rate?
    (A) F-18 fluoride
    (B) C-11 Pittsburg compound
    (C) C-11 acetate
    (D) F-18 fluorothymidine

30. Calculate the percent error using the following results obtained from the geometry test on the dose calibrator:
    Reference 4 ml volume reading is 1.9 mCi
    Actual 20 ml volume reading 1.68 mCi
    (A) 13.1%
    (B) 11.6%
    (C) −3.1%
    (D) −6.8%

31. Figure 3.3 is a routine cardiogram from a hospitalized patient. Interpret this tracing.
    (A) Normal sinus rhythm
    (B) Electronic ventricular pacemaker
    (C) Atrial fibrillation
    (D) Ventricular bigeminy

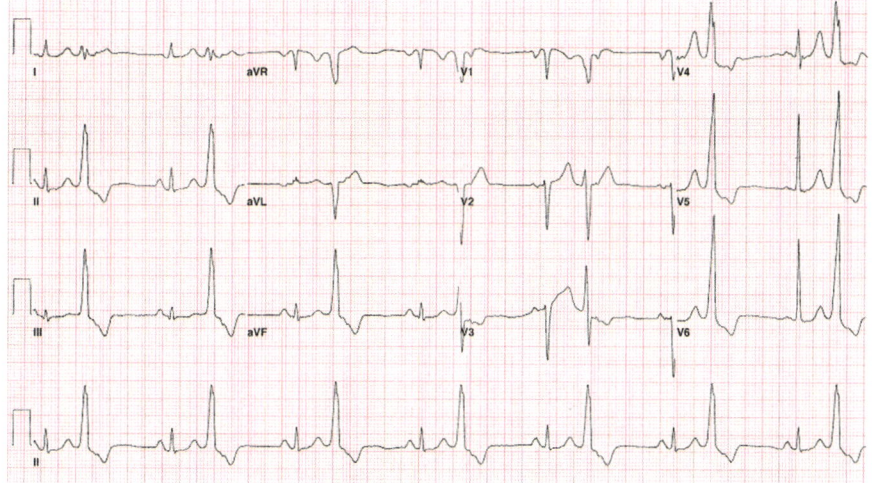

Fig. 3.3 ECG Sample Case: A 69-year-old woman with heart palpitations

32. An area of focal FDG uptake in the lungs, without corresponding finding on CT scan, can be caused by all of the following EXCEPT:
    (A) An injected blood clot
    (B) Motion artifact
    (C) Pulmonary infarction
    (D) Contamination

33. The main stream of X-ray photons generated in the X-ray tube is described as:
    (A) Braking radiation
    (B) Characteristic radiation
    (C) Compton scattering
    (D) Attenuation photons

34. A group of ROIs through planes, which define a three-dimensional region of relevance, is called:
    (A) Volume of interest
    (B) Maximum-intensity projection
    (C) Multiplanar reconstruction
    (D) Dose uptake ratio

35. Coincidence events registered in PET acquisition and defined as prompt counts include:
    (A) True and scatter events
    (B) Scatter and randoms
    (C) True and randoms
    (D) True, scatter, and randoms

36. An analytic reconstruction algorithm that assigns the values in the projection to all points along the line of acquisition through the image plane from which they were acquired is known as:
    (A) Filtered back projection
    (B) Back projection
    (C) Iterative reconstruction
    (D) Filtering

37. Quality control testing for PET agents that involves decay analysis in a dose calibrator for a defined period of time is called:
    (A) Specific activity analysis
    (B) Radiochemical purity
    (C) Radionuclidic identity
    (D) Bacterial endotoxin testing

38. The following are examples of oral hypoglycemic drugs EXCEPT:
    (A) Metformin
    (B) Glyburide
    (C) Dicumarol
    (D) Chlorpropamide

39. C-11 L-leucine, C-11 L-methionine, and C-11 L-tyrosine were developed as the PET tracers to assess:
    (A) Membrane synthesis
    (B) Lipids metabolism
    (C) Hypoxia extent
    (D) Protein synthesis

40. Which of the following patient's medications can be responsible for the findings presented on the coronal maximum-intensity projection PET image (Fig. 3.4)?
    (A) Metformin
    (B) Lasix
    (C) Propranolol
    (D) Valium

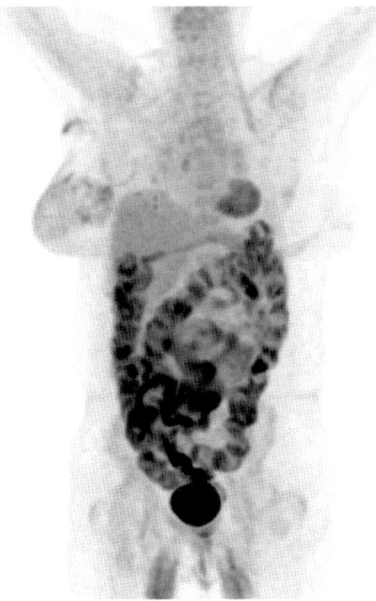

Fig. 3.4 PET/CT examination

41. Decreased myocardial blood flow combined with decreased myocardial glucose metabolism indicates the presence of:
    (A) Normal viable myocardium
    (B) Nonviable myocardium
    (C) Stunned myocardium
    (D) Hibernating myocardium

42. The parietal lobe of the brain is located behind the frontal lobe and controls:
    (A) Auditory information
    (B) Visual information
    (C) Smell sensation
    (D) Tactile sensation

43. The PET scanner quality control procedure in which data are used to compensate for the variation in efficiency in each line of response (LOR) in the sinogram is called:
    (A) Normalization
    (B) Calibration
    (C) Blank scan
    (D) Attenuation correction

44. The following statements correctly describe the standardized uptake value (SUV) in reconstructed PET images EXCEPT:
    (A) Quantitative accuracy for data acquired in the 2D is higher than that in the 3D
    (B) Emission data require correction for the presence of random coincidences
    (C) The background noise in data acquired in the 2D is higher than that in the 3D
    (D) Emission data require correction for the presence of scatter coincidences

45. The total attenuation is the sum of the attenuation due to different types of interactions and includes all of the following EXCEPT:
    (A) The photoelectric effect
    (B) The Compton scattering
    (C) The pair production
    (D) Bremsstrahlung radiation

46. If the collected data follow a Gaussian distribution, 68% of gathered values will be within:
    (A) One standard deviation
    (B) Two standard deviations
    (C) Three standard deviations
    (D) Mean +/−10

47. The parameter of the CT scanner defined as the ratio of the table feed per gantry rotation to the total X-ray beam width is called:
    (A) Pitch
    (B) Bed
    (C) Ring
    (D) Hybrid

48. A substitution radioactive for nonradioactive element in a biologically active PET tracer molecule without altering its biologic properties is called:
    (A) Hot-for-hot substitution
    (B) Cold-for-hot substitution
    (C) Hot-for-cold substitution
    (D) Cold-for-cold substitution

49. F-18 fluoroestradiol (FES) was developed as the PET tracer to assess:
    (A) Membrane synthesis
    (B) Estrogen receptor
    (C) Hypoxia extent
    (D) Protein synthesis

50. How many atoms disintegrating per second are measured by one becquerel?
    (A) 1,000
    (B) 100
    (C) 10
    (D) 1

51. Which of the following statements describing properties of the survey meters routinely used in the NM departments is FALSE?
    (A) A cutie-pie counter is an ionization chamber
    (B) A Geiger–Mueller counter is used for low level surveys
    (C) A Geiger–Muller counter output is proportional to the exposure rate
    (D) A cutie-pie output is proportional to the total energy deposited

52. The accessory organs of the digestive system include the:
    (A) Esophagus
    (B) Stomach
    (C) Liver
    (D) Small intestine

53. A linear transformation of the initial linear attenuation coefficient measurement into one in which the radiodensity of distilled water and the radiodensity of air at standard pressure and temperature (STP) is equal to 0 and −1,000 accordingly is called:
    (A) Hounsfield unit scale
    (B) Attenuation coefficient
    (C) Partial voluming
    (D) Beam hardening

54. The capacity to overlay data from distinct sources that will map a pixel from one source into a pixel from the other is called:
    (A) Image attenuation
    (B) Image registration
    (C) Filtering
    (D) Rebining

55. Two photons arising from two annihilation events and detected within each other's coincidence window are:
    (A) True coincidences
    (B) Random events
    (C) Scatter coincidences
    (D) Single events

56. The following tests can be used to assess the ability of the device to reproducibly records detected events EXCEPT:
    (A) Chi-square test
    (B) Poisson standard deviation
    (C) Gaussian standard deviation
    (D) Student's t-test

57. The dose calibrator quality control procedure performed with different sealed radionuclides is called:
    (A) Geometry
    (B) Accuracy
    (C) Linearity
    (D) Constancy

58. Which of the following radionuclides commonly used in PET imaging has the lowest positron range in water?
    (A) Carbon-11
    (B) Nitrogen-13
    (C) Oxygen-15
    (D) Fluorine-18

59. The Cotswold system (formerly the Ann Arbor Staging System) applies to both Hodgkin's disease (HD) and non-Hodgkin's lymphoma (NHL) and divides them into:
    (A) 2 stages
    (B) 4 stages
    (C) 6 stages
    (D) 8 stages

60. The diagram for the process of positron–electron annihilation is shown in the Fig. 3.5. Which of the following labels identifies the positron-emitting nucleus?
    (A) D
    (B) C
    (C) B
    (D) A

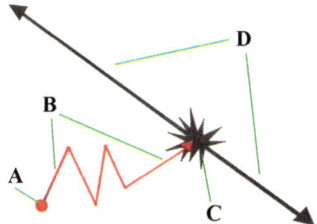

Fig. 3.5 Positron–electron annihilation diagram. *Illustration by Sabina Moniuszko*

61. When handling a minor radioactive spill the technologists should perform the following sequence of events:
    (A) Decontaminate personnel, survey the area, notify a supervisor
    (B) Write up report, contain the spill, notify the RSO
    (C) Clear the area, notify a supervisor, contain the spill
    (D) Decontaminate personnel, clear the area, write up report

62. Which of the following histopathological types of the gastric carcinoma is associated with the low F-18 FDG uptake?
    (A) Tubular carcinoma
    (B) Papillary carcinoma
    (C) Signet-ring cell carcinoma
    (D) Metastatic adenocarcinoma

63. Which of the following scintillators commonly used in PET has the highest light output?
    (A) LSO (lutetium oxyorthosilicate)
    (B) BaF2 (barium fluoride)
    (C) BGO (bismuth germinate)
    (D) GSO (gadolinium orthosilicate)

64. Low carbohydrate and a high protein diet favor the metabolism of:
    (A) Carbohydrates
    (B) Ketones
    (C) Amino acids
    (D) Fatty acids

65. The energy of the X-ray photons produced by the CT X-ray tube is controlled by the:
    (A) The tube voltage (kV)
    (B) The temperature of the anode
    (C) The tube current (mA)
    (D) The temperature of the cathode

66. Urinary bladder catheterization prior to PET imaging might be required for patients diagnosed with:
    (A) Pulmonary nodule
    (B) Brain tumor
    (C) Melanoma
    (D) Uterine carcinoma

67. Which of the following statements describing F-18 FDG uptake in gallbladder/biliary tract is FALSE?
    (A) No uptake is observed in normal GB wall
    (B) GB wall uptake is seen in acute cholecystitis
    (C) Focal GB uptake is observed in GB carcinoma
    (D) Cholestasis can cause false-negative liver lesions

68. In the process of differentiation between residual viable or recurrent tumor and radiation necrosis in patients with treated primary or metastatic CNS brain tumor, absence of FDG uptake in the region of interest indicates:
    (A) Brain tumor
    (B) Brain tumor and radiation necrosis
    (C) Radiation necrosis
    (D) Neither brain tumor nor radiation necrosis

69. Which of the following statements describing the clinical utility of PET/CT-FDG imaging vs. PET-FDG imaging is FALSE?
    (A) FDG-PET/CT has less of a tendency toward upstaging of patients than FDG-PET alone
    (B) FDG-PET/CT correctly downstages a number of patients compared with FDG-PET alone
    (C) FDG-PET/CT has more false-positive findings than FDG-PET alone
    (D) FDG-PET/CT is found to be more accurate for staging than FDG-PET alone

70. In the image in Fig. 3.6 shown below, what structure is depicted by line "c"?
    (A) Right ventricle
    (B) Liver
    (C) Left ventricle
    (D) Aorta

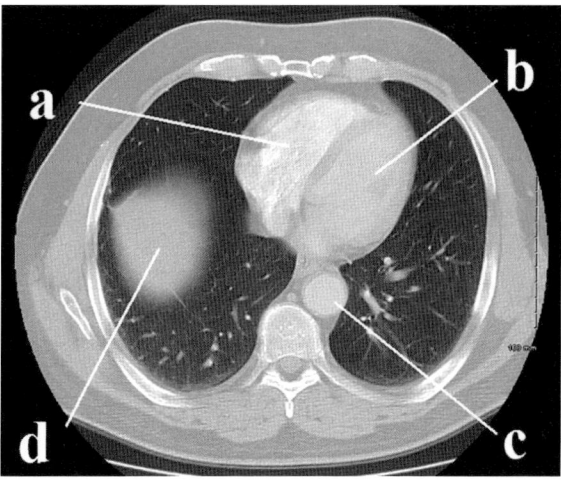

Fig. 3.6 CT anatomy, transaxial

71. What sign should be posted in an area accessible to personnel in which a major portion of the body of a person could receive a dose in excess of 100 mrem in 1 h?
    (A) Radioactive materials
    (B) Radiation area
    (C) High radiation area
    (D) Airborne radioactivity area

72. The three main divisions of the large intestine are the:
    (A) Duodenum, jejunum, and ileum
    (B) Cecum, colon, and rectum
    (C) Cecum, colon, and ileum
    (D) Duodenum, jejunum, and rectum

73. The following methods are employed in the quantitative PET F-18 FDG studies EXCEPT:
    (A) Tumor-to-background ratios
    (B) Signal-to-noise ratios
    (C) Standardized uptake values
    (D) Full kinetic analysis

74. A group of naturally occurring glycoproteins that regulates the production, differentiation, survival, and activation of hematopoietic cells are called:
    (A) Mucins
    (B) Immunoglobulins
    (C) Colony-Stimulating Factors (CSFs)
    (D) Thyroid-stimulating hormone (TSH)

75. PET images that are distinguished by "hot skin" and the manifestation of the lungs with high tracer uptake and the low tracer concentrations in the mediastinum are:
    (A) Non-attenuation-corrected (NAC) images
    (B) Attenuation-corrected (AC) images
    (C) Maximum-intensity projection (MIP) images
    (D) Attenuation-corrected (AC) or non-attenuation-corrected (NAC) images

76. The pharmacological effect of dipyridamole or adenosine can be reversed by the administration of:
    (A) Propranolol
    (B) Valium
    (C) Aminophylline
    (D) Nitroglycerine

77. Which of the following statements describing different methods of SUV normalization is FALSE?
    (A) SUV can be normalized to total body mass
    (B) SUV can be normalized to lean body mass
    (C) SUV can be normalized to body surface area
    (D) SUV normalization based on total body mass is the most dependable

78. The occipital lobe is located in the posterior part of the brain and is responsible for the processing of:
    (A) Auditory information
    (B) Visual information
    (C) Smell sensation
    (D) Tactile sensation

79. Which of the following histological types of thyroid carcinoma DOES NOT concentrate iodine?
    (A) Classic papillary
    (B) Classic follicular
    (C) Papillary encapsulated
    (D) Anaplastic

80. The energy imparted to a unit mass of matter by ionizing radiation is measured in:
    (A) Rad
    (B) Rem
    (C) Curie
    (D) Roentgen

81. N-13 ammonia demonstrates extended myocardial retention, by staying metabolically trapped within the myocytes. This is due to:
    (A) Activity of the Na/K-ATPase pumps
    (B) Binding to the mitochondrial complex
    (C) The glutamine synthetase pathway
    (D) Glucose transporters activity

82. Bilateral, symmetric decreased FDG uptake in the temporoparietal region of the brain is the prevailing pattern observed in:
    (A) Pick disease
    (B) Vascular dementia
    (C) Alzheimer's disease
    (D) Dementia with Lewy bodies

83. The presented PET-MIP image in the Fig. 3.7 was obtained in routine PET/CT examination. Which of the following expressions can be found in the body of the radiologist's report describing the exam's findings?
    (A) Hypermetabolic activity in the infracarinal region...physiologic bladder activity.....
    (B) Mass at the right lung base with rim of increased activity...increased activity in the left adrenal...
    (C) The chest demonstrates several punctate hypermetabolic foci....liver metastases
    (D) The chest demonstrates several punctate hypermetabolic foci...physiologic uptake in the abdomen and pelvis

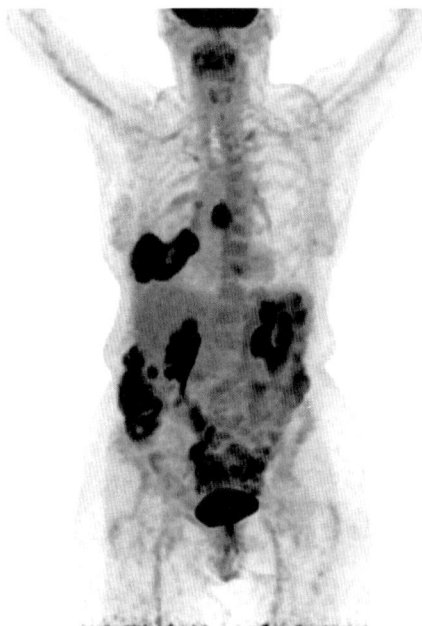

Fig. 3.7 PET/CT examination

84. A clinically significant incidence of febrile neutropenia after myelosuppressive chemotherapy is a common indication for treatment with:
    (A) Erythropoietin
    (B) Thrombopoietin
    (C) Macrophage colony-stimulating factor (M-CSF)
    (D) Granulocyte colony-stimulating factor (G-CSF)

85. According to the Response Evaluation Criteria in Solid Tumors (RECIST), complete response to therapy is defined as a disappearance of all tumor foci for at least:
    (A) 1 week
    (B) 2 weeks
    (C) 4 weeks
    (D) 8 weeks

86. Brain metabolism and blood flow are increased at the site of onset of the seizure in the:
    (A) Interictal state
    (B) Intraictal state
    (C) Inter and intraictal states
    (D) Neither inter or intraictal states

87. A type of beta decay in which a proton is converted to a neutron and the antimatter counterpart of an electron and a neutrino are released is called:
    (A) Positron emission
    (B) Isomeric transition
    (C) Electron capture
    (D) Beta (-) decay

88. Which of the following tests is the basis of screening as well as a useful tool in the diagnosis of colorectal cancer?
    (A) Barium enema
    (B) Occult blood testing
    (C) Sigmoidoscopy
    (D) Colonoscopy

89. Reimbursable by the Centers for Medicare & Medicaid Services oncologic applications for PET scanning in lymphoma management include all of the following EXCEPT:
    (A) Diagnosis
    (B) Staging
    (C) Therapy monitoring
    (D) Restaging

90. The event illustrated in the diagram in Fig. 3.8 is called:
    (A) A random event
    (B) A scatter event
    (C) A true event
    (D) An attenuated event

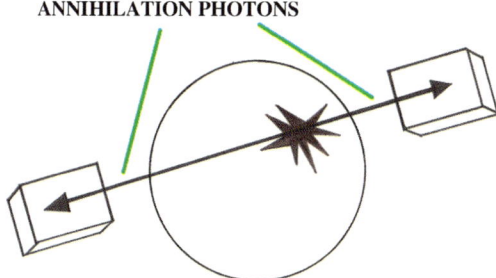

Fig. 3.8 Principle of positron emission imaging. *Illustration by Sabina Moniuszko*

91. The excretion of Ga-68 DOTA-peptides is primarily through the:
    (A) Skin
    (B) Bowel
    (C) Gallbladder
    (D) Kidney

92. Nigral degeneration and striatal dopamine deficiency are characteristic findings present in:
    (A) Parkinson's disease (PD)
    (B) Alzheimer's disease (AD)
    (C) Vascular dementia
    (D) Ictal epilepsy

93. The difference in the detection times between two coincidence photons that is used to determine most likely location of the annihilation event along LOR is applied in:
    (A) Hybrid imaging
    (B) Time-of-flight imaging
    (C) Image coregistration
    (D) Scatter correction

94. The single most important prognostic factor in patients with colon cancer is/are:
    (A) Metastases to regional lymph nodes
    (B) The location of the carcinoma
    (C) The size of the lesion
    (D) Coexisting diseases

95. Extending the axial FOV of the scanner to cover the patient more in a single-bed position results in:
    (A) Increased sensitivity
    (B) The decreased rates of scatter
    (C) The decreased rates of randoms
    (D) Increased resolution

96. Which of the following is the most common risk factor for colorectal cancer?
    (A) Smoking
    (B) Drinking
    (C) A family history
    (D) Uncontrolled diabetes

97. A pencil shape, a fan shape, and a cone shape are common terms used in radiography to describe:
    (A) CT detectors arrangements
    (B) CT detectors properties
    (C) X-ray beam
    (D) X-ray tube

98. A normal endometrial uptake F-18 FDG is most commonly seen:
    (A) During ovulation
    (B) During menstruation
    (C) A few days before the menstrual flow
    (D) A few days after the menstrual flow

99. F-18 flurpiridaz is a Positron Emission Tomography (PET) imaging tracer that has been explored in patients with:
    (A) Lymphoma
    (B) Malignant melanoma
    (C) Coronary artery disease
    (D) Non-small cell carcinoma

100. The presented images in Fig. 3.9 labeled A, B, C, and D were obtained during a routine CT of the head. The image described as A represents:
    (A) Lateral head localizer image
    (B) Coronal slice of the brain
    (C) Saggital slice of the brain
    (D) Tranverse slice of the brain

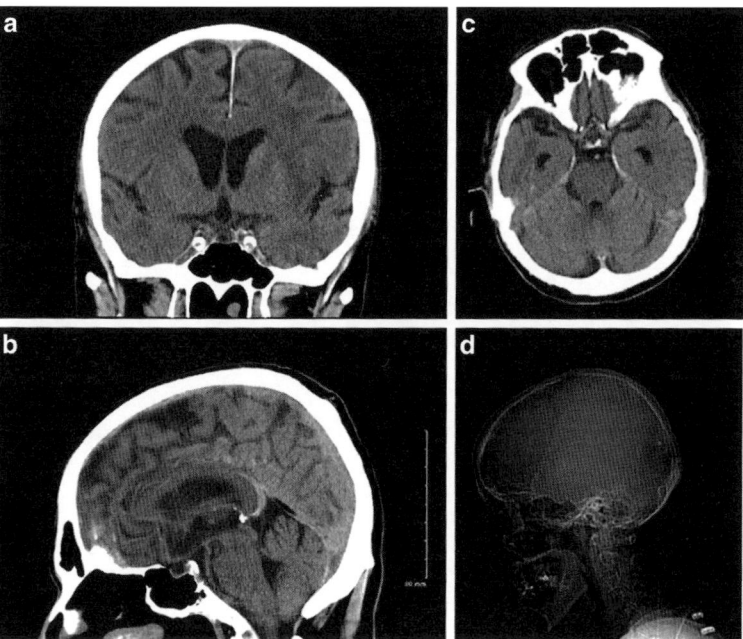

Fig. 3.9 Brain CT scans

101. A hypothetical aggregation of human physical and physiological characteristics arrived at by international consensus is called:
    (A) Average man
    (B) Average worker
    (C) Reference man

102. Diaphragmatic crus F-18 FDG uptake can be seen in patients with:
    (A) Tachycardia
    (B) Increased respiratory effort
    (C) Anxiety
    (D) Excessive sweating

103. In the test–retest setting, the reproducibility of quantitative PET parameters depends mainly on:
    (A) ROI and lesion size
    (B) Glucose correction factors
    (C) The reconstruction method
    (D) Body weight correction factors

104. The recommended time interval necessary to avoid increased FDG uptake in the spleen and bone marrow after granulocyte colony-stimulating factor (G-CSF) therapy is at least:
    (A) 1 day
    (B) 1 week
    (C) 10 days
    (D) 4 weeks

105. With regard to nodal lesions detection in patients with lymphoma, non-attenuation-corrected (NAC) PET images are superior to attenuation-corrected (AC) PET images in evaluating:
    (A) The deeply seated nodal lesions
    (B) The superficial nodal lesions
    (C) The anteriorly seated nodal lesions
    (D) The posterior nodal lesions

106. Segmental colon activity observed on PET F-18 FDG scan suggests:
    (A) Colon carcinoma
    (B) Colon polyp
    (C) Colon inflammation
    (D) Colon metastases

107. Which of the following preparations can be used if intravenous hydration before F-18 FDG imaging is indicated?
    (A) Dextrose
    (B) Lactose
    (C) Normal saline
    (D) Amino acids

108. The pattern of diffuse hypermetabolism in the skeleton and the spleen on PET-FDG study is most likely caused by:
    (A) Prolonged fasting
    (B) Bone metastases
    (C) Bone marrow hyperplasia
    (D) Excessive exercise

109. Which of the following radionuclides can be used in PET/CT scintigraphy to image the extent of disease in patients with differentiated thyroid carcinoma (DTC)?
    (A) I-131
    (B) F-18
    (C) C-11
    (D) I-124

110. A 15mCi dose of Nitrogen-13-ammonia, for myocardial perfusion imaging, is calibrated at 13:00 h. How many millicuries will be available at 12:55?
    (A) 11 mCi
    (B) 21 mCi
    (C) 38 mCi
    (D) 60 mCi

111. Decontamination must be performed if a wiped area EXCEEDS:
    (A) 2 dpm/100cm^2
    (B) 20 dpm/100cm^2
    (C) 200 dpm/100cm^2
    (D) 2,000 dpm/100cm^2

112. The display shown in Fig. 3.10 presents attenuation-corrected and reconstructed positron emission tomography (PET-FDG) viability study. The reoriented tomographic slices are:
    (A) The short axis slices
    (B) The vertical long axis slices
    (C) The oblique short axis slices
    (D) The horizontal long axis

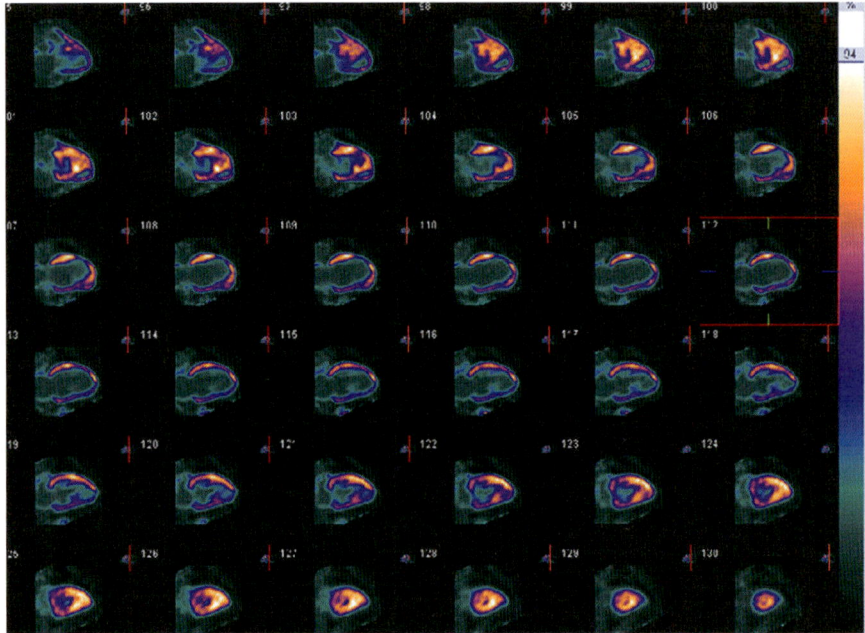

Fig. 3.10 PET/CT-FDG viability study

113. How increasing the administered activity will influence the scatter-to-true ratio?
    (A) The scatter-to-true ratio will stay the same
    (B) The scatter-to-true ratio will increase
    (C) The scatter-to-true ratio will decrease
    (D) The scatter-to-true ratio will decrease or increase

114. Non-attenuation-corrected (NAC) images can be differentiated from attenuation corrected (AC) images by the presence all of the following EXCEPT:
    (A) High noise
    (B) High skin activity
    (C) High lung activity
    (D) Low deep structures activity

115. If the pretest probability of disease is low, then a positive PET is more likely to be:
    (A) False negative
    (B) False positive
    (C) True negative
    (D) True positive

116. F-18 FDG uptake in tumors such as lipoma, neurofibroma, and desmoid tumor is best described as:
    (A) Absent
    (B) Low
    (C) Variable
    (D) High

117. Patients who need conscious sedation or general anesthesia should have their F-18 FDG dose administered:
    (A) Simultaneously with medication
    (B) Before the medication
    (C) 5 min after the medication
    (D) 30 min after the medication

118. A collaboration of the American College of Radiology Imaging Network (ACRIN), the American College of Radiology (ACR), and the Academy of Molecular Imaging (AMI) to ensure access to Medicare reimbursement for certain types of positron emission tomography (PET) scans is called:
    (A) The National Oncologic PET Registry (NOPR)
    (B) The Centers for Medicare and Medicaid Services (CMS) program
    (C) ACR accreditation program
    (D) ACR appropriateness criteria for imaging

119. The normal parathyroid glands on F-18 FDG-PET scintigraphy are:
    (A) Not visualized
    (B) Visualized but asymmetrical in appearance
    (C) Visualized and symmetrical in appearance
    (D) Visualized only if thyroid gland is present

120. If a 40 mCi dose of Rb-82 is needed for myocardial perfusion imaging at 8:00 A.M., how many millicuries will be available at 7:55 A.M?
    (A) 640 mCi
    (B) 360 mCi
    (C) 47.7 mCi
    (D) 33.6 mCi

121. The amount of radioactivity found in matter is measured in:
    (A) Rad
    (B) Rem
    (C) Curie
    (D) Roentgen

122. Elevated FDG activity observed on a PET scan performed further than 6 months after completion of radiation therapy most likely represents:
    (A) Tumor recurrence
    (B) Radiation necrosis
    (C) Flare phenomenon
    (D) Benign finding

123. Stage IV of the Cotswold system (formerly the Ann Arbor Staging System) is identified when:
    (A) The cancer affects lymph nodes on both sides of the diaphragm
    (B) The cancer spreads to extranodal sites
    (C) The cancer has only affected one lymph node region or organ
    (D) The cancer is either above or below the diaphragm

124. Selected tumors with low/variable FDG uptake include all of the following EXCEPT:
    (A) Prostate carcinoma
    (B) Mucinous adenocarcinoma
    (C) Renal cell carcinoma
    (D) Non-small cell lung carcinoma

125. PET and PET/CT have the highest sensitivity for the detection of:
    (A) Abdominal and pelvic lymph nodes involvement
    (B) Peripheral and thoracic lymph nodes involvement
    (C) Head and neck lymph nodes involvement
    (D) Bone involvement

126. Which of the following statements describing the usefulness of PET imaging in colorectal cancer is FALSE?
    (A) FDG-PET is useful for detecting both hepatic and extrahepatic metastases
    (B) FDG-PET is helpful in detecting nodal involvement
    (C) FDG-PET can differentiate local recurrence from scarring after radiation therapy
    (D) FDG-PET has no influence on surgical management of patients

127. If two Compton scattered photons add up simultaneously in the detector and the resultant peak falls within the window these events are called:
    (A) Randoms
    (B) Pulse pileups
    (C) Dead-time loss
    (D) Attenuation

128. Visceral functions, body temperature, and behavioral responses are controlled by:
    (A) The limbic system
    (B) The thalamus
    (C) The hypothalamus
    (D) The cerebellum

129. FDG-PET imaging of malignant mesotheliomas has been explored in all of the following clinical settings EXCEPT:
    (A) Evaluation of benign vs. malignant pleural disease
    (B) Radiotherapy planning
    (C) Assessment of intrathoracic disease extent
    (D) Monitoring metabolic response to therapy

130. The image in Fig. 3.11 is an example of what type of processing technique?
    (A) Maximum-intensity projection (MIP)
    (B) Minimum-intensity projection (mIP)
    (C) Volume-rendered display (VRT)
    (D) Multiplanar reconstruction (MPR)

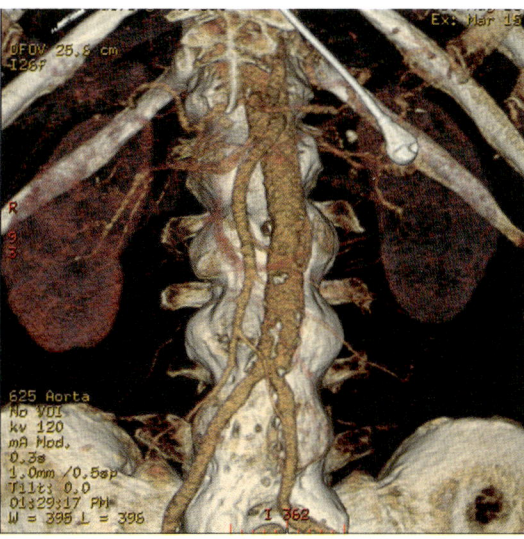

Fig. 3.11 Sample of reconstruction technique

131. The radiation sensitivity of a tissue is proportional to the:
    (A) Degree of cell differentiation
    (B) Distance from the source of radiation
    (C) Time of radiation exposure
    (D) Rate of cell proliferation

132. Signs and symptoms of hypoglycemia include all of the following EXCEPT:
    (A) Sweating
    (B) Palpitations
    (C) Confusion
    (D) Hyperthermia

133. Process in which positional information is gained from a coincidence event assigned to a line of response (LOR) joining the two relevant detectors is called:
    (A) Electronic registration
    (B) Rebinning
    (C) Electronic collimation
    (D) Filtering

134. If one were scanning a tumor that was found in the liver, the signal would be defined as the difference between the tumor and the surrounding tissue, while the noise would be the standard deviation of the signal level within:
    (A) The tumor
    (B) The surrounding tissue
    (C) The background
    (D) The whole image

135. Increasing the X-ray tube current (mA) will result in:
    (A) Increase in the number of X-ray photons produced
    (B) Decrease in the number of X-ray photons produced
    (C) Increase in the energy of X-ray photons produced
    (D) Decrease in the energy of X-ray photons produced

136. Metabolic, positron-emitter radiopharmaceuticals used in the diagnosis of neuroendocrine tumors, (NET), include PET tracers that allow investigating all of the following metabolic pathways EXCEPT:
    (A) Amine production and storage mechanism
    (B) Catecholamine transport
    (C) Cholesterol metabolic pathway
    (D) Serotonin production pathway

137. The benefit of 3D acquisition when compared to 2D is that the sensitivity of the scanner is improved by a factor:
    (A) 2–4
    (B) 4–6
    (C) 6–12
    (D) 12–24

138. The type of study where a given agent does not pass through a tissue bed but accumulates progressively in the organ of interest is called:
    (A) Perfusion study
    (B) Bolus study
    (C) Wash-in study
    (D) Wash-out study

139. FDG uptake in primary lesions is a direct function of all of the following EXCEPT:
    (A) The cellular proliferation
    (B) The cellular apoptosis
    (C) The number of cancer cells
    (D) The expression of GLUT receptors

140. A dose of F-18 FDG is calibrated to have 12 mCi at 8:15 A.M. If the patient comes 30 min late, how many milicuries will be remaining at 8:45?
    (A) 2.0 mCi
    (B) 12–24
    (C) 10 mCi
    (D) 14.5 mCi

141. The sealed sources inventory and leak test should be performed:
    (A) Every week
    (B) Every month
    (C) Every 6 months
    (D) Every year

142. Which of the following describes the finding, pointing with the arrow, on the PET/CT fused coronal image—Fig. 3.12a—and on the CT axial slice—Fig. 3.12b?
    (A) Pericardial effusion
    (B) The prosthetic mitral valve
    (C) A myxoma
    (D) A coronary stent

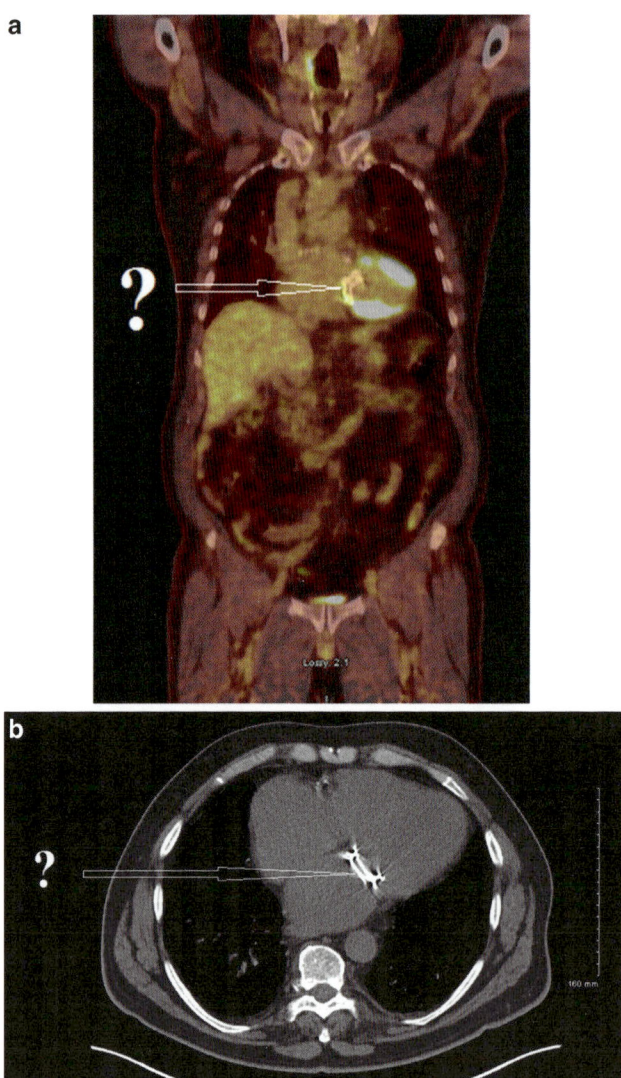

Fig. 3.12 (a) PET/CT coronal slice; (b) CT axial slice

143. The sensitivity of a PET scanner operating in 3D mode:
    (A) Is Equal across the field of view
    (B) Is highest in the axial center of the gantry
    (C) Rises up toward the periphery
    (D) Is the same as the sensitivity of 2D

144. Primary applications of PET and PET/CT in the brain imaging include all of the following EXCEPT:
    (A) Differentiation of dementias
    (B) Evaluation of primary brain tumors
    (C) Evaluation of brain injuries
    (D) Evaluation of seizure foci

145. A detailed specification standard for the exchange of digital images and data between imaging devices is called:
    (A) PACS
    (B) DICOM
    (C) DAC
    (D) NEMA

146. A direct-acting inotropic agent that increases myocardial contractility in a dose-dependent manner is called:
    (A) Adenosine
    (B) Dipyridamole
    (C) Dobutamine
    (D) Aminophylline

147. The reconstruction method incorporating the compensation for broadening of the point spread function (PSF) with increasing distance from the center of the scanner is called:
    (A) Ordinary Poisson (OP)–OSEM
    (B) Attenuation-weighted OSEM (AW-OSEM)
    (C) High-Definition PET
    (D) Fourier Rebinning (FORE)

148. The presented PET MIP images in Fig. 3.13 labeled a and b were obtained from the same patient five months apart from each other. Which of the following expressions can be found in the body of the radiologist's report describing findings from the most recent scan (a)?
    (A) Hypermetabolic activity in the right hemithorax…similar distribution… decreased SUV values
    (B) New areas of abnormal activity identified in liver….status post left nephrectomy
    (C) No new areas of abnormal activity identified…..status post right nephrectomy
    (D) Hypermetabolic activity…SUV 9.6 mediastinum…similar distribution

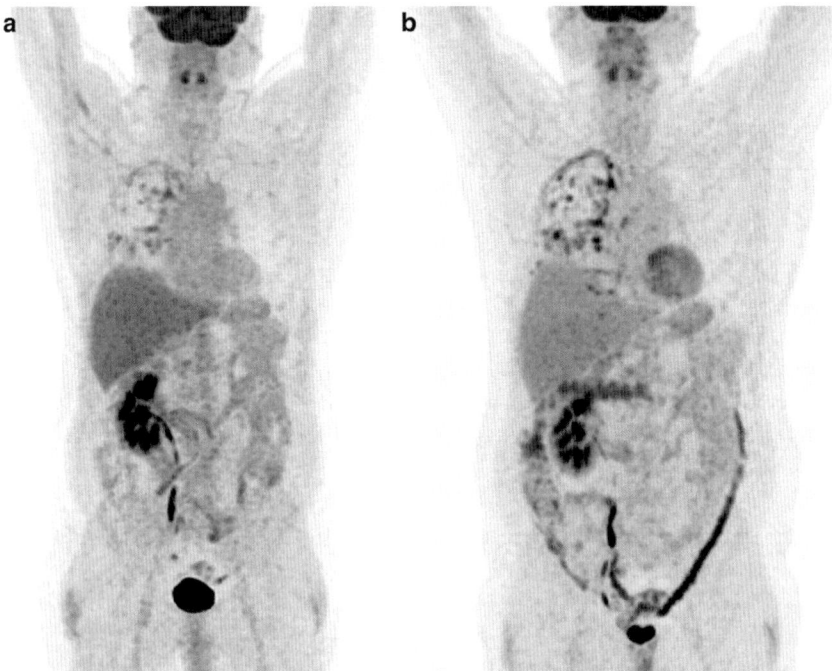

Fig. 3.13 (a) PET/CT examination-follow-up study; (b) PET/CT examination

149. All of the following statements describing the features of positron emission tomography (PET) and single-photon emission computed tomography (SPECT) are correct EXCEPT:
    (A) PET imaging has higher sensitivity then SPECT imaging
    (B) SPECT resolution is limited by technology
    (C) PET resolution is limited by positron range and photon non-collinearity
    (D) SPECT imaging can utilize higher doses of radionuclides

150. A Radiopharmacy has a vial of F-18 FDG, which contains 400 mCi in 5 ml at 7:00 A.M. If the radiopharmacy has two orders for 13 mCi each for myocardial viability studies at 9:00 A.M. and 10:00 A.M., respectively, what concentration will be remaining in the vial of F-18 FDG after drawing these two doses?
    (A) 3.9 mCi
    (B) 25.7 mCi/ml
    (C) 107 mCi
    (D) 107 mCi/ml

151. All of the following statements correctly describe FDG-PET imaging when compared with Ga-67 scintigraphy EXCEPT:
    (A) FDG-PET is a 1-day procedure vs. 2–7 days for Ga-67 scintigraphy
    (B) FDG-PET has superior spatial resolution to that of Ga-67 scintigraphy
    (C) FDG-PET is particularly useful in the follow-up of non-gallium-avid lymphoma scintigraphy
    (D) FDG-PET has much more radiation exposure to patients than that of Ga-67 scintigraphy

152. The X-axis of the data plotted on PET sinogram represents:
    (A) The angle of orientation of the LOR
    (B) The shift of the LOR from the center of gantry
    (C) The window of coincidence of the LOR
    (D) Displacement of the LOR from the center of FOV

153. The diagnostic performance of FDG-PET in the staging of patients with lymphoma is approximated as:
    (A) Sensitivity 90% and specificity 50%
    (B) Sensitivity 50% and specificity 50%
    (C) Sensitivity 50% and specificity 91%
    (D) Sensitivity 90% and specificity 91%

154. All of the following statements describing the epidemiology of breast cancer are true EXCEPT:
    (A) Breast cancer is the most frequently diagnosed cancer in women
    (B) Approximately 1 in 9 women will have breast cancer during their lifetime
    (C) The overall mortality from breast cancer has increased in recent years
    (D) The ratio of female to male breast cancer is approximately 100:1

155. Which of the following diagnosis should be considered first in patients presented with signs or symptoms related to nodal enlargement, and/or with other disease associated indicators, such as fevers or night sweats?
    (A) Multiple myeloma
    (B) Lymphoma
    (C) Lung carcinoma
    (D) Sarcoma

156. Fibroadenoma, gynecomastia, and ductal hyperplasia/adenoma are:
    (A) Breast cancers
    (B) Breast benign lesions
    (C) Breast cancer metastatic lesions
    (D) Breast chemo/ radiotherapy induced inflammation

157. A neoplastic disease of adipose tissues is called:
    (A) Lipoma
    (B) Osteosarcoma
    (C) Liposarcoma
    (D) Chondrosarcoma

158. The most important clinical tool in evaluating patients with suspected seizures is:
    (A) Magnetic resonance imaging (MRI)
    (B) Electromyography (EMG)
    (C) Electroencephalography (EEG)
    (D) Positron emission tomography (PET)

159. All of the following novel PET probes have been shown promising results in malignant pleural mesothelioma (MPM) evaluation EXCEPT:
    (A) F-18 fluorothymidine (FLT)
    (B) F-18 fluoromisonidazole (FMISO)
    (C) F-18 fluoro-dihydrotestosterone (FDHT)
    (D) C-11methionine (MET)

160. The NRC requires that all wipe tests be recorded in disintegrations per minute (dpm). If a reading of 103 net counts per minute (cpm) is obtained from the wipe test, and the well counter efficiency is 85%, what are the disintegrations per minute acquired from the wipe test?
    (A) 121 dpm
    (B) 88 dpm
    (C) 88 cpm
    (D) 1.2 cpm

161. In the image in Fig. 3.14, the descending aorta is labeled:
    (A) D
    (B) C
    (C) B
    (D) A

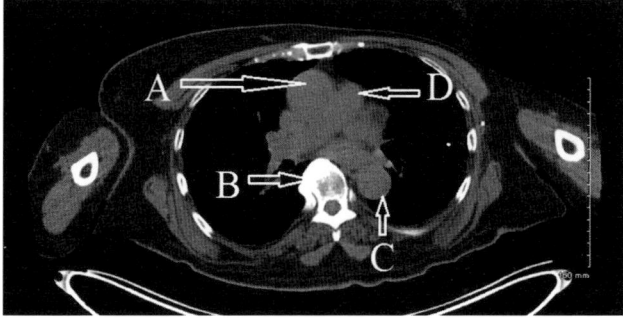

Fig. 3.14 Chest CT

162. A naturally occurring cyclic neuropeptide that inhibits several physiologic functions such as neurotransmission, the secretion of growth hormone, gastric acid production, gastrointestinal motility, and insulin secretion is called:
    (A) Cortisol
    (B) Epinephrine
    (C) Somatostatin
    (D) Norepinephrine

163. F-18 FDG focal uptake seen 6 months after completion of radiation therapy should be considered as:
    (A) Tumor recurrence
    (B) Normal findings
    (C) Radiation necrosis
    (D) Radiation pneumonitis

164. The posterior association cortex hypometabolism involving the posterior lateral, temporal lateral, and medial parietal and posterior cingulate cortices on FDG-PET images is reliable and an accurate finding for identifying:
    (A) Parkinson's disease
    (B) Dementia
    (C) Radiation necrosis
    (D) Alzheimer's disease

165. F-18 FDG uptake in fracture should normalize within:
    (A) 1 week
    (B) 1 month
    (C) 3 months
    (D) 6 months

166. The most common reaction to produce F-18 as fluoride ion (F— -18) is based on proton bombardment of:
    (A) Ne-20 (neon gas)
    (B) O-18 (oxygen enriched water)
    (C) Ne-18 (neon gas)
    (D) O-18 (oxygen enriched water)

167. The geometric efficiency of the PET scanner depends on all of the following EXCEPT:
    (A) The diameter of the ring
    (B) The distance between the source and the detector
    (C) The height of table
    (D) The number of detectors in the ring

168. A drug that reduces the metabolism of endogenous adenosine by inhibiting the enzyme called adenosine deaminaze is called:
    (A) Nitroglycerine
    (B) Dipirydamole
    (C) Propranolol
    (D) Aminophylline

169. The advantages of positron emission mammography (PEM) over whole-body positron emission tomography (PET-FDG) include all of the following EXCEPT:
    (A) The improvement in lesion detectability
    (B) Increase in the quantitative accuracy
    (C) Expansion of the staging capabilities
    (D) Improved delineation of the lesion

170. A wipe test on a dose package has produced 895 gross counts per minute (cpm). The daily background is 98 cpm and the well counter efficiency is 80%. What are the disintegrations per minute (dpm) produced by the wipe test?
    (A) 876 dpm
    (B) 996 dpm
    (C) 1,122 dpm
    (D) 1,241 dpm

171. In the image in Fig. 3.15 shown below, the area of physiologic F-18 FDG uptake is indicated by all of the following labels EXCEPT:
    (A) D
    (B) C
    (C) B
    (D) A

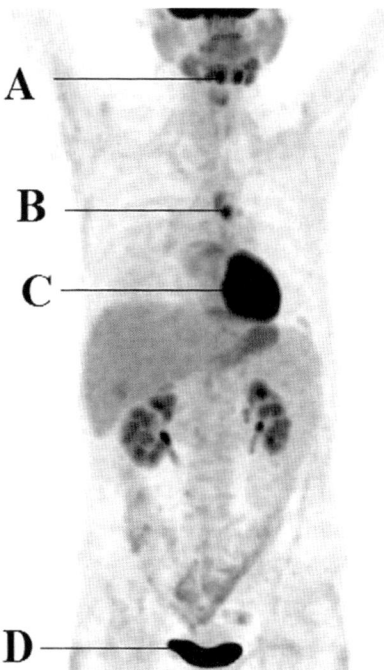

Fig. 3.15 PET/CT examination

172. What type of receptors is highly expressed on neuroendocrine tumors (NET) cells?
    (A) Cortisol receptors
    (B) Epinephrine receptors
    (C) Somatostatin receptors
    (D) Norepinephrine receptors

173. Laryngeal F-18 FDG uptake:
    (A) Is absent on normal scans
    (B) Is more pronounced if patient speaks after the scan completion
    (C) It can have an inverted T appearance
    (D) May be asymmetrical secondary to vocal cord paralysis

174. A PET-FDG scan performed in patients with esophagitis or Barrett esophagus can exhibit increased FDG uptake and will be classified as a:
    (A) False-negative study
    (B) True negative study
    (C) False-positive study
    (D) True positive study

175. The presence of intense F-18 FDG activity with a distribution that is not consistent with the site of surgery indicates the presence of:
    (A) Infarction
    (B) Foreign body
    (C) Infection
    (D) Artifact

176. The brain energy production depends solely on:
    (A) Anaerobic glycolysis
    (B) Aerobic glycolysis
    (C) Free fatty acids
    (D) Phosphocreatine

177. The number of counts per unit time detected by the device for each unit of activity present in a source is defined as:
    (A) The mean SUV
    (B) The scanner resolution
    (C) The scanner sensitivity
    (D) The scanner reproducibilty

178. The total uptake of the injected dose of F-18 FDG in the brain is approximately:
    (A) 3%
    (B) 6%
    (C) 9%
    (D) 12%

179. Physical property of the contrast media described as the measurement of the number of molecules and particles in a solution per kilogram of water is called:
    (A) Osmolality
    (B) Solubility
    (C) Viscosity
    (D) Integrity

180. The most frequently used clinical myocardial perfusion PET agent is:
    (A) F-18 FDG
    (B) Tc-99m Sestamibi
    (C) Rb-82
    (D) O-15 water

181. The presented images in Fig. 3.16 labeled A, B, C, and D were obtained during a routine PET/CT scan. The image labeled "D" is described as:
    (A) Topogram
    (B) Fused coronal
    (C) Non-attenuation-corrected
    (D) Maximum-intensity projection

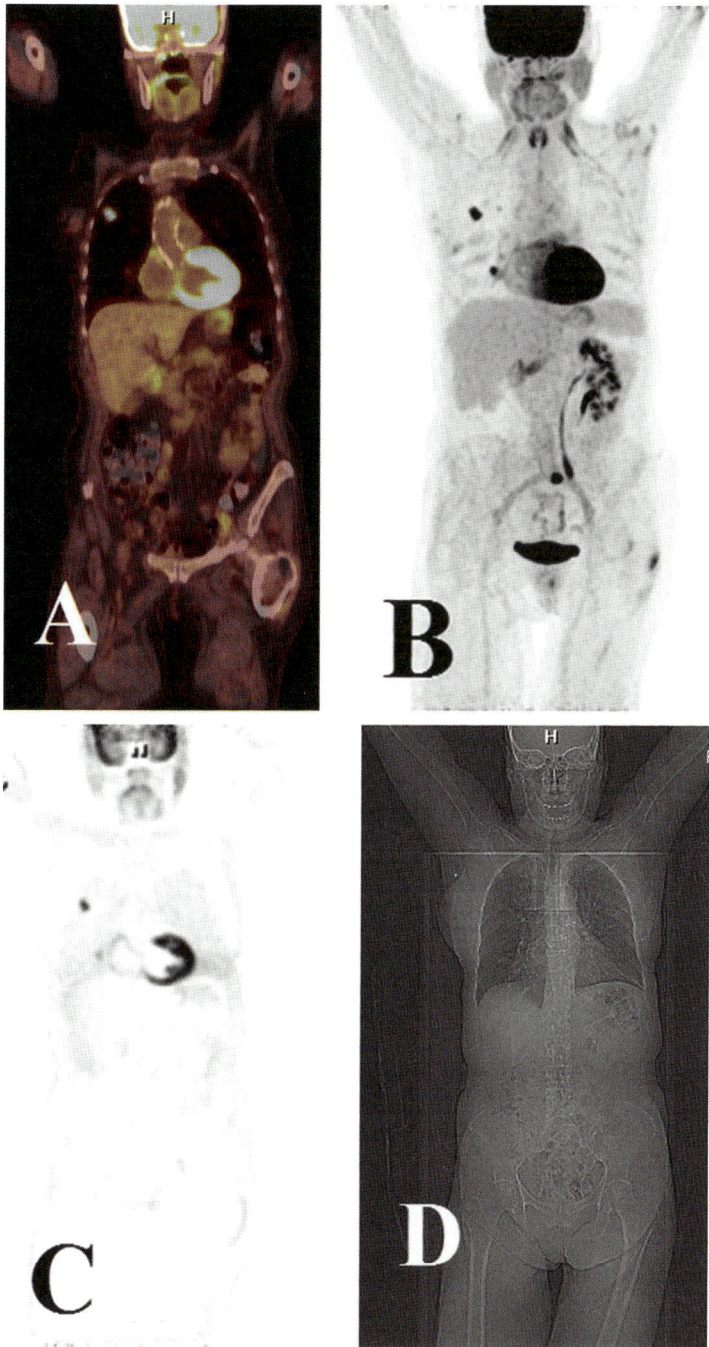

Fig. 3.16 (a–b) PET/CT images

182. Which of the following statements describing the characteristics of pulmonary nodules when differentiating benign from malignant lesions is FALSE?
    (A) The presence of cancer in small nodules is lower than that in large nodules
    (B) Benign nodules typically show a well-defined smooth and round contour
    (C) The presence of calcification in a pulmonary nodule increases the probability of a benign cause
    (D) Benign nodules typically have a volumetric doubling time range of 20 to 300 days

183. A vacuum tube that accelerates electrons against dynodes of increasing electric charge to amplify their signal is called:
    (A) Photomultiplier tube
    (B) X-ray tube
    (C) Photocathode
    (D) Digital–analog converter

184. Brain metabolism and blood flow are decreased at the site of onset of the seizure in the:
    (A) Interictal state
    (B) Intraictal state
    (C) Inter and intraictal states
    (D) Neither inter- or intraictal states

185. When the septa are removed, and coincidences are recorded between detectors lying in any ring combination the data are acquired:
    (A) In hybrid mode
    (B) In 2D mode
    (C) In 3D mode
    (D) In 4D mode

186. Epinephrine administered by IV bolus in patients with cardiac arrest will:
    (A) Induce bradycardia
    (B) Increase aortic diastolic blood pressure
    (C) Produce marked hypotension
    (D) Prevent tachyarrhythmia

187. Physical property of the contrast media is described as thickness or friction of fluid as it flows is called:
    (A) Osmolality
    (B) Solubility
    (C) Viscosity
    (D) Integrity

188. Posttraumatic breast hematoma, ruptured breast implant, and changes around breast prosthesis can lead to:
    (A) False-positive results in PET/CT scanning
    (B) False-negative results in PET/CT scanning
    (C) True negative results in PET/CT scanning
    (D) True positive results in PET/CT scanning

189. Sources of false-positive PET-FDG results in lung cancer imaging include all of the following EXCEPT:
    (A) Inflammatory pseudotumor
    (B) Histoplasmosis
    (C) Bronchioloalveolar carcinoma
    (D) Sarcoidosis

190. A radiation source is producing an exposure rate of 15 mR/h at a distance of 1 ft. How many feet away from the source should the technologist stand to achieve a background level of 0.03 mR/h?
    (A) 50 ft
    (B) 22.4 ft
    (C) 11.2 ft
    (D) 5 ft.

191. Which of the following PET/CT scanning protocols delivers the lowest radiation dose to the patient?
    (A) Topogram, low-dose CT, 370 MBq of F-18 FDG
    (B) Topogram, diagnostic CT with contrast, 370 MBq of F-18 FDG
    (C) Topogram, low-dose CT, 300 MBq of F-18 FDG, diagnostic CT with CA
    (D) Topogram, low-dose CT, 370 MBq of F-18 FDG, diagnostic CT with CA

192. A 60-year-old woman with concomitant obesity and strong family history of diabetes whose sugar level is well controlled with Metformin (Glucophage) is most likely to be diagnosed with:
    (A) Type I diabetes
    (B) Type II diabetes
    (C) Gestational diabetes
    (D) Malnutrition diabetes

193. Increasing the X-ray tube kV will result in:
    (A) Increasing the number of X-ray photons produced
    (B) Decreasing the number of X-ray photons produced
    (C) Increasing the energy of X-ray photons produced
    (D) Decreasing the energy of X-ray photons produced

194. Which of the following insulin preparations has the shortest serum half-life?
    (A) Lente insulin
    (B) Semilente insulin
    (C) Neutral protamine Hagedorn (NPH) insulin
    (D) Regular insulin

195. The small deviation away from a true 180° path that annihilation photons take is called:
    (A) Photon energy range
    (B) Photon non-collinearity
    (C) The lepton number
    (D) Photon collinearity

196. The 2010 Guidelines for Cardiopulmonary resuscitation (CPR) and Emergency Cardiovascular Care (ECC) of American Heart Association (AHA) recommend a change in the basic life support (BLS) sequence of steps for adults, children, and infants from A-B-C (Airway, Breathing, Chest compressions) to:
    (A) A-C-B (Airway, Chest compressions, Breathing)
    (B) B-C-A (Breathing, Chest compressions, Airway)
    (C) C-A-B (Chest compressions, Airway, Breathing)
    (D) C-B-A (Chest compressions, Breathing, Airway)

197. The process of applying a kernel to the raw data is called:
    (A) Fourier transformation
    (B) Convolution
    (C) Retrospective reconstruction
    (D) Windowing

198. In order to avoid any false-positive results, PET or PET/CT scans should be performed:
    (A) 1–2 weeks after the last cycle of chemotherapy
    (B) 2–4 weeks after the last cycle of chemotherapy
    (C) 4–6 weeks after the last cycle of chemotherapy
    (D) 6–8 weeks after the last cycle of chemotherapy

199. Focal increased F-18 FDG activity in the lungs is considered abnormal if is greater than activity in:
    (A) The myocardial wall
    (B) The liver
    (C) The mediastinal soft tissues
    (D) The thyroid

200. Hypoxia-mediated aggressive tumor behavior and resistance to therapy is mediated by the hypoxia inducible transcription factor called:
   (A) HIF-1
   (B) Choline
   (C) Integrin
   (D) CD-20

Answers

1. A – Rb-82 rest and stress

    Estimated effective radiation dose from Rb-82 rest and stress PET studies is ~12.6–13.5 mSv.
    (Einstein et al. 2007)

2. A – PVE is more prominent in smaller tumor

    Partial-volume effect (PVE) clearly depends on the extent (volume) of the tumor—the smaller the tumor, the greater underestimation of the SUV. PVE is also influenced by the shape of the tumor, surrounding tissues activity, and the spatial resolution of the system (scanner features, reconstruction parameters).
    (Soret et al. 2007)

3. A – Overestimates the attenuation coefficients

    Higher attenuation coefficients produce a rim of high activity at the truncation edge and can lead to misinterpretation of the PET scan.
    (Wahl 2009)

4. B – Partial-volume effect

    The partial-volume effect (PVE) is defined as quantitative bias resulting in the underestimation of counts density which differs from what they should be and influenced by the tumor size and shape, system resolution, and tissue sampling.
    (Soret et al. 2007)

5. A – The stopping power

    The stopping power depends on the type and energy of the particle and on the properties of the material it passes (density and effective atomic number (Z) of the material).
    (Saha 2005)

6. B – Convert the CT attenuation coefficients to those corresponding to PET

    The effects of contrast agents, metal implants, and respiratory motion should always be considered when quantitative protocols are applied with PET/CT.
    (Visvikis et al. 2004)

Answers

7. B – Iterative Reconstruction (IR)

    The feedback from this comparison is used to adjust the image estimate and to minimize the difference between these two datasets. In the ML-EM iterative method, the presumption is being made as to what the pixel count density will be in the reconstructed patient image. OS-EM uses only a subset of the projection data.
    (Wahl 2009)

8. B – Melanin content influences lesion detectability by PET

    PET can serve as particularly valuable tool for assessing the extent of disease in the follow-up of patients with more advanced melanoma. The role of PET imaging in the initial staging of melanoma without palpable lymph nodes remains controversial.
    (Karakousis and Czerniecki 2011)

9. C – Pharmacist

    During the last two decades FDG has been used by many investigators as an investigational New Drug (IND) in research studies. As of December 2011, all PET radiopharmaceuticals must have New Drug Application (NDA) or Abbreviated New Drug Application (or ANDA) for routine clinical use.
    (Vallabhajosula et al. 2011)

10. D – 1.4 h
    Formula 14

11. C – Atrial fibrillation

    Atrial fibrillation is the most common arrhythmia of the heart. On the EKG atrial fibrillation is recognized by an oscillating, irregular baseline (fibrillation waves) and the absence of P waves.

    The ventricular rhythm is unpredictable and the RR intervals irregular.
    (Goldberger 2006)

12. B – Myocardial viability

    Requirements for cellular viability include sufficient myocardial blood flow, intact sarcolemmal membrane function, and preserved metabolic activity.
    (Zaret and Beller 2005)

13. A – Stopping power

    The linear attenuation coefficient is a quantity that characterizes how easily a material or medium can be penetrated by X-rays or gamma rays and is measured in $cm-1$ (inverse of the mean distance).
    (Saha 2005)

14. B – Propranolol

    The brown fat deposits become more visible (increasing tracer uptake- more metabolically active) with cold exposure and less visible if an adrenergic beta blocker is given before the scan.
    (Cannon and Nedegaard 2004)

15. B – Misregistration artifacts

    Respiratory motion produces the misregistration—inaccurate localization—of lesion in the region of diaphragm (curvilinear artifacts along diaphragm).
    (Sureshbabu and Mawlawi 2005)

16. C – Staging of the disease

    The TNM (tumor, lymph nodes, metastasis) staging system is based on size, location, and number of lesions and does not depend on the degree of FDG uptake.
    (Lucignani et al. 2004)

17. D – LYSO

    Time-of-flight PET scanners were commercially available for a short time in the 1980s. (systems used BaF2 detectors which are very fast, but unluckily have very low detection efficiency). In 2006, a time-of-flight scanner based on LYSO- a variant of LSO in which some of lutetium is replaced by yttrium atoms- detectors was reintroduced and is now commercially available. (Philips Gemini TF)
    (Positron Emission Tomography 2011)

18. C – Doesn't affect SUV

    Water-equivalent contrast agents are called as negative contrast agents and they don't increase Hounsfield unit. Administration of the positive contrast medias, e.g., barium or iodine based agents leads to increase in HU.
    (Antioch and Bockish 2009): 131–138

19. D – The chest demonstrates several punctate hypermetabolic foci…physiologic uptake in the abdomen and pelvis

    Redemonstration of several small punctate foci of hypermetabolic activity within the hilar regions. Redemonstration of a patchy lobulated nodular density in the left mid lung zone with only mildly increased activity.
    (Radiology report frag)

20. C – 9.2 mCi

    Formula 19 B. Webster's formula does not use weight and height, therefore it should be disregarded when performing calculation.

Answers 123

21. D – Hibernatic myocardium

    Temporarily decreased contractile function of myocardial tissue, which follows an episode of ischemia, is described as myocardial stunning.
    (Zaret and Beller 2005)

22. C – 2 in.

    In adults, the recommended compression depth is 2 in. (5 cm); however, the recommended compression depth for infants and children is the depth of at least one-third of the anterior–posterior diameter of the chest (approximately 1.5 in. in infants and 2 in. in children).
    (American Heart Association 2012)

23. A – Underestimated

    Truncation artifacts seen in CT scans of large patients scanned with the arms down—scanning the patient with arms raised is a frequently applied technique.
    (Visvikis et al. 2004)

24. C – Hypothyroidism

    Decreased brain activity due to depression or hypothyroidism may be a cause of false-negative studies in patients with dementia.
    (Lin and Alavi 2009)

25. D – Following an inconclusive CCTA

    If a patient receives a FDG-PET study with inconclusive results, a follow-up SPECT test is not covered.
    (CMS 2011)

26. B – Alzheimer's disease

    A variety of biomarkers for amyloid plaque accumulation have been proposed—e.g., Pittsburgh compound B or PiB (11C-11PiB), stilbene derivative (C-11SB-13), florbetapir F-18 (F-18 AV-45).
    (Vallabhajosula et al. 2011)

27. A – A non-contrast low radiation dose scan

    The CT component is performed primarily for attenuation correction and anatomical correlation.
    (Sarji 2006)

28. B – Malignancy

    Increased ovarian uptake is related with malignancy in postmenopausal patients, but may be functional in premenopausal patients, e.g., around ovulation.
    (Lin and Alavi 2009)

29. D – F-18 fluorothymidine

    The DNA synthesis is a measure of cell proliferation and cytosine, guanine, adenine, and thymidine are the four nucleotides required for DNA synthesis.
    (Vallabhajosula et al. 2011)

30. B – 11.6%

    The given volume is additional information and must be disregarded, since the percent error formula does not utilize it.
    (Formula 8A)

31. D – Ventricular bigeminy

    Ventricular premature beats (VPBs) may occur normally or with organic heart disease. Ventricular bigeminy refers to the appearance of paired different ventricular complexes in the body-surface ECG. When a VPB occurs regularly after each normal beat, the grouping is called ventricular bigeminy.
    (Goldberger 2006)

32. C – Pulmonary infarction

    After no blood reaches a portion of the lung, that section of the lung suffers an infarct, meaning it dies because no blood or oxygen is reaching it.
    (Lin and Alavi 2009)

33. A – Braking radiation

    Almost all of the X-rays produced by the X-ray are bremsstrahlung or braking radiation type. If the bombarding electrons have sufficient energy, they can knock an electron out of an inner shell of the target metal atoms, and as a result, electrons from higher states drop down to fill the vacancy, emitting X-ray photons with precise energies determined by the electron energy levels (characteristic X-rays).
    (Wahl 2009)

34. A – volume of interest

    The purpose of a volume of interest (VOI) analysis is to calculate the distribution of pixel values within delineated tissue structures.
    (Lin and Alavi 2009)

35. D – True, scatter, and randoms

    Prompts represent coincidence events acquired in the standard coincidence window of a PET.
    (Turkington 2001)

Answers

36. B – Back projection

   Filtered back projection involves two steps: filtering the projections and back projecting them to create an image.
   (Christian et al. 2004)

37. C – Radionuclidic identity

   The half-life of the radionuclide is determined mathematically by mean of linear regression.
   (Mach and Schwarz 2010)

38. C – Dicumarol

   Oral hypoglycemic medications are used in the management of diabetes in patients diagnosed with non-insulin-dependent diabetes mellitus (NIDDM) whose blood sugar cannot be controlled by diet alone.
   (Mycek and Harvey 2008)

39. D – protein synthesis

   Since C-11 amino acids undergo metabolism in vivo, F-11 amino acids have been developed for imaging studies as tumor imaging agents.
   (Vallabhajosula et al. 2011)

40. A – Metformin

   Metformin significantly increases F-18 FDG uptake in the colon, and to a lesser extent, in the small intestine; however, diffuse uptake is rarely related to malignant disease, and therefore should not account for diagnostic impairment.
   (Soyka et al. 2010)

41. B – Nonviable myocardium

   When dysfunctional myocardium, with an intermediate decline in blood flow is encountered, the presence of myocardial viability myocardial is typically determined by evaluating myocardial metabolism (using FDG-PET imaging) in combination with myocardial blood flow (using PET or SPECT MPI). The extent of a blood flow/metabolism mismatch is correlated with the magnitude of the post-revascularization improvement in global left ventricular function.
   (Zaret and Beller 2005)

42. D – Tactile sensation

   The parietal lobe contains the primary sensory cortex that controls the body senses, such as touch or pain. Behind the primary sensory cortex is an area that controls fine sensation, such as weight, size, shape, or texture.
   (Christian et al. 2004)

43. A – Normalization

    Normalization calibration is used much like a high-count uniformity correction performed in the gamma cameras.
    (Christian et al. 2004)

44. C – The background noise in data acquired in the 2D is higher than that in the 3D

    The increased detection of scatter and random coincidences leads to a rise in the background noise compromising the accuracy of quantitative results derived from 3D images. The appearance of new scintillators, such as lutetium oxyorthosilicate (LSO) and gadolinium oxyorthosilicate (GSO) with a faster scintillation time and a better energy resolution, can lead to a reduction in the overall fraction of detected erroneous coincidences, and diminish their effect on quantitative accuracy of 3D PET.
    (Visvikis et al. 2004)

45. D – Bremsstrahlung radiation

    Bremsstrahlung is electromagnetic radiation produced by the deceleration of a charged particle when deflected by another charged particle, e.g., an electron by an atomic nucleus. The moving particle loses kinetic energy, which is converted into a photon because energy is conserved.
    (Early and Sodee 1995)

46. A – One standard deviation

    About 95% of the values lie within two standard deviations; and about 99.7% are within three standard deviations (68-95-99.7 rule).
    (Munro 2005)

47. A – pitch

    Typical pitch ratio is:–0.5, 1.0, and 1.5. The larger the pitch, the larger the axial coverage per unit time.
    (Prokop and Galanski 2003)

48. C – Hot-for-cold substitution

    C-11 for nonradioactive C-12 is an example of hot-for-cold substitution—the structure of the biologically active molecule has not been changed to introduce the PET radiolabel.
    (Mach and Schwarz 2010)

49. B – Estrogen receptor

    Estradiol is the most potent form of estrogen and it binds to estrogen receptor present in the cell nucleus of the female reproductive organs, breast, bone, liver, and also in various tissues in men.
    (Vallabhajosula 2007)

50. D – 1

As a result of having one Becquerel being equal to one transformation per second, there are $3.7 \times 1{,}010$ Bq in one curie.
(Lombardi 1999)

51. C – A Geiger–Muller counter output is proportional to the exposure rate

GM produces pulses that are independent from the energy deposited and consequently instrument's reading can be related to exposure rate only if the energy of the radiation is known.
(Christian et al. 2004)

52. C – Liver

Other accessory organs that aid in the digestion and absorption of nutrients include: salivary glands, teeth, gallbladder, pancreas, and appendix.
(Christian et al. 2004)

53. A – Hounsfield unit scale

CT number or Hounsfield number is a number that correlates to the Hounsfield scale which ranks various materials by their attenuation properties.
(Prokop and Galanski 2003)

54. B – Image registration

Misregistration is present when structures from one image dataset do not align correctly with structures from another image dataset.
(Wahl 2009)

55. B – Random coincidences

A random event occurs when two photons, which are not arising from the same annihilation event, are recorded by two opposite detectors within the coincidence time-window and erroneously recognized as nonexisting coincidence detection. Random coincidences are more probable at high count rates and/or with the wide coincidence window.
(Saha 2005)

56. D – Student's t-test

Student's t-test is used to check for differences between mean values by testing a null hypothesis that the two mean values are equal.
(Christian et al. 2004)

57. B – Accuracy

Accuracy testing is performed at installation and then annually, with at least two different sealed sources, e.g., Co-57, Cs-137, and Ba-133.
(Christian et al. 2004)

58. D – Fluorine-18

   F-18: half-life of 110 min, has the lowest mean positron energy from the listed radionuclides ~250 keV and consequently short positron range in H_2O ~2.4 mm.
   (Wahl 2009)

59. B – 4 stages

   The stages are described by Roman numerals I through IV (1–4), and each stage is characterized by the number and location of affected lymph nodes.
   (Jhanwar and Straus 2006)

60. D – A

   Positron-emitting radionuclides are typically produced in cyclotrons by the bombardment of stable elements with protons, deuterons, or helium nuclei. The radionuclides produced have an excess of protons and thus decay by the emission of positrons.
   (Wahl 2009)

61. C – Clear the area, notify a supervisor, contain the spill

   After initial steps the technologist should decontaminate the spill area using personnel and radiation safety precautions suitable for the radioactivity and type of radionuclide.
   (Christian et al. 2004)

62. C – Signet-ring cell carcinoma

   FDG uptake in gastric cancer depends on the glucose transporter GLUT-1 expression. One major reason for low FDG uptake in signet-ring cell carcinoma is the low GLUT-1 expression in this histological subtype of gastric cancer.
   (Lin and Alavi 2009)

63. A – LSO (lutetium oxyorthosilicate)

   LSO scintillator has the highest light output of all listed detectors (75% relative to NaI(Tl). Its poor energy resolution somewhat limits its application. BGO (bismuth germinate) is characterized by the high energy resolution; both scintillators BGO and LSO have comparable, high stopping power.
   (Lin and Alavi 2009)

64. C – Amino acids

   Dietary recommendations lead to better visualization of any areas in the hilum and carinal lymph nodes. Decreased uptake in the myocardium leads to better visualization of lesion in the left axilla.
   (Lin and Alavi 2009)

Answers

65. A – The tube voltage (kV)

    The tube voltage, across the cathode and the anode, accelerates the electrons, which then determines the energy of the electrons, and in the end, the energy of the photons produced.
    (Wahl 2009)

66. D – Uterine carcinoma

    PET/CT has the added advantage of anatomic imaging, which allows precise correlation of the abnormalities and minimizing the need to perform urinary bladder catheterization.
    (Lin and Alavi 2009)

67. D – cholestasis can cause false-negative liver lesions

    Cholestasis—any condition in which the flow of bile from the liver is blocked and inflammatory biliary tree uptake can cause false-positive liver lesions.
    (Lin and Alavi 2009)

68. C – Radiation necrosis

    CT and MRI have been proven deficient of accurate diagnosis on post-therapy residual or recurrent tumor. FDG uptake is low or absent in the region of necrosis and tumor presence is indicated by the area of hypermetabolism.
    (Miletich 2008)

69. C – FDG-PET/CT has more false-positive findings than FDG-PET alone

    In the deep nodal regions of the abdomen and the mediastinum, FDG-PET/CT has fewer false-positive findings than FDG-PET alone, presumably because of the improved distinction between malignant and nonmalignant FDG uptake, e.g., brown adipose tissue and muscle uptake.
    (Hutchings 2009)

70. D – Aorta

    (Madden 2007)

71. C – high radiation area

    Radiation area is the area accessible to personnel in which a major portion of the body of a person could receive a dose in excess of 5 mrem in 1 h.
    (Christian et al. 2004)

72. B – Cecum, colon, and rectum

    The large intestine is about 6 cm (3–4 in.) in diameter and approximately 1.5–1.8 m (5 ft) in length. The main function of the large intestine is to transport waste out of the body and to absorb water from the waste before it leaves.
    (Moore et al. 2010)

73. B – signal-to-noise ratios

   The signal-to-noise ratio (SNR) is one of the important measures of the performance of an imaging device and is defined as the ratio of the mean signal of a region of interest (ROI) to its standard deviation.
   (Boellaard 2011)

74. C – Colony-Stimulating Factors (CSFs)

   Granulocyte-colony stimulating factor (G-CSF), granulocyte-macrophage colony-stimulating factor (GM-CSF), and macrophage colony-stimulating factor (M-CSF), function as growth factors for specific cell types in the myeloid series (the term myeloid indicates an origin in the bone marrow or spinal cord, or a similarity to the marrow or spinal cord; "myeloid cell" is any leukocyte that is not a lymphocyte).
   (Mandell et al. 2010)

75. A – Non-attenuation-corrected (NAC) images

   The advantages of reconstructing images without AC include dodging of the noise amplification, reduction of the local background, and reduced patient scanning time.
   (Lin and Alavi 2009)

76. C – Aminophylline

   Aminophylline relaxes the smooth muscle of the bronchial airways and pulmonary blood vessels. In patients with asthma, aminophylline reduces airway responsiveness to adenosine, histamine, and allergen.
   (Mycek and Harvey 2008)

77. D – SUV normalization based on total body mass is the most dependable

   Body surface area and SUL-SUV normalized to lean body mass are less dependent on body habitus across populations than is SUV based on total body mass (F-18 FDG does not significantly accumulate in white fat in the fasting state).
   (Wahl and Jacene 2009)

78. B – Visual information

   In the occipital lobe the recognition of shapes and colors areas reside. The occipital lobe receives and processes visual information directly from the eyes and relates this information to the parietal and frontal lobes.
   (Christian et al. 2004)

79. D – Anaplastic

   Cancers that do not arise from follicular epithelium are not expected to trap iodine, e.g., anaplastic, medullary (arising from C cells).
   (Mosci and Iagaru 2011)

80. A – Rad

    The rad (radiation absorbed dose) is the measure of absorbed dose and relates to the amount of energy—100 ergs per gram—actually absorbed in some material, and is used for any type of radiation and any material. The unit can be used for any type of radiation, but it does not describe the biological effects of the different radiations.
    (Lombardi 1999)

81. C – The glutamine synthetase pathway

    Rb-82 chloride is transported into the cells by the active Na/K-ATPase pumps similar to potassium and thallium-201; flurpiridaz binds to the mitochondrial complex.
    (Takalkar et al. 2011)

82. C – Alzheimer's disease

    In advanced disease, the frontal lobe hypometabolism is observed, but temporoparietal abnormalities are always present.
    (Lin and Alavi 2009)

83. A – Hypermetabolic activity in the infracarinal region…physiologic bladder activity.

    The mass extends from the hilus through to the lateral chest wall…in the infracarinal region there is a moderate size area of hypermetabolic activity. The SUV value in his region has a maximum of 18.6.
    (Radiology report frag)

84. D – Granulocyte colony-stimulating factor (G-CSF)

    Granulocyte colony-stimulating factor G-CSF serves as a strong stimulus to both boost and speed up neutrophil production.
    (Mandell et al. 2010)

85. C – 4 weeks

    According to the RECIST, partial response is defined as a decline of at least 30% in tumor diameters for at least 4 wks.
    (Wahl and Jacene 2009)

86. B – Intraictal state

    In the course of the seizures (intraictal state) raised metabolism and blood flow are observed at the site of beginning of the seizures and in regions to which the seizure activity is spread.
    (Placantonakis and Schwartz 2009)

87. A – Positron emission

Proton-rich isotopes may decay via positron emission, in which a proton decays to a neutron, a positron, and a neutrino. The daughter isotope has an atomic number one less than the parent.
(Early and Sodee 1995)

88. D – Colonoscopy

Virtual colonography is being developed as a potential screening tool. A colonoscopy is considered the "gold standard" because of its ability to visualize, sample, and/or remove lesions from the entire colons. Screening is based on risk categories that take into account the patient's age, race, personal history of inflammatory bowel disease, polyps, cancer, family history of colon cancer, or presence of familial syndromes.
(Abeloff and Armitage 2008)

89. C – Therapy monitoring

Monitoring tumor response to treatment is only reimbursable for women with locally advanced and metastatic breast cancer when a change in therapy is anticipated.
(National Coverage Determination 2012)

90. C – A true event

A true event is recorded each time when both photons of an annihilation event are detected by two detectors in coincidence within the coincidence time-window, with neither photon undergoing any form of interaction prior to detection.
(Wahl 2009)

91. D – Kidney

Urinary bladder and spleen also receive high radiation doses, but the kidney is the critical organ.
(Castellucci et al. 2008)

92. A – Parkinson's disease (PD)

The nigrostriatal projection damage that characterizes PD is associated with striatal dopamine deficiency targeting the posterior putamen.
(Wahl 2009)

93. B – time-of-flight imaging

Taking into account the velocity of 511 keV photons a timing vagueness of 500 picoseconds translates to a position uncertainty of the positron decay ~7.5 cm.
(Saha 2005)

94. A – Metastases to regional lymph nodes

    Attributed mainly to the early detection overall 5-year disease-free survival rate has increased from 50–63% during the past 2 decades.
    (Ferrif 2012)

95. A – increased sensitivity

    A 33% increase in axial coverage from 16.2 to 21.6 cm results in a 78% increase in sensitivity for 3D acquisition. The greater axial coverage makes more efficient use of the radiation emitted from the patient and greater throughput and patient comfort.
    (Patton et al. 2009)

96. C – A family history

    Another risk factor is a personal history of the disease and polyps. Having inflammatory bowel disease for more than 10 years also increases risk for colon cancer.
    (Ferrif 2012)

97. C – X-ray beam

    First assembly of CT scanners had an X-ray tube which generated a thin, focused beam of X-rays called a pencil beam; second generation produced an X-ray beam that had a shape like an opened paper fan. The newest CT scanners, e.g., MDCT produce an X-ray beam which is no longer flat (fan) but rather three-dimensional (cone).
    (Prokop and Galanski 2003)

98. B – During menstruation

    Physiologic FDG accumulation in the uterus should be considered when focal FDG accumulation is observed in the pelvis in women of reproductive age. The PET/CT scan helps define physiologic accumulation of FDG in the uterus during menstruation.
    (Lin and Alavi 2009)

99. C – Coronary artery disease

    Awaiting FDA approval, F-18 flurpiridaz has completed a Phase 2 clinical trial and is a third agent—besides FDA-approved N-13 ammonia and Rb-82 chloride—utilized to assess myocardial perfusion. The first of two planned Phase 3 trials began in the second quarter of 2011.
    (Takalkar et al. 2011)

100. B – Coronal slice of the brain

    The coronal plane, also called the frontal plane, divides the body into front (anterior) and back (posterior).
    (Madden 2007)

101. D – Reference worker

    Reference man is defined as being between 20 and 30 years of age, weighing 70 kg, is 170 cm in height, and lives in a climate with an average temperature of from 10° to 20°C. He is a Caucasian and is a Western European or North American in habitat and custom. The vast majority of people, including women and children, fall outside the definition; it underestimates dose to children in a large number of situations, and to women in some situations.
    (U.S. NRC 2011)

102. B – Increased respiratory effort

    The crura of the diaphragm—right and left crus—are tendinous structures that extend inferiorly from the diaphragm to the vertebral column. On coronal images the crus uptake looks as a continuous vertical line.
    (Lin and Alavi 2009)

103. A – ROI and lesion size

    The size of the ROI affects the reproducibility of SUV uptake values obtained from larger, fixed ROIs and are more reproducible than single-pixel SUVs.
    (Wahl and Jacene 2009)

104. C – 10 days

    For a PET/CT study, an interval of 10 days after G-CSF administration is recommended to minimize the influence of G-CSF on the bone marrow. However, readers can find the variable recommended time interval ranging from 5 days to 1 month.
    (Hanaoka et al. 2011)

105. B – The superficial nodal lesions

    AC and NAC PET images are complementary to each other and should be jointly reviewed for the optimal assessment of these patients.
    (Lin and Alavi 2009)

106. C – Colon inflammation

    Focal colon activity is suggestive of colon carcinoma or polyp.
    (Lin and Alavi 2009)

Answers

107. C – Normal saline

    Hydration and frequent bladder voiding decrease the bladder (critical organ) radiation absorbed dose.
    (Lin and Alavi 2009)

108. C – Bone marrow hyperplasia

    Bone marrow hyperplasia is commonly seen in patients with malignancies who have been treated with chemotherapy and bone marrow stimulating agents, e.g., granulocyte colony-stimulating factor, erythropoietin.
    (Lin and Alavi 2009)

109. D – I-124

    I-124 is a positron-emitting radionuclide with a half-life of 4.2 days that can be used in PET/CT scintigraphy to image the extent of disease in patients with papillary and follicular carcinoma, similarly to I-131 whole-body scan.
    (Mosci and Iagaru 2011)

110. B – 21 mCi

    The pre-calibration formula and 10 min half-life of Nitrogen-13 is used to solve this problem.
    (Formula 16B)

111. C – 200 dpm/cm^2

    The wipe testing should be performed after the decontamination procedure.
    (Christian et al. 2004)

112. B – Vertical long axis slices

    In this view, the heart is in a horizontal position, and the apex of the heart is to the viewer's right. The tomogram is displayed with slices beginning at the septum, and progressing to the lateral wall of the left ventricle.
    (ACC/AHA/SNM 1992)

113. A – The scatter-to-true ratio will stay the same

    True and scatter rate coincidences vary linearly with the injected dose and as a result ratio does not change.
    (Saha 2005)

114. A – High noise

    Inhomogeneity of data transmission may lead to a noisy background and decrease the signal-to-noise ratio.
    (Lin and Alavi 2009)

115. B – False positive

    A negative PET scan in this circumstance is more likely to be true negative. A low pretest probability of disease allows easier acceptance of the hypothesis of absence of the disease.
    (Lin and Alavi 2009)

116. B – low

    Benign tumors as lipoma, neurofibroma, osteochondroma, and desmoid tumor are spotted on F-18 FDG-PET, mostly as secondary findings in the chest wall in patients being evaluated for other malignancies.
    (Hickeson 2011)

117. B – Before the medication

    If possible, the F-18 FDG injection should be performed before the medication, in order to avoid any drug-related alterations in F-18 FDG distribution.
    (Hamblen and Lowe 2003)

118. A – The National Oncologic PET Registry (NOPR)

    CMS at this time only pays for positron emission tomography (PET) scans for certain reasons and for certain types of cancer. In order to gather the information needed to decide which other types of cancer should be covered by Medicare, CMS will provide payment for the PET scans of patients who are properly registered with the National Oncologic PET Registry (NOPR).
    (The National Oncologic PET Registry 2011)

119. A – Not visualized

    Parathyroid adenomas and hyperplasia can cause focal increased uptake. The usefulness of C-11 methionine PET or PET-CT, particularly in cases of negative Tc-99m sestamibi SPECT examinations, is being investigated.
    (Lin and Alavi 2009)

120. A – 640 mCi

    The pre-calibration formula and 1.25 min half-life of Rb-82 is utilized to solve the problem.
    (Formula 16B)

121. C – Curie

    The curie is measured by the number of atomic disintegrations per second (1 Curie = $3.7 \times 1,010$ disintegrations /second). Often radioactivity is expressed in smaller units like: thousandths (mCi) and one millionths (uCi).
    (Lombardi 1999)

Answers

122. A – Tumor recurrence

Increased FDG uptake immediately after radiation therapy may be due to inflammatory change and not necessarily due to residual/recurrent tumor.
(Delbeke et al. 2002)

123. B – the cancer spread to extranodal sites

In stage IV, the disease is also present in extranodal sites, usually the lungs, liver, bone or bone marrow, and, more rarely, other sites.
(Jhanwar and Straus 2006)

124. D – Non-small cell lung carcinoma

This uptake becomes even more prominent as there is relatively low uptake in the surrounding aerated lung, as opposed to other soft tissues.
(Wahl and Buchanan 2002)

125. B – Peripheral and thoracic lymph nodes involvement

In the abdomen and pelvis, PET and CT provide comparable results in the detection of disease.
(Lin and Alavi 2009)

126. D – FDG-PET has no influence on surgical management of patients

PET changes the surgical management of patients either by identifying a resectable metastasis or by demonstrating unresectable extrahepatic metastases that were unsuspected clinically, not seen or equivocal on CT. Detection of unsuspected metastatic disease can spare patients futile attempts at curative resection of hepatic metastases.
(Wahl 2009)

127. B – Pulse pileups

The event will be counted but will be mispositioned with resulting image distortion.
(Lin and Alavi 2009)

128. C – The hypothalamus

The hypothalamus is a portion of the brain responsible for hormone production that manage body temperature, thirst, hunger, sleep, circadian rhythm, moods, sex drive, and the release of other hormones in the body.
(Christian et al. 2004)

129. B – Radiotherapy planning

   Tumor resectability, nodal involvement, guided needle or thoracoscopic biopsy, and prognosis in patients with malignant mesothelioma, have been also evaluated with FDG-PET.
   (Gerbaudo et al. 2011)

130. C – Volume-rendered display (VRT)

   Volume-rendered techniques (VRT) have become the standard method for quick display and evaluation of vascular disease in computed tomography angiography (CTA).
   (Prokop and Galanski 2003)

131. D – Rate of cell proliferation

   The sensitivity to radiation is proportional to the rate of growth of its cells, e.g., an embryo/fetus is more sensitive to radiation in the first three months than in later trimesters.
   (Lombardi 1999)

132. D – Hyperthermia

   Patient may also experience tremor, nervousness, hunger, headache, and seizures. Signs of hypoglycemia vary from person to person, but within an individual, they remain fairly constant.
   (Andreoli et al. 2001)

133. C – Electronic collimation

   With a physical collimator in place, directional data are obtained by preventing photons which are not normal or nearly normal to the collimator face from falling on the detector. In electronic collimation, these photons are not lost but may be detected and used as signal. This results in a important increase in detector sensitivity, e.g., by a factor of ~10 for 2D PET acquisition.
   (Wahl 2009)

134. A – The tumor

   The noise is described as the vagueness with which that tumor was recorded (described as the standard deviation).
   (Christian et al. 2004)

135. A – Increase the number of X-ray photons produced

   The tube current controls the temperature of the cathode and indirectly the number of X-ray photons produced.
   (Wahl 2009)

Answers

136. C – cholesterol metabolic pathway

The radiopharmaceuticals targeting the increased glucose but not cholesterol metabolic pathway have been used.
(Reubi and Maecke 2008)

137. B – 4–6

The increased count rate in 3D mode comes at the cost of increased scatter (from 10 to 40%), randoms from activity that are out of the field of view, and dead time.
(Fahey 2002)

138. C – Wash-in study

The example of the wash-in study is the intra-arterial administration of microspheres purposely engineered to be too large to pass through capillaries and which, as a result, mechanically embolize in a vascular bed.
(Miles et al. 2007)

139. B – The cellular apoptosis

Apoptosis is a multistep, programmed multi-pathway cell death that is genetically controlled in every cell of the body. In a number of diseases, the apoptosis cell-division ratio is altered. Labeled Anexin V has been employed to image apoptosis.
(Wahl 2009)

140. C – 10 mCi

The 12 mCi of F-18 FDG should be decayed 30 min to get the correct answer, using formula listed below.
(Formula 16A)

141. C – Every 6 months

The inventory and leak test must comprise all sources of activity greater than 100 µCi.
(Christian et al. 2004)

142. B – The prosthetic mitral valve

A myxoma is the most common primary tumor of the heart in adults, usually located in either the left—about 86 percent—or right atrium of the heart. Patients with atrial myxomas characteristically present in one of three ways: symptoms of atrioventricular valve obstruction (dyspnea, syncope, AF), signs of systemic embolization (CVA, PE), or with constitutional symptoms (fever, weight loss).
(Ferrif 2012)

143. B – Is highest in the axial center of the gantry

The sensitivity in 3D PET is highest in the axial center of the gantry and falls off toward the periphery; the sensitivity of the first and last few slices of a 3D acquisition is the same as the sensitivity of 2D.
(Fahey 2002)

144. C – evaluation of brain injuries

FDG-PET can be employed to evaluate a number of types of dementias including Alzheimer dementia (AD), frontotemporal dementia (FTD), and multi-infarct dementia, based on the display of FDG uptake/glucose metabolism. PET can help in the evaluation of patients who have temporal lobe epilepsy.
(Mittra and Quon 2009)

145. B – DICOM

DICOM-Digital Imaging and Communications in Medicine was developed by the American College of Radiology (ACR) and the National Equipment Manufacturers Association (NEMA).
(Christian et al. 2004)

146. C – Dobutamine

The beginning of action of dobutamine is within 1–2 min; still, as much as 10 min may be required to achieve the peak effect of a particular infusion rate. During the intravenous administration of dobutamine, the electrocardiogram (ECG, EKG) and blood pressure should be continuously monitored.
(Mycek and Harvey 2008)

147. C – High-Definition PET

HD-PET offsets for geometrical distortions arising from the increasingly oblique penetration into the detectors of annihilation photons away from the center of the scanner and results in improved intrinsic resolution and uniformity throughout the FOV.
(Patton et al. 2009)

148. A – Hypermetabolic activity in the right hemithorax...similar distribution... decreased SUV values

Patient with history of lung and renal carcinoma; hx of right lower lobe resection and left nephrectomy.
(Radiology report frag)

149. D – SPECT imaging can utilize higher doses of radionuclides

Radiotracers with shorter half-lives can be injected in higher activities to the patient without creating any additional radiation exposure to the patient.
(Rahmim and Zaidi 2008)

Answers

150. B – 25.7 mCi/ml

First, use formula 17A to obtain the specific concentration of 400 mCi/5ml, which is 80 mCi/ml. Decay this concentration to 10:00 A.M., which is 25.7 mCi/ml.

* Only concentration is needed; therefore, removed activity at specific time doesn't impact the concentration. If remaining volume is needed then decay initial concentration 80 mCi/ml to 9:00 A.M., which is 37.6 mCi/ml. Divide 13 mCi by concentration at 9:00 A.M. (13 mCi/37.6 mCi/ml), which is 0.35 ml (at 9:00A.M.). Decay 37.6 mCi/ml to 10:00A.M., which is 25.7 mCi/ml. Divide 13 mCi by concentration at 10:00 A.M. (13 mCi/25 mCi/ml), which is 0.5 ml. Added volume of 0.35 ml and 0.5 ml is 8.5 ml, which is subtracted from 5ml, that is, remaining 4.15 ml.
(Formula 16A and 17A)

151. D – FDG-PET has much more radiation exposure to patients than that of Ga-67 scintigraphy.

Radiation exposure from FDG-PET is about 10 mSv compared with approximately 44 mSv for standard Ga-67 scintigraphy.
(Spaepen et al. 2003)

152. B – The shift of the LOR from the center of gantry

The distance of the point from the center of the gantry can be determined from the amplitude of the sine wave (X-axis).
(Fahey 2002)

153. D – Sensitivity 90% and specificity 91%

The collective sensitivity and false-positive rate seem to be higher in patients diagnosed with Hodgkin disease, compared with patients diagnosed with non-Hodgkin lymphoma.
(Isasi et al. 2005)

154. C – The overall mortality from breast cancer has increased in recent years

Although its incidence has increased in the past decades, the overall mortality from this disease has decreased in recent years. This phenomenon is attributable to diagnostic efforts resulting in detection of many more early-stage cancers that are likely never to progress to become life-threatening.
(Kumar et al. 2009)

155. B – Lymphoma

As a result of the nonspecific nature of these findings, the diagnosis of lymphoma may be significantly delayed. Sometimes enlarged lymph nodes or splenomegaly may be accompanying findings in the course of evaluation for other medical issues.

(Cheson 2008)

156. B – breast benign lesions

    Benign breast lesions may show mild to moderate FDG uptake and can lead to false-positive results in PET/CT imaging.
    (Kumar et al. 2009)

157. D – Liposarcoma

    Liposarcomas are typically large bulky tumors at the time of diagnosis, and on FDG-PET imaging, appear as mildly hypermetabolic large masses.
    (Hickeson and Abikhzer 2011)

158. C – Electroencephalography (EEG)

    EEG, although it has several limitations, remains the most commonly used, and the easiest to perform, functional study in epileptic patients.
    (Placantonakis and Schwartz 2009)

159. C – F-18 fluoro-dihydrotestosterone (FDHT)

    Androgen receptors (ARs), principal components along the pathway to prostate cancer, are the target of FDHT, and they are not present in MPM.
    (Gerbaudo et al. 2011)

160. A – 121 dpm
    Formula 11

161. B – C

    The descending aorta is the main portion of the aorta, consisting of the thoracic aorta and the abdominal aorta, which continues from the aortic arch into the trunk of the body.
    (Andreoli et al. 2001)

162. C – Somatostatin

    The effects of somatostatin are mediated by interaction with somatostatin receptors on different target cells. Somatostatin receptors are found in the cells of neuroendocrine organs and in some non-neuroendocrine cells.
    (Castellucci et al. 2008)

Answers

163. A – Tumor recurrence

    Postradiation changes are characterized by mildly to moderately increased F-18 FDG uptake corresponding to the sites of radiation therapy, which gradually decreases in intensity.
    (Kazama et al. 2005)

164. D – Alzheimer's disease

    The crucial element of this hypometabolism is its magnitude relative to that of other cortices.
    (Miletich 2008)

165. C – 3 months

    The patient's medical and surgical history would be of utmost importance to the radiologists/nuclear medicine physicians who reads the scan. It is also critical to carefully correlate F-18 FDG uptake with the CT anatomy.
    (Zhuang et al. 2003)

166. B – O-18 (oxygen enriched water)

    A usual target form is made of tungsten, silver, or titanium and storage 0.3–3.0 ml of highly enriched O-18 water.
    (Vallabhajosula 2007)

167. C – The height of table

    Adding the distance between the detector and the source decreases the geometric efficiency of the scanner; increasing the diameter of the ring reduces the geometric efficiency and sensitivity. Sensitivity improves with increasing number of rings in the scanner.
    (Wahl 2009)

168. B – Dipirydamole

    Dipyridamole (Permole, Persantine) shares a common mechanism of action with adenosine, in that it indirectly increases the extracellular concentration of adenosine by blocking its cellular reuptake. Pharmacological effect of dipirydamole lasts for several hours after administration, while adenosine has a biological half-life of 10 s.
    (Mycek and Harvey 2008)

169. C – Expansion in staging capabilities

    Even though WB-PET can detect distant spread of breast cancer (TNM staging), dedicated PEM systems offer a higher spatial resolution and sensitivity, and as a result, improve the detectability of small lesions. Provided

tomographic images may further assist the surgeon in undertaking a more precise excision of involved breast tissue.
(Zaidi and Thompson 2009)

170. B – 996 dpm
    Formula 11

171. C – B
    Hypermetabolic activity within the mediastinum with SUV value of 9.6. The corresponding CT images show the soft tissue density in this region to measure 2 cm in diameter.
    (Radiology report frag)

172. C – Somatostatin receptors
    The majority of NETs express somatostatin receptors (SSTRs), so they can be effectively targeted and visualized with radiolabeled SST analogues in vivo. Among the five different SSTRs, most of the NETs express SSTR2.
    (Castellucci et al. 2008)

173. D – May be asymmetrical secondary to vocal cord paralysis
    Asymmetric uptake of FDG can be seen in the laryngeal muscles in patients with laryngeal nerve palsy contralateral to the side of the nerve dysfunction and secondary to postoperative changes.
    (Lin and Alavi 2009)

174. C – False-positive study
    It is recommended to advise the clinician of focal areas of increased FDG activity in the esophagus incidentally noted during a PET examination performed for other reasons, as this may represent early-stage esophageal malignancy.
    (Rohren et al. 2004)

175. C – Infection
    Increasing intensity of F-18 FDG uptake on follow-up FDG-PET imaging and CT findings, e.g., the presence of fat-stranding, fluid, and/or gas bubbles help to diagnose infection.
    (Hickeson and Abikhzer 2011)

Answers

176. B – Aerobic glycolysis

    The brain is the biggest energy user in the body attributable to the constant activity of the neurons. If the brain is deprived of oxygen for more than 3–5 min, permanent injury may result.
    (Newberg and Alavi 2010)

177. C – The scanner sensitivity

    The scanner sensitivity is ordinarily expressed in counts per second per microcurie (or megabecquerel).
    (Wahl 2009)

178. B – 6%

    In the brain, glucose is the primary substrate for brain metabolism, and very intense tracer uptake is observed in the normal cerebral cortex and basal ganglia.
    (Sarji 2006)

179. A – Osmolality

    Contrast agents are divided into two categories, high osmolar contrast media (ionic agents) and low osmolar contrast media (nonionic agents). An injection of high osmolar agents results in an immense increase in the number of particles contained in the vascular system. The introduction of particles into the vascular system causes water from body tissue to move into the vascular system in an effort to even out concentrations.
    (Prokop and Galanski 2003)

180. C – Rb-82

    It is likely that the clinical application of Rb-82 and PET for myocardial perfusion imaging will continue to grow.
    (Heller et al. 2009)

181. A – Topogram

    CT (computed tomography) projection radiograph, topogram, or scout view is defined as lateral or frontal image of patient reconstructed in rectangular grid from CT data.
    (Prokop and Galanski 2003)

182. D – Benign nodules typically have a volumetric doubling time range of 20 to 300 days

    Most malignant nodules have a volumetric doubling time—equivalent to a 26% increase in nodule diameter; less than 100 days and 2-year stability in the size of a nodule should suggest a benign cause.
    (Albert and Russell 2009)

183. A – Photomultiplier tube

The function of the photomultiplier tube (PMT) is to accept the light output from a scintillation crystal/photocathode, and additionally amplify this signal before transferring it to the computer of the PET system.
(Mittra and Quon 2009)

184. A – Interictal state

In general, interictal PET identifies focal areas of decreased metabolism; however, such hypometabolic areas are commonly considered to be bigger than the actual epileptogenic foci (surround inhibition following seizures).
(Placantonakis and Schwartz 2009)

185. C – in 3D mode

The sensitivity in 3D PET is highest in the axial center of the gantry and diminishes toward the periphery—the sensitivity of the first and last few slices of a 3D acquisition is the same as the sensitivity of 2D mode. The boost in sensitivity to true coincidences is the key motivation for the removal of septa. However, the sensitivity to scattered and random events in 3D mode also increases considerably.
(Fahey 2002)

186. B – Increase aortic diastolic blood pressure

The vasoconstrictor effect of epinephrine is the most important one in cardiac arrest. The effect of an IV bolus of epinephrine peaks in 2–3 min. Epinephrine should be used with caution in patients suffering from myocardial infarction, since epinephrine increases heart rate and raises blood pressure.
(Ferrif 2007)

187. C – Viscosity

The thickness of the contrast media is related to the concentration and the size of the molecules in a specific contrast agent. The thickness or viscosity affects the rate the contrast media can be injected. Heating the contrast media, usually to body temperature, reduces viscosity and it can be injected at a higher rate.
(Prokop and Galanski 2003)

188. A – false-positive results in PET/CT scanning

Chemo/radiotherapy induced inflammation, silicone injection, and inflammation/infection, e.g., mastitis/abscesses can also lead to false-positive results in PET/CT scanning.
(Kumar et al. 2009)

Answers 147

189. C – Bronchioloalveolar carcinoma

Fungal infection, rheumatoid nodule, lipoid pneumonia, and benign tumors can also be a frequent source of false-positive PET-FDG scans.
(Lin and Alavi 2009)

190. B – 22.4 ft
(Formula 12)

191. A – Topogram, low-dose CT, 370 MBq of F-18 FDG

An average effective patient dose from the whole-body 18F-FDG PET/CT examinations is about 25 mSv.
(Brix et al. 2005)

192. B – Type II diabetes

In type 2 diabetes (non-insulin-dependent diabetes mellitus or NIDDM), either the body does not produce enough insulin or the cells ignore the insulin. Type 2 diabetes is the most common form of diabetes.
(Andreoli et al. 2001)

193. C – Increasing the energy of X-ray photons produced

Kilovoltage (kV) controls the energy level of the X-ray photons—the higher the kV, the higher the energy of the photons.
(Wahl 2009)

194. D – Regular insulin

Regular insulin (crystalline zinc insulin), given subcutaneously, lowers blood sugar in minutes. Regular insulin is suitable, in emergencies for I.V. administration.
(Mycek and Harvey 2008)

195. B – Photon non-collinearity

The intrinsic physical limitations of positron range and photon non-collinearity degrade the spatial resolution of the scanner and deteriorate with the distance between the two detectors.

The contribution from non-collinearity amounts to 1.8–2 mm for 80–90 cm PET scanners.
(Saha 2005)

196. C – C-A-B (Chest compressions, Airway, Breathing)

The highest survival rates from cardiac arrest are reported among patients who have a witnessed arrest and an initial rhythm of ventricular fibrillation (VF) or pulseless ventricular tachycardia (VT). In these patients, the critical initial elements of BLS are chest compressions and early defibrillation. By changing the sequence to C-A-B, chest compressions will be initiated sooner and the delay in ventilation should be minimal.
(American Heart Association 2012)

197. B – Convolution

Convolution is a mathematical operation on two functions producing a third function that is typically viewed as a modified version of one of the original functions. Reconstruction filter or kernel is applied to improve the essential characteristics of the image, e.g., to augment definition of the edges, minimize noise etc.
(Groch and Erwin 2000)

198. B – 2–4 weeks after the last cycle of chemotherapy

Postchemotherapy- or postradiotherapy-induced inflammation and increased FDG uptake is not uncommon in patients who underwent chemotherapy or radiotherapy.
(Lin and Alavi 2009)

199. C – the mediastinal soft tissues

Nodules should not be compared to surrounding aerated lung, but rather to other solid soft tissue to evaluate for relatively increased uptake. Evaluation usually can be made with mediastinal soft tissues or blood pool.
(Wahl 2009)

200. A – HIF-1

Hypoxia inducible factor-1 (HIF-1) stimulates events that allow for the adaptation of tumor cells to hypoxia, such as unregulated glycolysis, angiogenesis, and p53 mutation. Choline, a phosphatedylcholine precursor, can be targeted to the cell membrane to image proliferation in cancer cells; an integrin is implicated in metastasis, angiogenesis, and proliferation.
(Rice et al. 2011)

References and Suggested Readings

Albert RH, Russell JJ. Evaluation of the solitary pulmonary nodule. Am Fam Physician. 2009;80(8):827–31.
Abeloff DM, Armitage OJ. Abeloff's clinical oncology. 4th ed. Philadelphia, PA: Churchill Livingstone Elsevier; 2008.

ACC/AHA/SNM policy statement. Standardization of cardiac tomographic imaging. J Nucl Med. 1992;33:1434–5.
American Heart Association. http://www.heart.org/idc/groups/heart.public/@wcm/@ecc/documents/downloadable/ucm_317350.pdf. Accessed 3 Jan 2012.
Andreoli TE, Bennett JC, et al. Cecil essentials of medicine. 5th ed. Philadelphia, PA: WB Saunders Company; 2001.
Antioch G, Bockish A. How to optimize CT/for PET/CT. In: Wahl R, editor. Principles and practice of PET and PET/CT. 2nd ed. Philadelphia, PA: Lippincott and Williams, a Walter Kluwer business; 2009. p. 131–8.
Boellaard R. Need for standardization of F-18 FDG PET/CT for treatment response assessments. J Nucl Med. 2011;52:93S.
Brix G, Lechel U, Glatting G, et al. Radiation exposure of patients undergoing whole-body dual-modality 18F-FDG PET/CT examinations. J Nucl Med. 2005;46:608–13.
Cannon B, Nedegaard J. Brown adipose tissue: function and physiological significance. Physiol Rev. 2004;84(1):277–359.
Castellucci P, Valentina Ambrosini V, et al. PET/CT in neuroendocrine tumors. PET Clin. Vol. 3, No. 2, April 2008.
Cheson DB. Staging and evaluation of the patient with lymphoma. Hematol Oncol Clin North Am. 2008;22:825–7.
Christian PE, Bernier DR, Langan JK. Nuclear medicine and PET: Technology and techniques. 5th ed. St. Louis, MO: Mosby; 2004.
CMS. National Coverage Determination.https://www.cms.gov/medicare-coverage-database/details/ncd. Accessed 25 Dec 2011.
Delbeke D, Martin WH, Sandler MP. Colorectal, pancreatic, and hepatobiliary. In: Wahl RL, Buchanan JW, editors. Principles and practice of positron emission tomography. Philadelphia, PA: Lippincott Williams & Wilkins; 2002. p. 217–33.
Early PJ, Sodee BD. Principles and practice of nuclear medicine. 2nd ed. Mosby: St. Louis, MO; 1995.
Einstein AJ, Moser KW, Thompson RC, et al. Radiation dose to patients from cardiac diagnostic imaging. Circulation. 2007;116:1290–305.
Fahey HF. Data Acquisition in PET Imaging. J Nucl Med Technol. 2002;30:2.
Ferrif F. Ferri's clinical advisor. 14th ed. Philadelphia, PA: Elsevier Mosby; 2012.
Ferrif F. Practical guide to the care of the medical patient. 7th ed. St Louis, Mo: Mosby; 2007.
Gerbaudo HV, Katz IS, Nowak KA, et al. Multimodality imaging review of malignant pleural mesothelioma diagnosis and staging. PET Clin. 2011;6:275–97.
Goldberger LA. Clinical electrocardiography: a simplified approach. 7th ed. St. Louis, MO: Mosby; 2006.
Groch WM, Erwin WDJ. SPECT in the year 2000: basic principles. J Nucl Med Technol. 2000;28(4):233–44.
Hamblen MS, Lowe JV. Clinical F-18 FDG oncology patient preparation techniques. J Nucl Med Technol. 2003;31:3–7.
Hanaoka K, Hosono M, et al. Fluorodeoxyglucose uptake in the bone marrow after granulocyte colony-stimulating factor administration in patients with non-Hodgkin's lymphoma. Nucl Med Commun. 2011;32(8):678–83.
Heller GV, Calnon D, Dorbala S. Recent advances in cardiac PET and PET/CT myocardial perfusion imaging. J Nucl Cardiol. 2009;16:962–9.
Hickeson M, Abikhzer G. Review of physiologic and pathophysiologic sources of fluorodeoxyglucose uptake in the chest wall on PET. PET Clin. 2011;6:339–64.
Hutchings M. PET Imaging in Lymphoma. Expert Rev Hematol. 2009;2(3):261–76.
Isasi CR, Lu P, Blaufox MD. A meta analysis of 18F-2-deoxy-2-fluoro-D-glucose positron emission tomography in the staging and restaging of patients with lymphoma. Cancer. 2005;104(5):1066–075.
Jhanwar SY, Straus JD. The role of PET in Lymphoma. J Nucl Med. 2006;47:1326–34.
Karakousis CG, Czerniecki JB. Diagnosis of melanoma. PET Clin. 2011;6:1–8.

Kazama T, Faria SC, et al. FDGPET in the evaluation of treatment for lymphoma: clinical usefulness and pitfalls. Radiographics. 2005;25(1):191–207.

Kumar R, Rani N, et al. False-negative and false-positive results in FDG-PET and PET/CT in breast cancer. PET Clin. 2009;4:289–98.

Lin CE, Alavi A. PET and PET/CT: a clinical guide, 2 nd ed. New York, NY: Thieme; 2009.

Lombardi MH. Radiation safety in nuclear medicine. Boca Raton, FL: CRC Press; 1999.

Lucignani G, Paganelli G, Bombardieri E. The use of standardized uptake values for assessing FDG uptake with PET in oncology: a clinical perspective. Nucl Med Commun. 2004;25(7):651–7.

Mach HR, Schwarz SW. Challenges for developing PET tracers: isotopes, chemistry, and regulatory aspects. PET Clin. 2010;5:131–53.

Madden EM. Introduction to sectional anatomy workbook and board review guide (Point). 2nd ed. Philadelphia, PA: Lippincott Williams & Wilkins; 2007.

Mandell LG, Bennett EJ, Dolin R. Mandell, Douglas, and Bennett's principles and practice of infectious diseases. 7th ed. Philadelphia, PA: Churchill Livingstone Elsevier; 2010.

Miles AK, Blomley JKM, et al. Functional and physiological imaging in Grainger & Allison's diagnostic radiology. Philadelphia, PA: Churchill Livingstone; 2007.

Miletich SR. Positron emission tomography for neurologists. Neurol Clin. 2008;27:61–8.

Mittra E, Quon A. Positron emission tomography/computed tomography: the current technology and applications. Radiol Clin N Am. 2009;47:147–60.

Moore LK, Dalley FA, Agur RMA. Clinically oriented anatomy. 6th ed. Philadelphia, PA: Lippincott Williams & Wilkins, a Walters Kluwer business; 2010.

Mosci C, Iagaru A. PET/CT imaging of thyroid cancer. Clin Nucl Med. 2011;36(12):180–5.

Munro HB. Statistical methods for health care research. 5th ed. Philadelphia, PA: Lippincott Williams & Wilkins; 2005.

Mycek MJ, Harvey RA. Lippincott's illustrated reviews: pharmacology. 3rd ed. Philadelphia, PA: Lippincott; 2008.

National Coverage Determination (NCD) for PET Scans (220.6). https://www.cms.gov/medicare-coverage-database/details/ncd-details.aspx?NCDId=211&ver=2. Accessed 14 Jan 2012

Newberg BA, Alavi A. Normal patterns and variants in PET brain imaging. PET Clin. 2010;5:1–13.

Patton JA, Townsend WD, Brian F, Hutton FB. Hybrid imaging technology: from dreams and vision to clinical devices. Semin Nucl Med. 2009;39:247–63.

Placantonakis GD, Schwartz HT. Localization in Epilepsy. Neurol Clin. 2009;27:1015–30.

Positron Emission Tomography (PET) – Nuclear medicine imaging technology. http://EzineArticles.com/6314268. Accessed 20 Sep 2011

Prokop M, Galanski M. Spiral and multislice computed tomography of the body. New York, NY: Thieme; 2003.

Rahmim A, Zaidi H. PET versus SPECT: strengths, limitations and challenges. Nucl Med Commun. 2008;29:193–7.

Reubi JC, Maecke HR. Peptide-based probes for cancer imaging. J Nucl Med. 2008;49:1735–8.

Rice LS, Roney AS, et al. The next generation of positron emission tomography radiopharmaceuticals in oncology. Semin Nucl Med. 2011;41:265–82.

Rohren EM, Turkington TG, Coleman RE. Clinical application of PET in oncology. Radiology. 2004;231:305–32.

Saha GB. Basics of PET imaging. New York, NY: Springer; 2005.

Sarji AS. Physiological uptake in FDG PET simulating disease. Biomed Imaging Interv J. 2006;2(4):e59.

Soret M, Bacharach SL, Buvat I. Partial-volume effect in PET tumor imaging. J Nucl Med. 2007;48:932–45.

Spaepen K, Stroobants S, Verhoef G, et al. Positron emission tomography with [18F]FDG for therapy response monitoring in lymphoma patients. Eur J Nucl Med Mol Imaging. 2003;30:S97–S105.

Sureshbabu W, Mawlawi O. PET/CT imaging artifacts. J Nucl Med Technol. 2005;33:156–61.

Soyka DJ, Strobel K, Veit-Haibach P, et al. Influence of bowel preparation before 18F-FDG PET/CT on physiologic 18F-FDG activity in the intestine. J Nucl Med. 2010;51(4):507–10.

Takalkar A, Agarwal A, Adams S, et al. Cardiac Assessment with PET. PET Clin. 2011;6:313–26.

The National Oncologic PET Registry (NOPR) http://clinicaltrials.gov/ct2/show/NCT00868582. Accessed 25 Dec 2011.

Turkington GT. Introduction to PET Instrumentation. J Nucl Med Technol. 2001;29(1):4–11.

U.S.NRC.http://www.nrc.gov/reading-rm/doc-collections/cfr/part020/part020-1003.html. Accessed 27 Sep 2011

Vallabhajosula S. 18F-labeled positron emission tomographic radiopharmaceuticals in oncology: an overview of radiochemistry and mechanisms of tumor localization. Semin Nucl Med. 2007;37:400–19.

Vallabhajosula S, Solnesn L, Vallabhajosula B. Broad overview of positron emission tomography radiopharmaceuticals and clinical applications: what is new? Semin Nucl Med. 2011;41:246–64.

Visvikis D, Turzo A, et al. Technology related parameters affecting quantification in positron emission tomography imaging. Nucl Med Commun. 2004;25(7):637–41.

Wahl RL, Buchanan JW, editors. Principles and practice of positron emission tomography. Philadelphia, PA: Lippincott Williams & Wilkins; 2002.

Wahl LR, Jacene H. From RECIST to PERCIST: evolving considerations for PET response criteria in solid tumors. J Nucl Med. 2009;50(5):122s–50s.

Wahl RL. Principles and practice of PET and PET/CT. 2nd ed. Philadelphia, PA: Lippincott and Wilkins; 2009.

Zaidi H, Thompson C. Evolution and developments in instrumentation for positron emission mammography. PET Clin. 2009;4:317–27.

Zaret BL, Beller GA. Clinical nuclear cardiology: state of the art and future directions. 3rd ed. Philadelphia, PA: Mosby; 2005.

Zhuang H, Sam JW, Chacko TK, et al. Rapid normalization of osseous FDG uptake following traumatic or surgical fractures. Eur J Nucl Med Mol Imaging. 2003;30(8):1096–103.

Chapter 4
Practice Test # 3: Difficulty Level-Hard

Questions

1. Which of the following cardiac imaging studies deliver the lowest estimated effective radiation dose?
   (A) Rb-82 rest and stress
   (B) CT attenuation correction
   (C) N-13 ammonia rest and stress
   (D) O-15 water rest and stress

2. Recovery coefficient, Geometric Transfer Matrix, and Deconvolution technique are modification methods employed in:
   (A) Attenuation calculation
   (B) Scatter correction
   (C) Partial-volume effect correction
   (D) Attenuation measurement

3. The number of electrons discharged from the cathode filament is controlled by the:
   (A) The tube voltage (kV)
   (B) The temperature of the anode
   (C) The tube current (mA)
   (D) The distance from the target

Answers to Test #3 begin on page 191

4. Which of the following are the most common artifacts in PET/CT imaging?
   (A) Truncation artifacts
   (B) Motion artifacts
   (C) Contrast medium artifacts
   (D) Metallic implants artifacts

5. The PET scanner quality control procedure in which data are used to convert the reconstructed image pixel values into activity concentration is called:
   (A) Normalization
   (B) Calibration
   (C) Blank scan
   (D) Attenuation correction

6. Post-processing technique performed on CT images that involves reformatting of cross-sectional images to produce images of the outsides of anatomical structures is called:
   (A) Multiplanar reconstruction
   (B) 3D surface rendering
   (C) Cone beam reconstruction
   (D) Back projection

7. ALL of the following statements describing the usefulness of PET-FDG imaging in renal cell carcinoma (RCC) are correct EXCEPT:
   (A) High physiologic background activity in urine limits scan interpretation accuracy
   (B) Metastatic RCC has more intense FDG uptake compared with the primary
   (C) Primary RCC has more intense FDG uptake compared with the metastatic
   (D) The administration of furosemide can be beneficial for reducing false-negative scan results

8. The reconstruction algorithm that reduces the unnecessary 3D data to a stack of independent 2D sonograms, which can then be reconstructed using either 2D filtered back projection (FBP) or 2D iterative algorithms, is called:
   (A) Fourier transform
   (B) Convolution
   (C) Filtering
   (D) Fourier rebinning

9. The patented PET tracers that have been developed by a radiopharmaceutical developer or manufacturer are called:
   (A) Proprietary agents
   (B) Research agents
   (C) Nonproprietary agents
   (D) Contrast agents

10. A patient is scheduled to have PET myocardial perfusion imaging using Rb-82 as a tracer of choice. The technologist draws up a 42-mCi dose of Rb-82 for the resting injection at 10:00 A.M. If the injection is delayed 3 min, how many milicuries of Rb-82 will be remaining in the syringe at 10:03 A.M.?
    (A) 48 mCi
    (B) 26 mCi
    (C) 8 mCi
    (D) 6 mCi

11. The display shown in Fig. 4.1 presents attenuation-corrected and reconstructed positron emission tomography (PET-FDG) viability study. The reoriented tomographic slices are:
    (A) Short-axis slices
    (B) Vertical long-axis slices
    (C) Oblique short-axis slices
    (D) Horizontal long axis

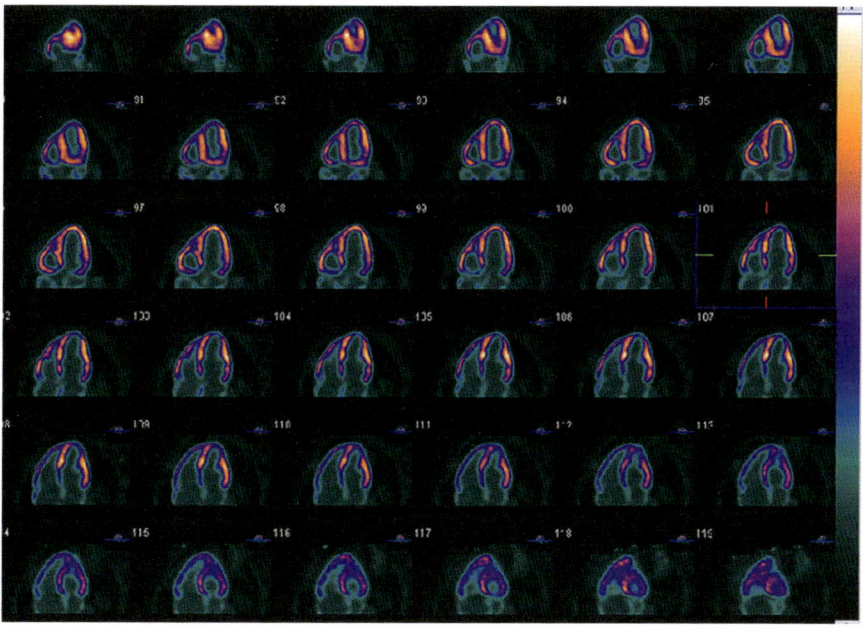

Fig. 4.1 PET/CT-FDG viability study

12. The following are examples of molecular and functional alterations occurring in cancer tissue EXCEPT:
    (A) Increased protein synthesis
    (B) Increased angiogenesis
    (C) Increased oxygen tension
    (D) Increased glucose metabolism

13. Which of the following types of cardiac scanning processing requires performance of blood pool subtraction?
    (A) Imaging using water O-15
    (B) Imaging using rubidium Rb-82
    (C) Imaging using acetate C-11
    (D) Imaging using ammonia N-13

14. Which of the following halogens most closely mimics the size of the hydrogen atom?
    (A) Br-2
    (B) Cl-2
    (C) F-2
    (D) I-2

15. Two photons arising from the same annihilation event and detected along two different lines of response (LOR) are:
    (A) True coincidences
    (B) Random events
    (C) Scatter coincidences
    (D) Single events

16. PET/CT imaging artifact described as a liver lesion that can inaccurately become visible at the base of the lung and mimics a lung nodule is produced by:
    (A) Contrast medium
    (B) Respiratory motion
    (C) Patient motion
    (D) Dose extravasation

17. Which of the following physical properties of different scintillators describe LSO (lutetium oxyorthosilicate) detector?
    (A) Attenuation coefficient—0.96, relative light output—15, decay time—300 ns
    (B) Attenuation coefficient—0.87, relative light output—75, decay time—40 ns
    (C) Attenuation coefficient—0.35, relative light output—100, decay time—230 ns
    (D) Attenuation coefficient—0.44, relative light output—5, decay time—0.6 ns

18. Which of the following statements describing brown adipose tissue (BAT) is TRUE?
    (A) BAT is richly innervated by parasympathetic nerves
    (B) BAT is not present in newborns
    (C) BAT primary function is to generate body heat
    (D) BAT contains cells rich in ribosomes

19. Which of the following radiopharmaceuticals has been developed as the PET tracer to measure a membrane lipid synthesis?
    (A) F-18 fluoride
    (B) F-18 fluorocholine
    (C) F-18 fluoroestradiol
    (D) F-18 fluorothymidine

20. The molecular imaging strategy that replicates the downstream physiological effects of one or more molecular or genetic processes is called:
    (A) Direct molecular imaging
    (B) Surrogate molecular imaging
    (C) Indirect molecular imaging
    (D) Reporter gene imaging

21. Which of the following detectors that have been used in PET imaging is intrinsically radioactive?
    (A) LSO (lutetium oxyorthosilicate)
    (B) BaF2 (barium fluoride)
    (C) BGO (bismuth germinate)
    (D) GSO (gadolinium orthosilicate)

22. In which of the following types of seizures consciousness is not impaired?
    (A) Partial complex seizures
    (B) Partial simple seizures
    (C) Petit mal seizures
    (D) Grand mal seizures

23. Mean sensitivity and specificity of PET myocardial perfusion studies for the detection of coronary artery disease (CAD) are accordingly:
    (A) 93% and 50%
    (B) 93% and 92%
    (C) 50% and 92%
    (D) 50% and 50%

24. Hot-for-cold substitution is applied in the development process of all of the following PET tracers EXCEPT:
    (A) Carbon-11
    (B) Oxygen-15
    (C) Nitrogen-13
    (D) Fluorine-18

25. The pattern of FDG uptake in multi-infarct dementia is characterized by:
    (A) The parietotemporal hypometabolism
    (B) The visual cortices involvement
    (C) The frontotemporal regions involvement
    (D) Scattered regions of hypometabolism

26. The presented PET MIP, fused PET/CT, and CT axial images in Fig. 4.2 were obtained from the patient referred for the evaluation of abdominal mass. Based on the findings the abdominal mass represents:
    (A) Metastatic cancer of the liver
    (B) Solid tumor of the left kidney
    (C) Cavitary mass arising from the left kidney
    (D) Cavitary mass adjacent to small bowel

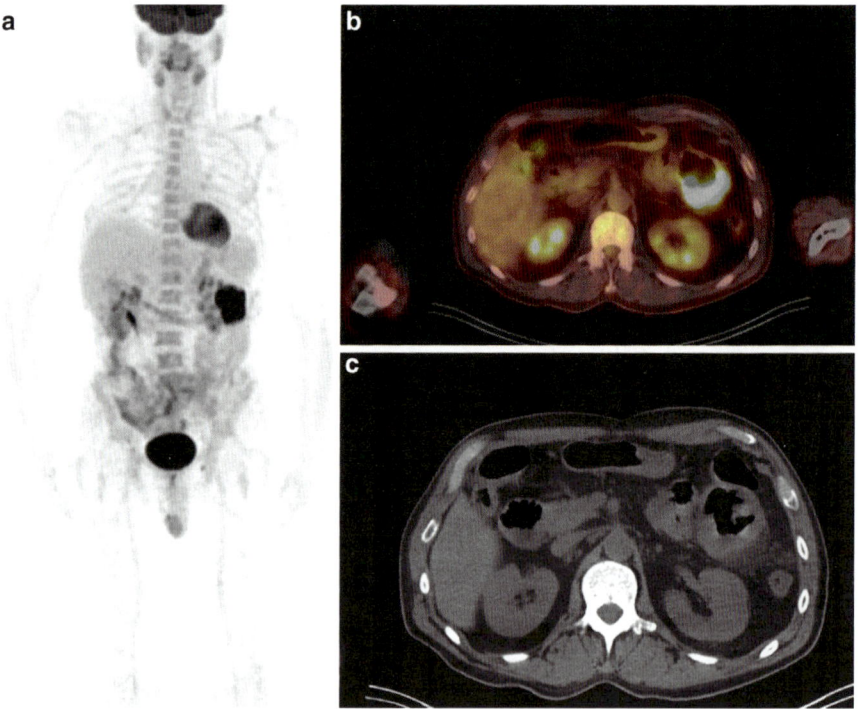

Fig. 4.2 (a) PET MIP image; (b) PET/CT image; (c) CT image

27. Any chest area that specially attenuates the x-ray beam and as a result appears more dense than the surrounding region is called:
    (A) Plaque
    (B) Opacity
    (C) Atelectasis
    (D) Pneumonia

28. The area of maximal electrophysiological interictal activity is called:
    (A) The brain infarct
    (B) The epileptic focus
    (C) The epileptogenic lesion
    (D) The brain ischemia

29. Fluoromisonidazole (F-18 MISO) was developed as the PET tracer to assess:
    (A) Membrane synthesis
    (B) Lipids metabolism
    (C) Hypoxia extent
    (D) Protein synthesis

30. Two patients are scheduled to have PET myocardial perfusion imaging at 8:00 A.M. and 8:20 A.M., each with dose of 15 mCi Nitrogen-13-ammonia. What is the total millicurie amount that should be available at 7:30 A.M. to accommodate these two studies?
    (A) 600 mCi
    (B) 480 mCi
    (C) 120 mCi
    (D) 36 mCi

31. Which of the following statements describing hypoxia in a growing tumor is FALSE?
    (A) Hypoxia inhibits cell proliferation
    (B) Hypoxia promotes cells adaptive responses
    (C) Hypoxia "guards" cells from the cytotoxic effects of radiation
    (D) Hypoxia is independent from the local vasculature

32. Normal, focal ureteral activity can be seen in:
    (A) The lower pelvis
    (B) The lower abdomen
    (C) The superior pelvis
    (D) The superior abdomen

33. Computed tomography acquisition (CT) performed by acquiring unenhanced CT images first, followed by a series of CT images after intravenous injection of contrast medium, is called:
    (A) Unenhanced CT with a low-dose technique
    (B) Dynamic contrast-enhanced (DCE) CT
    (C) Dual energy CT
    (D) Multislice CT

34. Dementia with Lewy bodies (DLB) has bilateral temporoparietal decreased FDG uptake similar to that present in patients with Alzheimer's disease (AD), and also involves:
    (A) The frontal lobe
    (B) The occipital lobe
    (C) The cerebellum
    (D) The basal ganglia

35. The main objective of Bayesian analysis is to combine both clinical and imaging-based characteristics to obtain an assessment of the:
    (A) Cost of treatment
    (B) Time of recovery
    (C) Probability of disease
    (D) Longtime prognosis

36. Radiation effects on bone marrow affecting FDG uptake can be described as:
    (A) Increased uptake in the area of spine
    (B) Increased area of uptake corresponding to the radiation field
    (C) Decreased uptake in the area of spine
    (D) Decreased area of uptake corresponding to the radiation field

37. Hybrid PET-CT scanners, equipped with multislice CT, can be used to perform the following types of cardiac diagnostic imaging EXCEPT:
    (A) PET myocardial perfusion study
    (B) Coronary angiography
    (C) Echocardiography
    (D) Calcium scoring

38. The sphincter muscle that protects the opening of the esophagus into the stomach is called the:
    (A) Pyloric sphincter
    (B) Esophageal sphincter
    (C) Sphincter of Oddie
    (D) Sphincter ani

39. The consequences of the mesothelioma stage on treatment selection depend entirely on whether:
    (A) Chemotherapy will be a treatment possibility
    (B) Surgical intervention will be a treatment possibility
    (C) Radiotherapy will be a treatment possibility
    (D) Radioimmunotherapy will be a treatment possibility

40. A package of several F-18 FDG unit doses is reading 19.5 mR/h. How many half value layers of lead (Pb) should be placed in front of the package to reduce the exposure to a background level of 0.03 mR/h?
    (A) 38.5 HVLs
    (B) 9.4 HVLs
    (C) 4-1 HVLs
    (D) 2.8 HVLs

41. The amount of radioactivity, for gamma and beta radiation, measured with wipe tests on the packages designated White I, Yellow II, or Yellow III Department of Transportation DOT labels, should not EXCEED:
    (A) 2.2 dpm/cm^2
    (B) 22 dpm/cm^2
    (C) 222 dpm/cm^2
    (D) 2,222 dpm/cm^2

42. The most common site for distant metastases of the colorectal cancer is:
    (A) The lung
    (B) The brain
    (C) The liver
    (D) He spleen

43. According to the Cotswold system (formerly the Ann Arbor Staging System), involvement of lymph nodes on both sides of the diaphragm describes:
    (A) Stage I of lymphoma
    (B) Stage II of lymphoma
    (C) Stage III of lymphoma
    (D) Stage IV of lymphoma

44. The main physicochemical property of a PET radiotracer that decides its ability to enter the brain and label the target receptor or enzyme is:
    (A) The lipophilicity of the complex
    (B) The hydrophilicity of the complex
    (C) The molecular mass of the complex
    (D) The electrical charge of the complex

45. Cardiac PET quantification of myocardial blood flow (MBF) and coronary flow reserve (CFR) may be useful for detection and evaluation of all of the following EXCEPT:
    (A) Left ventricle ejection fraction
    (B) Balanced ischemia on qualitative images
    (C) Evaluation of collateral flow
    (D) Identification of endothelial dysfunction

46. Diffusely increased marrow FDG uptake may be secondary to all of the following EXCEPT:
    (A) Radiation therapy
    (B) Anemia
    (C) Inflammation
    (D) G-CSF therapy

47. Malignant attributes of pulmonary nodules on computed tomography (CT) include:
    (A) Small size
    (B) Decrease in size over time
    (C) Round margins
    (D) Mixed attenuation

48. PET has been shown to have reduced sensitivity in patients with colorectal:
    (A) Mucinous adenocarcinoma
    (B) Carcinoma in situ
    (C) Metastatic carcinoma
    (D) Poorly differentiated adenocarcinoma

49. According to the Cotswold system (formerly the Ann Arbor Staging System), involvement of a single lymph node region or involvement of a single extra-lymphatic organ outlines:
    (A) Stage I of lymphoma
    (B) Stage II of lymphoma
    (C) Stage III of lymphoma
    (D) Stage IV of lymphoma

50. According to a facility's protocol, the maximum F-18 FDG dose that could be injected to a patient is 14 mCi. A 12 mCi dose of F-18 FDG is calibrated for 8:00 A.M. If the patient comes an hour early, what is the earliest time the dose will be under 14 mCi?
    (A) 7:45 am
    (B) 7:30 am
    (C) 7:15 am
    (D) 7:00 am

51. In rooms with a negative pressure, the direction of airflow at the boundaries of the room is:
    (A) Out of the room
    (B) Into the room
    (C) Around the room
    (D) Below the room

52. Clinical semiology of seizures, one of the main areas of study in patients with epilepsy, evaluates:
    (A) Signs and symptoms
    (B) Electroencephalograms
    (C) Magnetoencephalograms
    (D) Autopsy findings

53. Which of the following statements correctly explains the influence of FDG-PET imaging on staging in patients with Hodgkin's lymphoma (HL)?
    (A) Upstaging of approximately 15–25% of patients
    (B) Downstaging in a small minority of patients
    (C) Upstaging in a small minority of patients
    (D) Downstaging of approximately 15–25% of patients

54. A substance that forms a complex with a biomolecule and by binding to a site on a target protein serves as a signal triggering molecule is called:
    (A) Enzyme
    (B) Ligand
    (C) Tracer
    (D) Isotope

55. Within the broad group of malignant lymphomas, the Hodgkin's disease is set apart from other lymphomas by the presence of:
    (A) Splenomegaly
    (B) The Reed–Sternberg cells
    (C) The Schwann cells
    (D) Lymphadenopathy

56. The brain structure described as a "sensory relay" is called:
    (A) The limbic system
    (B) The thalamus
    (C) The hypothalamus
    (D) The cerebellum

57. A pencil shape, a fan shape, and a cone shape are commonly used terms in radiography to describe:
   (A) CT detector
   (B) PET crystal
   (C) X-ray beam
   (D) PET/CT fusion

58. The tumors that arose from cells that stem from the neural crest cells, and share a characteristic feature to produce peptide hormones, as well as synthesize amines from certain precursors are called:
   (A) Sarcomas
   (B) Fibroid tumors
   (C) Adenocarcinomas
   (D) Neuroendocrine tumors

59. All of the following statements appropriately describe the usefulness of FDG-PET imaging in malignant pleural mesothelioma (MPM) EXCEPT:
   (A) FDG-PET reduces the number of futile surgical procedures
   (B) FDG-PET imaging is useful for guiding needle biopsy
   (C) FDG-PET/CT increases the accuracy of overall MPM staging
   (D) High levels of FDG uptake are associated with a favorable prognosis

60. The radiation exposure rate at a distance of 12 inches from radioactive source is 12.5 mR/h. How many feet away should the technologist stand to reduce the exposure level to 3.0 mR/h?
   (A) 2 ft
   (B) 4.2 ft.
   (C) 24.5 ft.
   (D) 60 ft.

61. The annual allowable limit for radiation exposure for the total effective dose equivalent (TEDE) to the whole body is less than or equal to:
   (A) 10 mSv (1 rem)
   (B) 20 mSv (2 rem)
   (C) 50 mSv (5 rem)
   (D) 500 mSv (50 rem)

62. The amount of F-18 FDG uptake in atherosclerotic lesions correlates with:
   (A) The density of eosinophils in the lesions
   (B) The density of erythrocytes in the lesions
   (C) The density of macrophages in the lesions
   (D) The density of basophils in the lesions

63. The attenuation-corrected (AC) PET, images when compared to the non-attenuation-corrected (NAC):
    (A) Have less noise
    (B) Require additional time
    (C) Are prone to artifacts
    (D) Don't allow SUV measurement

64. Selected tumors with low/variable FDG uptake include all of the following EXCEPT:
    (A) Bronchoalveolar carcinoma
    (B) Iodine-avid differentiated thyroid cancer
    (C) Metastatic liver carcinoma
    (D) Hepatocellular carcinoma

65. Increased synthesis of monoclonal immunoglobulins in multiple myeloma functions as a straightforward approach for functional imaging with:
    (A) F-18 fluorodeoxyglucose
    (B) C-11 methionine
    (C) C-11 raclopride
    (D) F-18 fluoride

66. When compared with Ga-68 DOTA-peptides, F-18DOPA may offer advantages for the detection of neuroendocrine tumors with:
    (A) A high expression of SSR
    (B) A low or absent expression of SSR
    (C) A decreased glucose metabolism
    (D) An increased glucose metabolism

67. Cancer that starts in antibody producing white blood cells is called:
    (A) Lymphocytic leukemia
    (B) Multiple myeloma
    (C) Hodgkins lymphoma
    (D) Monocytic leukemia

68. Hypometabolic area seen after radiation therapy in patients with treated CNS brain tumor, adjacent to or distant from the tumor is secondary to:
    (A) Inflammation
    (B) Edema
    (C) Stroke
    (D) Metastases

69. The ECG records normal electrical currents as specific waves in the following order:
    (A) P wave, QRS complex, ST segment, T wave, and U wave
    (B) QRS complex, P wave, ST segment, T wave, and U wave
    (C) QRS complex, U wave, P wave, ST segment, and T wave
    (D) P wave, QRS complex, ST segment, U wave, and T wave

70. The difference among the daily blank sinogram, and a reference blank sinogram acquired at some point in the last setup of the scanner, is called:
    (A) Average variance
    (B) Streak artifact
    (C) Scatter correction
    (D) Calibration factor

71. Radiation dose equivalency is measured in:
    (A) Rad
    (B) Rem
    (C) Curie
    (D) Roentgen

72. PET F-18 FDG findings commonly observed in patients with chronic obstructive pulmonary disease (COPD) include:
    (A) Diffusely increased F-18 FDG activity in the lungs
    (B) Decreased lung volume
    (C) Prominent right ventricle F-18 FDG uptake
    (D) Decreased anteroposterior thoracic diameter

73. The main advantage of the Straton x-ray tube over the traditional x-ray tube results mainly from:
    (A) More effective shielding
    (B) More effective cooling and heat dissipation
    (C) Lower price and energy use
    (D) User-friendly interface

74. All of the following statements correctly describe the postsurgical F-18 FDG uptake at the intervention site EXCEPT:
    (A) Postsurgical F-18 FDG uptake is mainly diffuse
    (B) Postsurgical F-18 FDG uptake corresponds to the site of surgery
    (C) Postsurgical F-18 FDG uptake increases in intensity with time
    (D) Postsurgical F-18 FDG uptake decreases in size with time

75. The manifestation of hypermetabolic lesions in architecturally unchanged trabecular bone in patients with multiple myeloma suggests the presence of:
    (A) Scar tissue
    (B) Bone metastases
    (C) Active lesions
    (D) Avascular necrosis

76. All of the following types of medications are affecting fluorodeoxyglucose (FDG) uptake in patients with brain tumors EXCEPT:
    (A) Corticosteroids
    (B) Mineralocorticoids
    (C) Sedatives
    (D) Anticonvulsants

77. The incremental prognostic value of PET myocardial perfusion imaging:
    (A) Predicts recovery time after cardiac events
    (B) Predicts time to hospital discharge
    (C) Predicts adverse cardiac events
    (D) Predicts cost of treatment

78. The most common sites of neuroendocrine tumor (NET) onset are:
    (A) The bronchus/lungs and gastroenteropancreatic tract
    (B) The brain and the skin
    (C) The thyroid and urinary tract
    (D) Adrenal glands and genital tract

79. All of the following findings have been observed on FDG-PET scans of patients with Cystic Fibrosis (CF) EXCEPT:
    (A) The higher focal activity was seen during disease exacerbation
    (B) The higher focal activity disappeared on the PET scan after antibiotic therapy
    (C) The PET foci showed corresponding CT scan findings
    (D) The higher focal activity disappeared on the CT scan after antibiotic therapy

80. The following values were obtained from a Cs-137 measurement on a dose calibrator during a Monday to Friday workweek. What is the standard sample deviation of the series of measurements listed below?
    490 µCi, 503 µCi, 482 µCi, 507 µCi, 514 µCi
    (A) 499.2
    (B) 675
    (C) 168.7
    (D) 13

81. Ring dosimeters should be issued to individuals who are likely to exceed a minimum extremity dose of:
    (A) 1,000 mrem/year (10 mSv/year)
    (B) 2,000 mrem/year (20 mSv/year)
    (C) 5,000 mrem/year (50 mSv/year)
    (D) 10,000 mrem/year (100 mSv/year)

82. Pattern of F-18 FDG uptake in the normal tonsils, soft palate, mylohyoid muscle, and sublingual glands observed on sagittal images is described as:
    (A) C shape
    (B) T shape
    (C) An inverted C shape
    (D) An inverted T shape

83. The Society of Nuclear Medicine recommends that F-18 FDG-PET should be routinely performed on patients previously treated for differentiated thyroid cancer (DTC) when the findings of radioactive iodine whole-body scintigraphy (WBS) are negative and:
    (A) The thyroglobulin (Tg) levels are more than 10 ng/mL
    (B) The thyroglobulin (Tg) levels are less than 10 ng/mL
    (C) The thyroid-stimulating hormone (TSH) levels are more than 30 mIU/L
    (D) The thyroid-stimulating hormone (TSH) levels are less than 30 mIU/L

84. The following are amino acids EXCEPT:
    (A) Leucine
    (B) Methionine
    (C) Choline
    (D) Tyrosine

85. A profile of the counts across the point source image is called:
    (A) System resolution
    (B) System sensitivity
    (C) Point spread function
    (D) Line spread function

86. The most important single prognostic factor for survival and prognosis in patients diagnosed with neuroendocrine tumors is the presence of:
    (A) Brain metastasis
    (B) Lung metastasis
    (C) Liver metastasis
    (D) Lymph node metastasis

87. The interaction between penetrating radiation and matter when the incident x-ray photon deflected from its original path loses energy but continues to travel through the material along an altered path is called:
    (A) The photoelectric effect
    (B) The Compton scattering
    (C) The pair production
    (D) Bremsstrahlung radiation

88. Frontotemporal dementia is a clinical syndrome known as:
    (A) Pick's disease
    (B) Vascular dementia
    (C) Alzheimer's disease
    (D) Dementia with Lewy bodies

89. All of the following positron emission tomography myocardial perfusion tracers are used for noninvasive myocardial blood flow (MBF) quantitation EXCEPT:
    (A) Water O-15
    (B) Rubidium Rb-82
    (C) Acetate C-11
    (D) Ammonia N-13

90. Which of the following axial CT images in Fig. 4.3 matches the findings presented on the Fig. 4.4 coronal maximum-intensity projection PET image ?
    (A) Fig. 4.3a
    (B) Fig. 4.3b
    (C) Fig. 4.3c
    (D) Fig. 4.3d

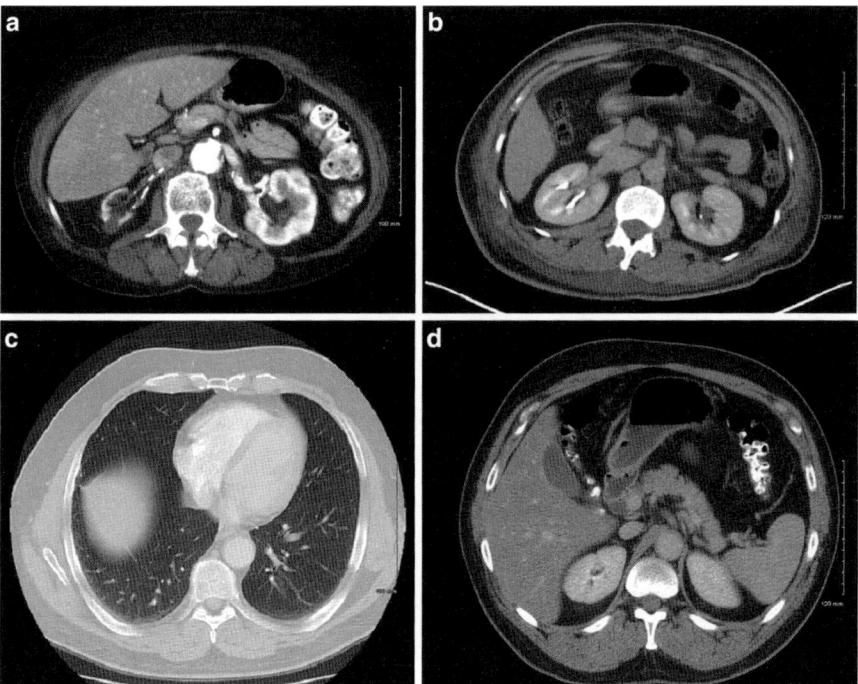

Fig. 4.3 (a) CT axial slice; (b) CT axial slice; (c) CT axial slice; (d) CT axial slice

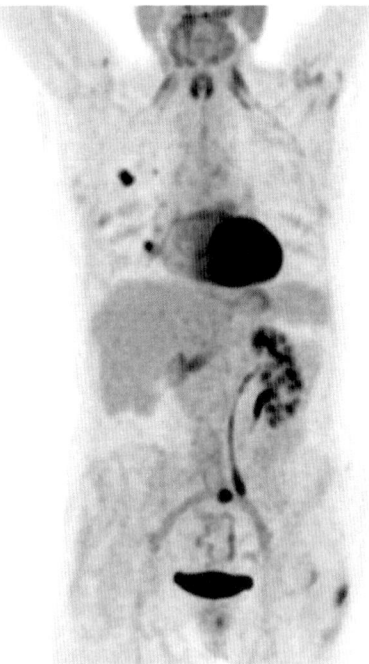

Fig. 4.4 PET/CT MIP image

91. In the resting myocardium, and under normal conditions, 15% to 20% of the energy is delivered by:
    (A) Vitamin C
    (B) Glucose
    (C) Choline
    (D) Fatty acids

92. Interictal PET scans are most valuable in the management of the patient with:
    (A) Partial complex seizures
    (B) Partial simple seizures
    (C) Petit mal seizures
    (D) Grand mal seizures

93. PET/CT findings in anaplastic thyroid cancer scintigraphy can be described by all of the following EXCEPT:
    (A) PET and PET/CT define the local extent of disease and the presence of metastases
    (B) A positive PET/CT scan after therapy is linked with longer survival
    (C) PET and PET/CT have an impact on patients' management
    (D) Intense FDG uptake and volume are prognostic for a bad outcome

94. The FDG-PET sensitivity and specificity in restaging and follow-up of melanoma are accordingly:
    (A) 56% and 45%
    (B) 70% and 74%
    (C) 92% and 94%
    (D) 100% and 100%

95. All of the following radiopharmaceuticals can be used for the evaluation of recurrent or residual medullary thyroid carcinoma (MTC) EXCEPT:
    (A) In-111 Octreoscan
    (B) C-11 acetate
    (C) F-18 DOPA
    (D) Ga-68 DOTATOC

96. Possible explanations of relative insensitivity of FDG-PET for the detection of regional nodal metastases in patients with esophageal carcinoma include:
    (A) The mediastinal proximity
    (B) The primary tumor mass proximity
    (C) Esophagitis
    (D) Barrett esophagus

97. The signal-to-noise ratio (SNR) is the ratio obtained when the signal in an image is:
    (A) Divided by the background in the image
    (B) Multiplied by the background in the image
    (C) Divided by the noise in the image
    (D) Multiplied by the background in the image

98. The following statements describing PET and PET/CT for the management of patients with breast cancer are true EXCEPT:
    (A) PET has limited sensitivity in detecting lesions less than 10 mm
    (B) PET/CT cannot detect a lesion beyond the resolution of CT
    (C) In situ carcinoma shows higher FDG uptake than invasive ductal cancer
    (D) Dense breast may mask small and low-grade tumors

99. 6-[F-18]fluoro-L-DOPA was developed as the PET tracer to visualize:
    (A) Neurons in the basal ganglia
    (B) Amyloid in the brain cortex
    (C) Viable myocardium
    (D) Sentinel node

100. Which of the following structures function as the normal pacemaker of the heart?
    (A) Atrioventricular node
    (B) Sinoatrial node
    (C) Right bundle branches
    (D) Ventricular myocardium

101. In the image in Fig. 4.5, the ascending aorta is labeled:
    (A) D
    (B) C
    (C) B
    (D) A

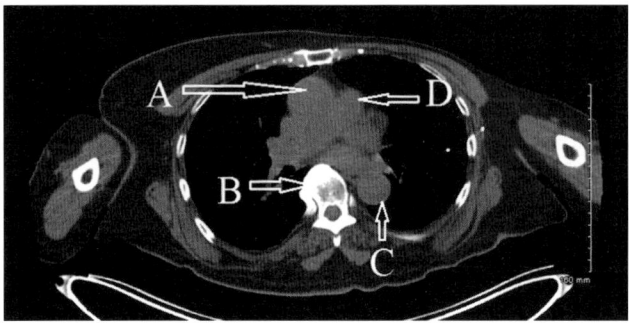

Fig. 4.5 Chest CT

102. The single most important factor in determining initial prognosis and the need for adjuvant chemotherapy for patients diagnosed with breast cancer is/are:
    (A) Axillary lymph node metastasis
    (B) Histologic tumor type
    (C) Tumor size
    (D) Mediastinal lymph node metastasis

103. The primary difference between NEMA performance measurements, defined as NU 2-2007 and NU 2-2001, is:
    (A) NU 2-2007 addresses spatial resolution measurement using a point source
    (B) NU 2-2007 addresses the intrinsic radioactivity in LSO and LYSO crystals
    (C) NU 2-2001 addresses intrinsic scatter fraction measurement
    (D) NU 2-2001 addresses the intrinsic radioactivity in LSO and LYSO crystals

104. The physiological breast uptake in postmenopausal women, who are NOT on hormone replacement therapy (HRT), should be:
    (A) Absent
    (B) Less than the liver
    (C) More than the liver
    (D) More than the heart

105. All of the following factors contribute to degradation of resolution in the reconstructed images in positron emission tomography (PET) imaging EXCEPT:
    (A) Positron range
    (B) Inter-crystal scattering
    (C) The width of scintillation crystals
    (D) Photon collinearity

106. In the evaluation of malignancy, misinterpreting normal uptake of F-18 FDG within the thymus results in a potential pitfall in the evaluation of the:
    (A) Posterior mediastinum
    (B) Anterior mediastinum
    (C) Pericardium
    (D) Pleura

107. Scatter events comprise _____ in 3D positron emission tomography (PET):
    (A) 10–20% of all events
    (B) 20–30% of all events
    (C) 30–40% of all events
    (D) 40–60% of all events

108. F-18 fluorodeoxyglucose (FDG) use in patients with suspected primary and residual/recurrent gliomas is limited by:
    (A) The low F-18 FDG uptake in normal brain tissue
    (B) The high F-18 FDG uptake in normal brain tissue
    (C) The low F-18 FDG uptake in tumor tissue
    (D) The high F-18 FDG uptake in tumor tissue

109. The most important problem with the PET/MR scanner is:
    (A) Correcting for attenuation of gamma rays
    (B) Correcting for scatter of gamma rays
    (C) Correcting for patient motion
    (D) Correcting for breathing artifacts

110. The path distance required for a positron to find an electron for annihilation depends on:
    (A) The number of positrons and number of electrons in the immediate area of decay
    (B) The energy of positron and number of electrons in the immediate area of decay
    (C) The energy of positron and energy of electron in the immediate area of decay
    (D) The number of positrons and charge of electron in the immediate area of decay

111. Abnormal bone FDG uptake by tumor cells is proportional to:
    (A) Blood flow
    (B) Osteoblastic activity
    (C) Glucose metabolism
    (D) Cell wall synthesis

112. Which of the following thyroid carcinomas is the most aggressive form of thyroid malignancy?
    (A) Papillary
    (B) Follicular
    (C) Medullary
    (D) Anaplastic

113. Which of the following tissues has the lowest CT number?
    (A) Fat
    (B) Blood
    (C) Muscle
    (D) Bone

114. Coronary vasodilator reserve (CVR) is defined as the ratio between:
    (A) Peak hyperemic and rest myocardial blood flow
    (B) Rest myocardial and peak hyperemic blood flow
    (C) Peak hyperemic and post-stress myocardial blood flow
    (D) Rest myocardial and post-stress myocardial blood flow

115. The spatial resolution in normal breast tissue in the WB PET scanner is negatively impacted by lying down because of:
    (A) Cardiac motion
    (B) Respiratory motion
    (C) Table motion
    (D) Gantry motion

116. All of the following interventions enhance myocardial FDG uptake EXCEPT:
    (A) Oral glucose loading
    (B) Oral fatty acids loading
    (C) Infusion of insulin and glucose
    (D) Nicotinic acid derivatives administration

117. Registration of images affected by respiratory or cardiac motion, tumor growth or shrinkage, and weight gain or loss can only be performed using:
    (A) Deformable registration technique
    (B) Rigid registration technique
    (C) Segmented coregistration
    (D) Intensity-based coregistration

118. Warping, a technique to improve registration accuracy over a larger region of the patient's body, is an example of:
    (A) Rigid coregistration
    (B) Segmented coregistration
    (C) Deformable coregistration
    (D) Intensity-based coregistration

119. What percentage of the injected dose of F-18 sodium fluoride is taken up by bone?
    (A) 25%
    (B) 50%
    (C) 75%
    (D) 100%

120. A 13 mCi dose of F-18 FDG is calibrated for 9:00 A.M. What time will the dose of F-18 FDG be less than 8 mCi?
    (A) 45 min
    (B) 60 min
    (C) 75 min
    (D) 85 min

121. Copper-diacetyl-bis(N4-methylthiosemicarbazone) (Cu-ATSM) and copper-pyruvaldehyde-bis(N4-methylthiosemicarbazone) (Cu-PTSM) are being studied as potential markers of:
    (A) Hypoxia and perfusion
    (B) Angiogenesis and cell proliferation
    (C) Protein synthesis and myocardial oxidation
    (D) Movement disorders and chemotherapy response

122. Which of the following statements correctly describes the concept of the positron emission mammography (PEM)?
    (A) Two planar detectors capable of detecting the 511-keV annihilation photons in a conventional mammography unit
    (B) Four planar detectors capable of detecting the 1,022-keV annihilation photons in a conventional mammography unit
    (C) Two planar detectors capable of detecting the 511-keV annihilation photons in a conventional CT unit
    (D) Four planar detectors capable of detecting the 1,022-keV annihilation photons in a conventional MRI unit

123. Which of the following PET radiotracers is the preferred method of measuring Myocardial Oxygen Consumption (MVO2) noninvasively?
    (A) C-11 palmitate
    (B) C-11 glucose
    (C) C-11 acetate
    (D) C-11 lactate

124. Normal thymic activity on a F-18 FDG scan will appear:
    (A) V shaped
    (B) O shaped
    (C) T shaped
    (D) H shaped

125. Lower sensitivity of F-18 L-Thymidine (FLT) PET for tumor detection when compared to that of FDG-PET is explained by the FLT uptake:
    (A) Lower in tumors and higher background activity in the liver and bone marrow
    (B) Lower in tumors and lower background activity in the liver and bone marrow
    (C) Higher in tumors and higher background activity in the liver and bone marrow
    (D) Higher in tumors and lower background activity in the liver and bone marrow

126. A highly aggressive tumor that develops from transformed cells originating in the protective lining that covers many of the internal organs of the body is called:
    (A) Sarcoma
    (B) Glioblastoma
    (C) Mesothelioma
    (D) Adenocarcinoma

127. The enormous decrease in photons detection efficiency by SPECT, when compared to that of PET, is caused by:
    (A) Shorter imaging time
    (B) Lower injected dose
    (C) Use of collimator
    (D) Use of shielding

128. A group of the brain structures responsible for behavior and emotions is called:
    (A) The basal ganglia
    (B) The corpus callosum
    (C) The limbic system
    (D) The reticular formation

129. A cyclic RGD-based radiotracer introduced by GE Healthcare F-18 AH111585 (Fluciclatide/GE 135) was developed as the PET tracer to measure:
    (A) Membrane synthesis
    (B) Estrogen receptor
    (C) Hypoxia
    (D) Angiogenesis

130. The presented images in Fig. 4.6 labeled A, B, C, and D were obtained during a routine CT of the brain. The image described as B represents:
    (A) Lateral brain localizer image
    (B) Coronal slice of the brain
    (C) Sagittal slice of the brain
    (D) Tranverse slice of the brain

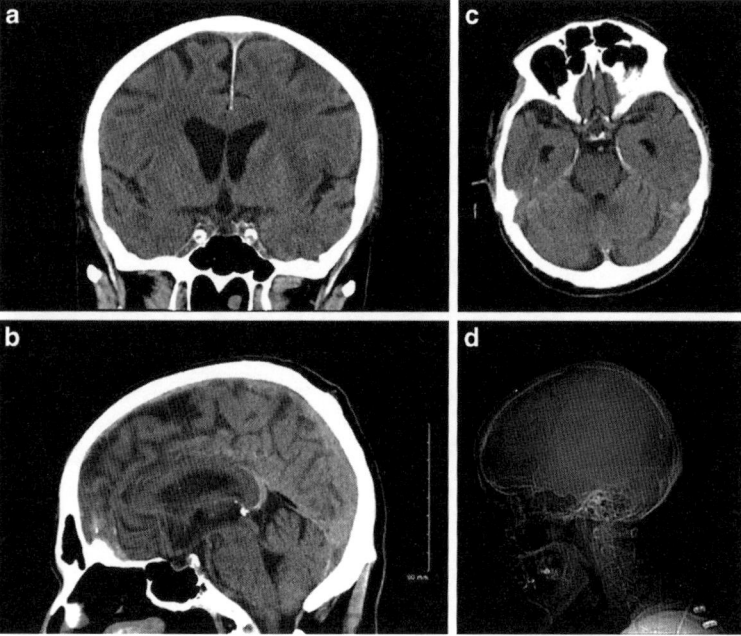

Fig. 4.6 (a–d) Brain CT scans

131. The non-collinearity that arises from the deviation of the two annihilation photons from the exact 1,800 position degrades the spatial resolution of the scanner by between:
    (A) 0.5 and 1 mm
    (B) 1 and 1.8 mm
    (C) 1.8 and 2 mm
    (D) 2 and 2.5 mm

132. All of the following tracers have been developed and validated for the assessment of cardiac metabolism EXCEPT:
    (A) F-18 fluorodeoxyglucose
    (B) C-11 palmitate
    (C) C-11 epinephrine
    (D) C-11 acetate

133. Techniques known as convolution-subtraction, Monte Carlo modeling, direct measurement, "Gaussian fit" techniques, methods described as multiple energy window, and model-based correction algorithms have been proposed for:
    (A) Random correction
    (B) Scatter correction
    (C) Dead-time correction
    (D) Detector normalization

134. The molecular imaging strategy that involves uninterrupted interaction between the imaging probe and the molecular target (e.g., a specific enzyme or receptor) is called:
    (A) Direct molecular imaging
    (B) Surrogate molecular imaging
    (C) Indirect molecular imaging
    (D) Reporter gene imaging

135. Detecting the depth of interaction (DOI) within a longer scintillation PET crystal improves the scanner:
    (A) Sensitivity
    (B) Resolution
    (C) Non-collinearity
    (D) Reproducibility

136. The normal distribution of a blood perfusion radiopharmaceutical in the brain:
    (A) Is asymmetric uptake in both hemispheres
    (B) Flow ratio the gray matter–to–white matter is approximately 1:4
    (C) Pattern of radiopharmaceutical distribution can be affected by auditory stimuli
    (D) Flow ratio the gray matter–to–white matter is approximately 1:1

137. Breast-Specific Gamma Imaging (BGSI) physiologic approach to breast imaging is employing:
    (A) A high-resolution gamma camera and Tc-99 m Sestamibi
    (B) A low-resolution gamma camera and Tc-99 m Sestamibi
    (C) A high-resolution gamma camera and Tc-99 m sulfur colloid
    (D) A low-resolution gamma camera and Tc-99 m sulfur colloid

138. The overall glucose metabolism in early-onset versus late-onset Alzheimer's disease is characterized as:
    (A) Greater in magnitude and lesser in extent
    (B) Greater in magnitude and greater in extent
    (C) Lesser in magnitude and greater in extent
    (D) Lesser in magnitude and lesser in extent

139. In time-of-flight imaging (TOF), the measurements of the time delay between detection of the coincident annihilation photons allow:
    (A) More accurate SUV measurements
    (B) More precise localization of the source
    (C) To avoid motion artifacts
    (D) To reduce scanning time

140. The molecular imaging strategy involving reporter gene methods is called:
    (A) Direct molecular imaging
    (B) Surrogate molecular imaging
    (C) Indirect molecular imaging
    (D) Delay molecular imaging

141. According to the Society of Nuclear Medicine practice guidelines, when using a 10 mCi (370 MBq) dose of F-18 sodium fluoride for PET imaging, the effective radiation dose to the patient is:
    (A) 270 mRem (2.7 mSv)
    (B) 530 mRem (5.3 mSv)
    (C) 890 mRem (8.9 mSv)
    (D) 120 mRem (11.2 mSv)

142. The nitrogen-13 (N-13) isotope returns with a beta positive decay scheme to:
    (A) Oxygen-18
    (B) Boron-11
    (C) Carbon-13
    (D) Nitrogen-15

143. Avalanche photodiodes (APDs), semiconductor devices, are:
    (A) Light detectors
    (B) X-ray detectors
    (C) Magnetic field detectors
    (D) Ultrasound detectors

144. Lidocaine, procainamide, or intravenous amiodarone is used in cardiopulmonary resuscitation to:
    (A) Induce vasoconstriction
    (B) Increase aortic diastolic blood pressure
    (C) Produce hypotension
    (D) Prevent tachyarrhythmias

145. In receiver operating characteristic curve (ROC) analysis, the true positive fraction of a diagnostic test is plotted against:
    (A) True negative fraction
    (B) True positive plus true negative fraction
    (C) False-positive fraction
    (D) True positive plus false-positive fraction

146. Each sinogram of the raw data acquired in PET represents:
    (A) The data acquired at the projection angles across all slices
    (B) The data acquired from the center of gantry
    (C) The data for the slice across all projection angles
    (D) The data acquired from the center of FOV

147. Which of the following statements describing positron emission mammography (PEM) imaging is FALSE:
    (A) Scan is performed in sitting up position
    (B) Scan mimics mammographic views
    (C) Scan provides tomographic views
    (D) Scan provides resolution ~ 5 mm

148. PET myocardial perfusion imaging is the most beneficial for the group of patients described as:
    (A) Young and hypotensive
    (B) Obese and women
    (C) Hypertensive and men
    (D) Smokers and diabetics

149. Which of the following PET radiopharmaceuticals is directly produced out of the target without further chemistry?
    (A) F-18 fluorodeoxyglucose
    (B) N-13 ammonia
    (C) F-18 fluorine gas
    (D) C-11 choline

150. The event illustrated in the diagram in Fig. 4.7 is called:
    (A) A random event
    (B) A scatter event
    (C) A true event
    (D) An attenuated event

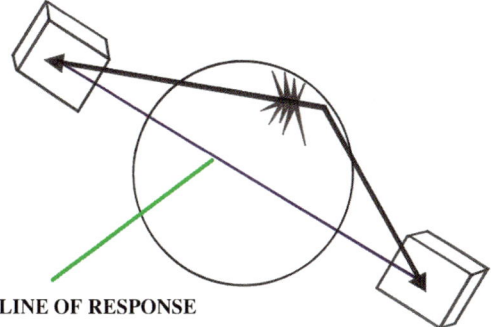

Fig. 4.7 Principle of positron emission tomography. *Illustration by Sabina Moniuszko*

151. The theory of using metabolic tracers for viability evaluation is based on the concept that:
    (A) Viable myocytes are metabolically inactive, whereas scarred or fibrotic tissue is metabolically active
    (B) Viable myocytes are metabolically active, whereas scarred or fibrotic tissue is metabolically inactive
    (C) Viable myocytes and scarred or fibrotic tissue are metabolically inactive
    (D) Viable myocytes and scarred or fibrotic tissue are metabolically active

152 Which of the following statements describing F-18 FDG-PET imaging in thyroid carcinoma is FALSE?
    (A) PET can be negative in well-differentiated types
    (B) PET negative lesions are more likely to be resistant to I-131 treatment
    (C) FDG uptake is proportional to iodine uptake
    (D) PET may not be accurate in patients with Tg levels below 2 ng/dL

153. The positron-emitting imaging agents [F-18]-fluoro-L-thymidine (FLT) and F-18, or C-11-2'-fluoro-5-methyl-1-beta-d-arabinofuranosyluracil (FMAU), are markers of:
    (A) Tumor hypoxia
    (B) Cell proliferation
    (C) Angiogenesis
    (D) Glucose metabolism

154. Breast cancer imaging with positron emission tracers can include all of the following approaches EXCEPT:
    (A) Perfusion imaging
    (B) Proliferation imaging
    (C) Vasculature imaging
    (D) Neurotransmitters imaging

155. What fraction of energy generated in X-ray tube system is converted to x-ray?
    (A) 1%
    (B) 5%
    (C) 10%
    (D) 15%

156. Which of the following medications should be withheld in patients undergoing pharmacological stress test with dipyridamole?
    (A) Albuterol
    (B) Aspirin
    (C) Aggrenox
    (D) Advair

157. According to the PERCIST—PET Response Criteria in Solid Tumors—criteria for treatment response evaluation, the changes in SUVs should be assessed as:
    (A) Percentage change in the same lesion
    (B) Percentage change in the "hottest" lesion
    (C) Value change in the same lesion
    (D) Value change in the "hottest" lesion

158. A group of nuclei associated with voluntary motor control is called:
    (A) The basal ganglia
    (B) The corpus callosum
    (C) The limbic system
    (D) The reticular formation

159. The spread of electrical stimuli through the atria and ventricles is called:
    (A) Repolarization
    (B) Depolarization
    (C) Agitation
    (D) Initiation

160. Clinical categories of non-Hodgkin lymphomas (NHLs) include all of the following EXCEPT:
    (A) Acute
    (B) Indolent
    (C) Aggressive
    (D) Highly aggressive

161. The PET quality control procedure that corrects for nonuniformities in images due to variations in the gain of PM tubes, location of the detector in the block, and the physical variation of the detector is called:
    (A) Blank scan
    (B) Calibration
    (C) Normalization
    (D) Resolution

162. The rate of brain metabolism is measured by the consumption of:
    (A) Oxygen and free fatty acids
    (B) Insulin
    (C) Oxygen and glucose
    (D) Phosphocreatine

163. According to the PERCIST-criteria for treatment response evaluation, the following requirements of PET scans performance have to be met EXCEPT:
    (A) SUV should be corrected for lean body mass
    (B) SUV should be corrected for serum glucose levels
    (C) Evaluation for proper PET and CT registration should be performed
    (D) The right hepatic lobe background should be determined

164. Left ventricular ejection fraction (LVEF) measurements during gated PET perfusion imaging are assessed:
    (A) At rest only
    (B) At rest and during peak stress
    (C) At rest and post-stress
    (D) Post-stress only

165. The tumor's total glycolytic volume (TGV) is defined as:
    (A) SUV × injected activity
    (B) SUV × tumor volume
    (C) Tumor volume × glucose level
    (D) Injected activity × glucose level

166. The intensity of FDG uptake in the majority of mesotheliomas:
    (A) Ranges from absent to low
    (B) Ranges from low to moderate
    (C) Ranges from moderate to high
    (D) Is always high

167. The pattern of myocardial blood flow, combined with myocardial glucose metabolism called a reverse mismatch pattern, is defined as:
    (A) Decreased myocardial blood and decreased myocardial glucose metabolism
    (B) Decreased myocardial blood and retained myocardial glucose metabolism
    (C) Normal myocardial blood and decreased myocardial glucose metabolism
    (D) Normal myocardial blood and retained myocardial glucose metabolism

168. Melanomas that develop from cells that do not contain pigment are called:
    (A) Metastatic melanomas
    (B) Amelanotic melanomas
    (C) Melanomas in situ
    (D) Primary melanomas

169. Under conditions of mild to moderate myocardial ischemia:
    (A) Anaerobic metabolism stops and fatty acid oxidation turns up
    (B) Fatty acid oxidation stops and anaerobic metabolism turns up
    (C) Fatty acid oxidation and anaerobic metabolism stops
    (D) Anaerobic metabolism and fatty acid oxidation turns up

170. The relative amount of damage caused by a particular type of radiation is called:
    (A) Distribution factor
    (B) Quality factor
    (C) Damage factor
    (D) Dose rate factor

171. When PET/CT is used instead of either alone, overall accuracy of diagnosis:
    (A) Is decreased by 20% to 25%
    (B) Is the same
    (C) Is increased by 20 to 25%
    (D) Is increased by 90 to 95%

172. PET-FDG studies in patients diagnosed with Huntington's disease demonstrate:
    (A) Decreased uptake in the caudate nucleus and putamen
    (B) Decreased uptake in the hypothalamus and cerebellum
    (C) Increased uptake in the caudate nucleus and putamen
    (D) Increased uptake in the hypothalamus and cerebellum

173. The Response Evaluation Criteria in Solid Tumors (RECIST) defines all of the following categories of tumor response to therapy EXCEPT:
    (A) Complete response
    (B) Partial response
    (C) Stable disease
    (D) Recurrent disease

174. Clinical characteristics of a lesion that raise concern for the possibility of melanoma include all of the following EXCEPT:
    (A) Asymmetry of the lesion
    (B) The lesion borders irregularity
    (C) The lesion color homogeneity
    (D) The lesion thicker than 6 mm

175. The following statements describing different techniques of image registration are true EXCEPT:
    (A) Warping is an example of deformable image registration technique
    (B) Rigid registration methods are less complex than deformable ones
    (C) Deformable registration techniques should be performed before rigid registration
    (D) Rigid registration methods allow transformations such as translation, rotation

176. The chronic complications of diabetes include the following EXCEPT:
    (A) Retinopathy
    (B) Nephropathy
    (C) Dyslipidemia
    (D) Ketoacidosis

177. The delayed coincidence channel technique is commonly implemented method for:
    (A) Random correction
    (B) Scatter correction
    (C) Dead-time correction
    (D) Detector normalization

178. The paroxysmal, synchronous, rhythmic firing of a population of pathologically interconnected neurons is called:
    (A) Ictal events
    (B) Rapid eye movement
    (C) Interictal events
    (D) Non-rapid eye movement

179. A package contains several doses of F-18 FDG. The half value layer of F-18 is 4.1 mm of lead (Pb). How many millimeters of lead shielding should be put in place to reduce an exposure rate from 16 mR/h to 2 mR/h?
    (A) 3.0 mm
    (B) 10 mm
    (C) 12.4 mm
    (D) 16.8 mm

180. The coronal computed tomography multiplanar reconstruction (MPR) image in Fig. 4.8 demonstrates the presence of:
    (A) An extra spleen
    (B) Riedel's lobe
    (C) Wilms' tumor
    (D) An extra kidney

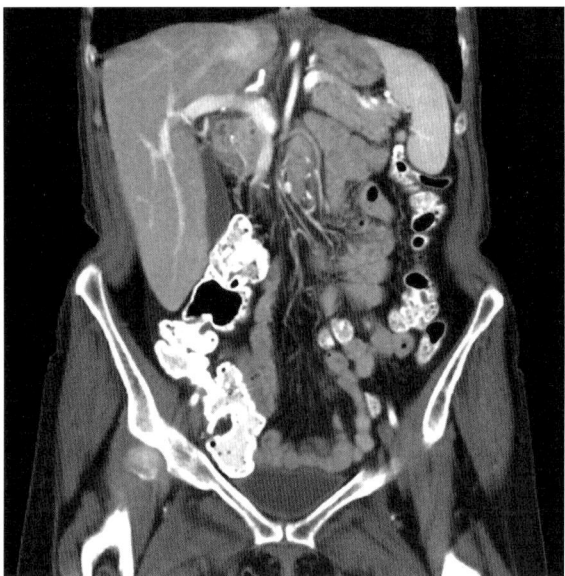

Fig. 4.8 CT MPR coronal image

181. The F-18 sodium fluoride uptake mechanism in bone is dependent on:
    (A) Cell proliferation
    (B) Osteoblastic activity
    (C) Glucose metabolism
    (D) Cell wall synthesis be similar to

182. Cold pressor testing with PET MPI has been used for the noninvasive assessment of:
 (A) Fatty acids metabolism
 (B) Adrenergic receptors imaging
 (C) Endothelial function assessment
 (D) Myocardial blood flow

183. According to the Response Evaluation Criteria in Solid Tumors (RECIST), progressive disease is defined as an increase in the sum of all tumor diameters from the lowest tumor size for at least:
 (A) 10%
 (B) 20%
 (C) 30%
 (D) 40%

184. According to the Centers of Medicare and Medicaid Services, an inconclusive test is a test whose results can be designated by all of the following EXCEPT:
 (A) Equivocal
 (B) Unpredictable
 (C) Technically uninterpretable
 (D) Discordant with a patient's clinical data

185. The PET/CT quality control procedure performed daily to ensure proper 511 keV attenuation coefficient measurements is called:
 (A) Registration
 (B) Calibration
 (C) Normalization
 (D) Singles

186. Increased expression of the insulin-independent glucose transporter, GLUT-1, and absence of the insulin dependent transporter, GLUT-4, in the lactating breast is responsible for:
 (A) Physiologic high uptake of FDG
 (B) Pathologic low uptake of FDG
 (C) Pathologic high uptake of FDG
 (D) Physiologic low uptake of FDG

187. A registration technique that employs two images as inputs, and creates the displacement field which specifies the transformations that should be applied to pixels of one of the images so that it can be aligned with the other, is called:
 (A) Deformable registration technique
 (B) Rigid registration technique
 (C) Segmented coregistration
 (D) Intensity-based coregistration

188. Which of the following patient/lesion characteristics supports benign nature of lung disease?
    (A) PET SUV >2.5
    (B) Patient age 20–29 years
    (C) Upper/middle lobe location
    (D) History of malignancy

189. The arrangement of detectors in positron emission mammography (PEM) results in spatial resolution of:
    (A) 1.5–2 mm FWHM
    (B) 2–4 mm FWHM
    (C) 4–6 mm FWHM
    (D) 6–8 mm FWHM

190. A 15 mCi dose of F-18 FDG is prepared for a patient that is scheduled for 12:00 P.M.; however, the patient is late and shows up at 13:00 hours. If you have a bulk F-18 FDG vial with a concentration of 200 mCi/4 ml at 10:00 A.M., what volume should be added to the above dose from the bulk F-18 FDG vial to make it a 15 mCi dose at 13:00 hours?
    (A) 0.07 ml
    (B) 0.2 ml
    (C) 0.3 ml
    (D) 0.6 ml

191. Which of the following PET cardiac tracers has been used to assess regional myocardial consumption of oxygen?
    (A) F-18 fluorodeoxyglucose
    (B) C-11 palmitate
    (C) C-11 epinephrine
    (D) C-11 acetate

192. Which of the following statements describing properties of contrast agents is FALSE?
    (A) Ionic agents cause fewer adverse reactions than nonionic medias
    (B) Water-equivalent contrast agents are negative medias
    (C) Allergic reactions to intravenous contrast agents may occur up to 48 hrs post administration
    (D) Contrast agent can cause thyrotoxic effects

193. The most common indication for use of granulocyte colony-stimulating factor (G-CSF) is for the treatment of:
    (A) Anemia after cancer chemotherapy or radiotherapy
    (B) Thrombocytopenia after cancer chemotherapy or radiotherapy
    (C) Neutropenia after cancer chemotherapy or radiotherapy
    (D) Alopecia after cancer chemotherapy or radiotherapy

194. The striatum, globus pallidus, substantia nigra, and subthalamic nucleus are the main components of:
    (A) The basal ganglia
    (B) The corpus callosum
    (C) The limbic system
    (D) The reticular formation

195. A procedure that causes the membranes around the lung to stick together and prevents the buildup of fluid in the space between the membranes is called:
    (A) Thoracocentesis
    (B) Pleurodesis
    (C) Aspiration
    (D) Biopsy

196. A glycoprotein that regulates the production, differentiation, survival, and activation of neutrophils (polymorphonuclear leukocytes), and neutrophilic precursors, is called:
    (A) Erythropoietin
    (B) Thrombopoietin
    (C) Macrophage colony-stimulating factor (M-CSF)
    (D) Granulocyte colony-stimulating factor (G-CSF)

197. The World Health Organization (WHO) criteria and the Response Evaluation Criteria in Solid Tumors (RECIST) provide standardized methodologies for assessing treatment response based on:
    (A) Morphological evaluation
    (B) Metabolic evaluation
    (C) Functional assessment
    (D) Quantitative assessment

198. Which of the following is an example of molecular and functional alterations occurring in cancer tissue?
    (A) Decreased amino acid transport
    (B) Decreased DNA synthesis
    (C) Increased oxygen tension
    (D) Increased membrane synthesis

199. A major advantage of N-13 ammonia PET MPI, as compared with Rb-82 PET MPI, is the ability to perform a/an:
    (A) Shorter study
    (B) Exercise-induced stress MPI study
    (C) Pharmaceutical stress MPI studies
    (D) Low-cost studies

200. A 13 mCi unit dose of F-18 FDG in 2.5 ml is calibrated for 13:00 hours. What would be the concentration at 14:30 hours?
    (A) 7.4 mCi/ml
    (B) 5.6 mCi/ml
    (C) 2.9 mCi/ml
    (D) 2.2 mCi/ml

Answers

1. B – CT attenuation correction

   Estimated effective radiation dose from CT attenuation correction is ~0.35 mSv.
   (Di Carli and Lipton 2007)

2. C – Partial-volume effect correction

   Correction methods do not generate partial volume effect-corrected images but rather produce only PVE-corrected regional SUV. These methods are not suitable for visual tumor assessment.
   (Soret et al. 2007)

3. C – The tube current (mA)

   The number of electrons that stream from the cathode to the anode is controlled by the temperature of the cathode, which is controlled by the mA.
   (Wahl 2009)

4. B – Motion artifacts

   Respiratory motion artifacts are caused by the "recorded" different breathing features: during PET acquisition the final image is an average of many breathing cycles and during short CT scan the final image is representing a specific stage of the breathing cycle. This 'freezing' of the respiratory cycle by the CT and blurring of the respiratory cycle during PET produces a mis-match between the PET and CT data.
   (Sureshbabu and Mawlawi 2005)

5. B – Calibration

   Normalization and calibration corrections are applied to the PET data after acquisition.
   (Christian et al. 2004)

6. B – 3D surface rendering

   3D rendering does not generate images of anatomical slices, but the surfaces of, e.g., anatomical structures. Generated images can be used in, e.g., craniofacial surgery, radiation therapy, and orthopedics. Maximum-Intensity Projection (MIP) is a 3D rendering technique.
   (Calhoun et al. 1999)

7. C – Primary RCC has more intense FDG uptake compared with the metastatic RCC

   Metastatic RCC has more intense FDG uptake than the primary, perhaps secondary to the more aggressive character of the metastases.
   (Mittra and Quon 2009)

8. D – Fourier rebinning

   The reconstruction of 3D PET data is a computationally intensive task since 3D imaging increases scanner sensitivity by a factor of 6–8 or more. The introduction of Fourier rebinning (FORE) made the job of processing large data much easier.
   (Wahl 2009)

9. A – Proprietary agents

   Imaging agents developed in academic settings are often not patented and, therefore, have no attached intellectual property (generic, nonproprietary agents). Often the academic developer publishes the research without obtaining a patent, moving that knowledge into the public domain and companies cannot own the exclusive right to market these agents.
   (Graham 2010)

10. C – 8 mCi

    It is necessary to know the half-life of Rb-82 to solve this problem. The half-life of Rb-82 is 1.25 min (75 sec). One important thing to remember is that, when decaying the activity, the answers will always be a smaller number then the activity being decayed. The reverse of this is true when a pre-calibration of activity is performed.
    (Formula 16A)

11. D – Horizontal long axis

    This view is displayed with the cardiac apex at the top and the cardiac base at the bottom, with the left ventricle to the viewer's right and the right ventricle to the viewer's left; serial slices are beginning at the inferior surface of the heart and progressing toward the superior surface.
    (ACC/AHA/SNM 1992)

12. C – Increased oxygen tension

    Increased protein synthesis, increased angiogenesis, and increased glucose metabolism in the end lead to the expansion of mass lesions.
    (Wahl 2009)

13. A – Imaging using water O-15

    Water -15, metabolically inactive and freely diffusible across cell membranes, is not accumulated in myocardium and instead reaches equilibrium between extra- and intravascular compartments.
    (Di Carli and Lipton 2007)

14. C – F-2

    In any given organic molecule, the C-F bond closely mimics the biological behavior of the C-H bond-what is more, the C-F bond is more stable than C-H bond and is chemically unrecognizable by hexokinase.
    (Vallabhajosula et al. 2011)

15. C – Scatter coincidences

    A scatter coincidence occurs when at least one of the two detected photons has undergone at least one Compton scatter preceding detection. As a consequence the coincident event will be assigned to a wrong line of response and will increase the image noise. Scatter fraction reflects the scatter for the entire PET system and is defined as the ratio between scatter and the total number of counts.
    (Saha 2010)

16. B – Respiratory motion

    Anatomic misregistration of the liver in PET/CT may be considerable. Although breathing protocols for CT, e.g., the breath-hold protocol, the shallow breathing protocol has some bearing on these issues, but no protocol is ideal. Recognition of the level of misregistration and attenuation correction artifacts is requisite for reviewing and can be improved by consequent comparison of uncorrected PET and CT images.
    (Sureshbabu and Mawlawi 2005)

17. B – Attenuation coefficient—0.87, relative light output—75, decay time—40 ns

    A—high-density BGO (bismuth germinate) crystals, C—high light yielding NaI(Tl) crystals (thallium-doped sodium iodide), and D—the shortest decay time but rarely used BaF2 (barium fluoride) crystals.
    (Saha 2010)

18. C – BAT primary function is to generate body heat

    Brown adipose tissue (BAT) or brown fat is one of two types of fat—the other being white adipose tissue—especially abundant in newborns and in hibernating mammals. Its primary function is to transfer energy from food into heat in animals or newborns that do not shiver. Brown fat cells contain a higher number of mitochondria rich in iron (brown appearance). BAT is acutely cold-induced and is stimulated by sympathetic nervous system.
    (Cannon and Nedegaard 2004)

19. B – F-18 fluorocholine

    The uptake of radiolabeled choline reflects the cell proliferative activity by estimating membrane lipid synthesis (cells with high proliferation rate have high uptake of choline).
    (Roivainen et al. 2000)

20. B – Surrogate molecular imaging

    Vascular dilatation, increased permeability, and new vessel formation (angiogenesis) are secondary physiological effects of increased nitric oxide activity and vascular endothelial growth factor (VEGF) expression, respectively.
    (Miles et al. 2007)

21. A – LSO (lutetium oxyorthosilicate)

    The LSO is intrinsically radioactive—Lu-176—and is not useful, e.g., for SPECT imaging, contaminates the SPECT data, and can generate image artifacts and introduce quantification error, but can be used for PET (lower photon energy than 511 keV and low activity level).
    (Saha 2010)

22. B – Partial simple seizures

    Grand mal seizures and partial simple seizures are generalized seizures that involve loss of consciousness.
    (Placantonakis and Schwartz 2009)

23. B – 93% and 92%

    For detection of myocardial ischemia, myocardial perfusion PET is considered to have higher diagnostic accuracy when compared with the more frequently used SPECT (sensitivity: 85%; specificity: 72%).
    (Machac 2005)

24. D – Fluorine-18

    Even though fluorine is the most abundant halogen in soil samples, there are no naturally occurring organofluorine complexes in animals.
    (Mach and Schwarz 2010)

25. D – Scattered regions of hypometabolism

    Alzheimer dementia (AD) is characterized by parietotemporal hypometabolism. Lewy body dementia (LBD) has a similar pattern to AD, but additionally involves the visual cortices. Frontotemporal dementia (FTD) predominantly affects the frontotemporal regions.
    (Wahl 2009)

26. D – Cavitary mass adjacent to small bowel

   A large cavitary mass likely extending to an adjacent small bowel loop with no evidence to suggest bowel obstruction.
   Radiology report frag

27. B – Opacity

   Opacity is a nonspecific term that does not indicate the size or pathologic nature of the abnormality. The radiopacity of various objects and tissues depends on atomic number, thickness, and physical opacity and results in radiographs showing different opacities. Radiopaque tissues/objects result in a whiter image; less radiopaque objects result in a blacker image.
   Hansell et al. 2008

28. B – The epileptic focus

   The epileptogenic lesion is responsible for the epileptic state.
   Placantonakis and Schwartz 2009

29. C – Hypoxia extent

   F-18 MISO binds selectively to hypoxic cells both in vitro and in vivo and has been used to measure hypoxia in brain, lung, and in the hearts of patients with myocardial ischemia.
   (Vallabhajosula et al. 2011)

30. A – 600 mCi

   Pre-calibrate the activity needed for 8:00 A.M. dose (pre-calibration of 15 mCi N-13 for 30 min), which is 120 mCi. Then pre-calibrate the activity needed for the 8:20 A.M. dose (pre-calibration of 15 mCi N-13 for 50 min), which is 480 mCi. Add both activities to receive total 600 mCi activity needed at 7:30 A.M. Remember to use the proper half-life of N-13(10 min) and not use the half-life of F-18 by mistake.
   (Formula 16B)

31. D – Hypoxia is independent from the local vasculature

   Hypoxia occurs in tumors as a result of tumor expansion (cell proliferation) exceeding the rate of local vasculature development (angiogenesis) beyond the maximum range of oxygen diffusion in tissue. Hypoxia stimulates angiogenesis by release of hypoxia-inducible factor-1, which controls transcription of vascular endothelial growth factor.
   (Vallabhajosula et al. 2011)

32. C – The superior pelvis

   The ureter crosses the iliac vessels in the superior pelvis, and urine retention can be responsible for the increased uptake.
   (Lin and Alavi 2009)

33. B – Dynamic contrast-enhanced (DCE) CT

   The method usually involves scanning with high temporal frequency on fixed CT slices over 3–5 min followed by analysis using the arterial input function (AIF) and time intensity of contrast enhancement in the tissue (tissue curve), e.g., absence of enhancement strongly suggests a benign cause, with a 96.5% negative predictive value.
   (Houseni et al. 2011)

34. B – The occipital lobe

   Like Alzheimer's disease and Parkinson's disease, DLB is a neurodegenerative disorder that results in progressive intellectual and functional deterioration. The most notorious difference between DLB and AD is decline in visual cortex activity in patients with DLB responsible for recurrent visual hallucinations.
   (Lin and Alavi 2009)

35. C – Probability of disease

   The combination of advanced imaging techniques such as FDG-PET and clinical parameters such as hemoptysis, a history of malignancy, and a history of tobacco use in Bayesian models is suggested for more precise evaluation of, e.g., pulmonary nodules.
   (Houseni et al. 2011)

36. D – Decreased area of uptake corresponding to the radiation field

   Radiation therapy reduces bone marrow activity almost to background in the area exactly corresponding to the radiation field.
   (Wahl 2009)

37. C – Echocardiography

   Data indicate that CT calcium scoring and PET perfusion imaging are complementary for the evaluation of cardiovascular risk, and can be combined to stratify patients into different risk-based categories.
   (Bengel et al. 2009)

38. B – Esophageal sphincter

   Esophageal sphincter is also referred to as the cardiac sphincter. The pyloric sphincter guards the opening of the pylorus into the duodenum.
   (Moore et al. 2010)

39. B – Surgical intervention will be a treatment possibility

   Vigilant staging is imperative in reducing the risk of finding unresectable tumor during surgery, or of performing unsuccessful surgery on a patient with extrapleural disease.
   (Zielinski et al. 2010)

Answers

40. B – 9.4HVLs

$0.03 \text{ mR/h} = 19.5 \text{ mR/h} \times e^{-0.693(X/4.1\text{HVL})}$ (divide 0.03 mR/h by 19.5 mR/h).

$0.0015 = e^{-0.693(X/4.1\text{HVLs})}$ (to move x out of exponent take natural log (ln) of each side of equation).

$\ln(0.0015) = e^{-0.693(X/4.1\text{HVLs})}$ (remember inverse of e^x is natural log (ln) of e).

−6.5×4.1 mm HVL/−0.693 = 38.5 mm.

The answer is required in HVLs; therefore, 38.5 mm/4.1 mm(HVL of F-18FDG) = 9.4HVLs.
(Formula 13)

41. B – 22 dpm/cm^2

For alpha radiation the measured amount of radioactivity should not exceed 2.2 dpm/cm^2.
(Christian et al. 2004)

42. C – The liver

Direct invasion of adjacent structures, particularly in the pelvis, and lymph node spread occur early.
(Abeloff and Armitage 2008)

43. C – Stage III of lymphoma

For each stage, extranodal cancers that have spread beyond the lymph nodes into other tissues or organs are indicated by the letter "E." The subscript "S" indicates spread to the spleen.
(Jhanwar and Straus 2006)

44. A – The lipophilicity of the complex

Lipophilicity describes the ability of a chemical compound to dissolve in fats, oils, and lipids.
(Mach and Schwarz 2010)

45. A – left ventricle ejection fraction

Microcirculation and endothelial functions are key mediators of coronary disease progression, and they can be evaluated with MBF and CFR.
(Bengel et al. 2009)

46. A – Radiation therapy

Bone marrow is a frequent site of lymphomatous involvement and metastatic tumors from breast, lung, and prostate cancers, and they may present either as diffuse or focal marrow uptake on FDG-PET imaging.
(Inoue et al. 2006)

47. D – Mixed attenuation

   Cavitation with thick or irregular walls, endobronchial location, and amorphous calcification patterns also indicates malignancy.
   (Prokop and Galanski 2003)

48. A – Mucinous adenocarcinoma

   Adenocarcinomas that are comprised of at least 60% mucus are referred to as mucinous adenocarcinomas.
   (Fong et al. 1999)

49. A – stage I of lymphoma

   For each stage, the absence of systemic symptoms is designated by the subscript "A"; the subscript "B" is used if any of the following symptoms are present: unexplained weight loss, drenching night sweats, or fever.
   (Jhanwar and Straus 2006)

50. A – 7:45 am

   This problem is calculated by using given time as elapse time in the pre-calibration formula

   For example $12 \text{ mCi} = I_o \times e^{-(0.693)(15 \text{ min}/110 \text{ min})} = 13.2 \text{ mCi}$

   The maximum injectable dose is 14 mCi; therefore, 13.2 mCi at 7:45 am is the correct answer.

51. B – Into the room

   The exhaust system should not allow for passive circulation of airborne radioactivities into the surrounding nonrestricted areas.
   (Christian et al. 2004)

52. A – Signs and symptoms

   Semiologic signs can be grouped into positive or negative motor signs, automatisms, autonomic manifestations, and speech signs. Although several semiologic signs of seizures can foresee the hemispheric lateralization of seizures, they are commonly not considered dependable predictors lobar localization of foci.
   (Placantonakis and Schwartz 2009)

53. A – Upstaging of approximately 15–25% of patients

   FDG-PET has a considerable influence on staging in HL, and upstaging is important, as HL is a disease in which early and advanced stages are treated very differently.
   (Hutchings 2009)

Answers

54. B – Ligand

    A number of biologically PET ligands have been developed and utilized in PET investigations to study various biochemical functions in healthy and diseased subjects, e.g., to evaluate drug effects and receptor occupancies in the living human brain. Determining the usefulness of a PET ligand for human applications necessitates the expertise of several scientists including radiochemists, pharmacologists, and clinicians who work in a close partnership in an interdisciplinary environment.
    (Mach and Schwarz 2010)

55. B – The Reed–Sternberg cells

    These large, malignant cells are found in diseased tissues, and are thought to be a type of malignant B lymphocyte. Although the presence of Reed–Sternberg cells is essential to the diagnosis of Hodgkin's disease, R-S cells are not unique to HD.
    (Kumar V. Abbas K.A.Robbins and Cotran Pathologic Basis of Disease. 8th ed. Saunders Elsevier, Philadelphia, PA. 2010).

56. B – The thalamus

    The thalamus, part of a limbic system, refines sensory information—thalamocortical loop—into a more interpretable and manageable form for higher brain sections. It also modulates arousal mechanisms, maintains alertness, and directs attention to sensory events.
    (Christian et al. 2004)

57. C – X-ray beam

    In fan-beam scanners, an x-ray source and detector are mounted on a rotating gantry are acquired using a fan-shaped x-ray beam transmitted through the patient. The patient is scanned slice by slice, in the axial plane, and the images are obtained by piling up the slices to obtain multiple 2D representations.

    The cone-beam technique implies a single 360° scan in which the x-ray source and a corresponding area detector synchronously move around the patient.
    (Prokop and Galanski 2003)

58. D – Neuroendocrine tumors

    These cells were referred to as Amine Precursor Uptake and Decarboxylation (APUD) cells. As a group, the tumors that arose from these cells were classified as APUDomas; currently more frequently referred to as neuroendocrine tumors (NET).
    (Castellucci et al. 2008)

59. D – High levels of FDG uptake are associated with a favorable prognosis

FDG-PET/CT imaging accurately detects the presence or absence of systemic metastases, and accurately diagnoses and estimates the extent of locoregional and distant MPM recurrence.
(Gerbaudo et al. 2011)

60. A – 2 ft.
12.5 mR/hr × $(1)^2$ = 3.0 mR/hr × $(x)^2$ (12inches = 1foot)
12.5 mR/hr/3.0 mR/hr = $(x)^2$
4.2 = $((x)^2$ (remember to take square root of 4.2 to remove exponent from x)
$\sqrt{4.2}$ = 2.0 foot
* You must remember to obtain the square root in a situation like the problem above, since you are looking for D (distance) not D 2 (not distance squared). Also, present the answer in the requested units.
Formula 12

61. C – 50 mSv (5 rem)

The annual allowable limits for radiation exposure for the TEDE for the lens of eye—150 mSv(15 rem), for a fetus—5 mSv (0.5 rem), and for the skin—500 mSv (50 rem).
(Christian et al. 2004)

62. C – The density of macrophages in the lesions

F-FDG uptake seems to also be related to the size of plaques. Large plaques build up more FDG than do smaller or less bulky lesions.
(Lin and Alavi 2009)

63. C – Are prone to artifacts

The misregistration artifacts are distinctive to the use of CT-based attenuation correction; other artifacts are generated at areas of high-density material, e.g., metal and iodine, and are most noticeable with CT-based AC.
(Lin and Alavi 2009)

64. C – Metastatic liver carcinoma

Well-differentiated cells, e.g., hepatocytes have a relatively high glucose-6-phosphatase activity, which allows dephosphorylation of FDG and subsequent leakage of the tracer from cells. Metastatic liver cells do not share this characteristic and for that reason F-18 FDG is of very limited value in diagnosing hepatocellular carcinoma (HCC) but is useful in suspected metastatic liver carcinoma imaging.
(Wahl and Buchanan 2002)

Answers

65. B – C-11 methionine

Carbon-11-methionine PET is a novel approach in which this radiolabeled amino acid is rapidly taken up and integrated into newly synthesized immunoglobulins. Fluorine-18-fluoro-deoxy-L-thymidine (F-18FLT) PET, where F-18 FLT is incorporated into DNA in the place of thymidine, can be also employed to analyze the bone marrow component in hematological disorders.
(Wahl 2009)

66. B – A low or absent expression of SSR

F-18 FDG targets the glycolytic pathway; tumors with a low or absent expression of SSR, such as medullar thyroid carcinoma and undifferentiated NETs, cannot be successfully visualized with octreotide-based radiopeptides.
(Castellucci et al. 2008)

67. B – Multiple myeloma

Multiple myeloma originates in plasma cells, a type of white blood cell normally responsible for the production of antibodies. The common symptoms of multiple myeloma include elevated calcium, renal failure, anemia, and bone lesions.
(Kumar and Abbas 2010)

68. B – Edema

Radiation necrosis is a portion of a progression of clinical syndromes related to central nervous system (CNS) complications of radiotherapy. The term radiation necrosis is used to refer to radiation injury, but pathology is not limited to necrosis and a spectrum of injury patterns may occur.
(Lin and Alavi 2009)

69. A – P wave, QRS complex, ST segment, T wave, and U wave

For the reason that cardiac depolarization and repolarization normally occur in a synchronized fashion, the ECG is able to register these electrical currents as specific waves.
(Goldberger 2006)

70. A – Average variance

The average variance is a sensitive indicator of various detector problems, and if the average variance exceeds 2.5, recalibration of the PET scanner is recommended.
(Saha 2010)

71. B – Rem

    The rem (roentgen equivalent man) measures the biological effect of radiation and is calculated from the energy imparted to matter by ionizing radiation. To determine equivalent dose (rem), you multiply absorbed dose (rad) by a quality factor (Q) that is unique to the type of incident radiation.
    (Lombardi 1999)

72. C – Prominent right ventricle F-18 FDG uptake

    Flattening of the diaphragm, diffusely diminished F-18 FDG activity in the lungs, increased lung volume, and increased anteroposterior thoracic diameter are commonly seen in patients with COPD.
    (Hickeson and Abikhzer 2011)

73. B – More effective cooling and heat dissipation

    The Straton tube cooling rates are 5–10 times greater than for conventional tubes, which result in shorter rotation times and faster scans.
    (Patton et al. 2009)

74. C – postsurgical FDG uptake increases in intensity with time

    Additionally, postsurgical F-18 FDG uptake is often not related to any discrete space-occupying lesion on the matching CT images.
    (Hickeson and Abikhzer 2011)

75. C – Active lesions

    PET can detect early marrow involvement of multiple myeloma, and is useful in assessing the extent of active disease at the time of initial presentation. PET can also be useful in evaluating treatment response.
    (Wahl 2009)

76. B – Mineralocorticoids

    Mineralocorticoids are hormones that regulate salt and water balances .They are produced in the adrenal glands and their secretion is regulated by other hormones such as adrenocorticotropic hormone (ACTH).
    (Lin and Alavi 2009)

77. C – Predicts adverse cardiac events

    Three groups of patients with normal, mild, and moderate to severe PET perfusion scans had annual rates of hard events of 0.4%, 2.3%, and 7%, respectively, and PET data were the strongest predictors of total cardiac events.
    (Yoshinaga et al. 2006)

78. A – The bronchus/lungs and gastroenteropancreatic tract

    Neuroendocrine tumors include such tumors as adenomas from the pituitary gland, islet cell tumors from the pancreas, pheochromocytoma and neuroblastoma from the adrenal medulla, medullary thyroid carcinoma from the C-cells of the thyroid gland, and carcinoid tumors from the gastrointestinal tract from the lung.
    (Castellucci et al. 2008)

79. D – The higher focal activity disappeared on the CT scan after antibiotic therapy

    The coregistered CT scan showed many additional findings that were not seen on PET scans. Although foci seen on PET scans during exacerbations disappeared after the resolution of exacerbation, the corresponding CT scan findings remained unchanged.
    (Klein et al. 2009)

80. D – 13

    Obtain the mean (n) value by adding all five values and dividing by five, which are 499. Now obtain the sum, ($n,$) of all five values, which will give you 81, 16, 289, 64, and 225 respectively, and added together equals to 675.

    $$SD = \sqrt{\frac{675}{5-1}} = \sqrt{169} = 13.$$

    (Formula 10)

81. C – 5,000 mrem/year (50 mSv/year)

    The ring dosimeter should be worn with the label on the inside of workers preferred hand.
    (Lombardi 1999)

82. C – An inverted C shape

    Symmetry on coronal images is helpful in evaluating FDG uptake in the head and neck.
    (Lin and Alavi 2009)

83. A – The thyroglobulin (Tg) levels are more than 10 ng/

    Publications provide data that support that the patients with high levels of Tg (>10 ng/mL) are more likely to have positive PET scans.
    (Fletcher et al. 2008)

84. C – Choline

   Choline is a quaternary ammonium base and is a precursor for phospholipids synthesis.
   (Vallabhajosula et al. 2011)

85. C – Point spread function

   The image of the point object is always blurred by the imaging system and the amount of blurring can be characterized in terms of the full-width-at-half-maximum (FWHM) of the point spread function.
   (Christian et al. 2004)

86. C – Liver metastasis

   If the tumor diameter is less than 1 cm, secondary lesions in the liver are present in more or less 15% to 25% of neuroendocrine tumors (NETs), and greater than 75% if the tumor size is greater than 2 cm.
   (Jensen 2005)

87. A – The photoelectric effect

   Photoelectric effect (PE) of x-rays, prevailing at low X-ray energies, occurs when the x-ray photon is absorbed, and electrons from the outer shell of the atom are ejected; as a result the ionized atom returns to the neutral state with the emission of an x-ray characteristic of the atom.
   (Early and Sodee 1995)

88. A – Pick's disease

   People with Pick's disease have abnormal substances (called Pick bodies and Pick cells) inside nerve cells in the damaged areas of the brain. Frontal and temporal decreased FDG uptake is the prevailing pattern.
   (Lin and Alavi 2009)

89. C – Acetate C-11

   C-11 is used for the quantification of regional myocardial oxidative metabolism, which is useful to demarcate the extent and distribution of viable myocardium in patients with left ventricular dysfunction.
   (Al-Mallah et al. 2010)

90. A – Fig. 4.3a

   The right kidney appears to be hypotrophic and nonfunctioning.
   (Radiology report frag)

Answers

91. B – Glucose

The breakdown of fatty acids in the mitochondria by b-oxidation is exquisitely sensitive to oxygen deprivation. The myocardium has a unique ability to switch substrates according to the metabolic needs and conditions.
(Bashir and Gropler 2009)

92. A – Partial complex seizures

In partial complex seizures (temporal lobe epilepsy), the source of the seizures is localized. This is the most common form of epilepsy referred for epilepsy surgery. Interictal FDG-PET studies have reduced value in the presence of multiple hypometabolic regions in patients with multifocal brain syndromes. Grand mal and petit mal are generalized seizures.
(Christian et al. 2004)

93. A – A positive PET/CT scan after therapy is linked with longer survival

Longer survival is related to a negative PET scan after completion of therapy. PET/CT improves detection of all sites of cancer and provides a better staging than CT or bone scintigraphy.
(Mosci and Iagaru 2011)

94. C – 92% and 94%

FDG-PET is more accurate than conventional imaging modalities in restaging and follow-up of melanoma (92% and 94%, vs 56% and 45% for conventional imaging).
(Valk et al. 2003)

95. B – C-11 acetate

Somatostatin receptor scintigraphy using predominantly In-111-labeled tracers has been used to evaluate DTC that has reduced or absent uptake of radioiodine. Other radiopharmaceuticals such as Ga-68 DOTATOC and F-18 DOPA may provide complementary information to F-18 FDG-PET/CT.
(Mosci and Iagaru 2011)

96. B – The primary tumor mass proximity

The small size and the close proximity of periesophageal lymph nodes to the primary tumor mass are responsible for lower sensitivity—ranging from 22 to 57%—of FDG-PET for the detection of regional nodal metastases.
(Rohren et al. 2004)

97. C – Divided by the noise in the image

The signal is described as the difference between an object and its background and the noise as the ambiguity with which that object is recorded.
(Christian et al. 2004)

98. C – In situ carcinoma shows higher FDG uptake than invasive ductal cancer

    False-negative results are reported in slow-growing and well-differentiated tumors such as tubular carcinoma and in situ carcinoma.
    (Kumar et al. 2009)

99. A – Neurons in the basal ganglia

    6-[F-18]fluoro-L-DOPA was the first FDOPA PET agent. First brain imaging was performed in 1984 to visualize the dopamineric neurons in basal ganglia.
    (Becherer et al. 2004)

100. B – Sinoatrial node

    Typically, the signal for cardiac electrical stimulation fires up in the sinus node, also called the sinoatrial (SA) node. This node is located in the right atrium near the opening of the superior vena cava (SVC).
    (Goldberger 2006)

101. D – A

    The ascending aorta is the first section of the aorta, which starts from the left ventricle of the heart and extends to the aortic arch. The right and left coronary arteries that supply blood to the heart muscle arise from the ascending aorta.
    (Andreoli et al. 2001)

102. A – Auxillary lymph node metastasis

    Sentinel lymph node biopsy is a well-established procedure for differentiating axillary lymph node metastasis from primary breast cancer. PET and PET/CT scanning as an independent imaging modality for detecting axillary lymph node status showed lower sensitivity (approximately 40%) nevertheless high specificity in detecting axillary lymph node metastases.
    (Kumar et al. 2009)

103. B – NU 2-2007 addresses the intrinsic radioactivity in LSO and LYSO crystals

    NEMA provides recommended procedures for measuring system sensitivity, spatial resolution, scatter correction, accuracy of attenuation correction, and overall clinical image quality.
    National Electrical Manufacturers Association 2007

104. B – Less than the liver

    Postmenopausal women receiving HRT have SUVs similar to those of the premenopausal women. Breasts of premenopausal women had a higher SUV than breasts of postmenopausal women not receiving HRT.
    (Lin and Alavi 2009)

Answers

105. D – Photon collinearity

Differences from 180º between the two trajectories of the emitted photons, known as photon **non-collinearity**, may result in ~1.54–1.76 mm FWHM blurring in a typical scanner.
(Sanchez-Crespo and Larsson 2006)

106. B – Anterior mediastinum

The thymus is composed of two identical lobes and is located anatomically in the anterior superior mediastinum, in front of the heart and behind the sternum.
(Lin and Alavi 2009)

107. D – 40–60% of all events

Scatter effects become a significant problem, especially in 3D PET, due to the fact that the lead septa are removed to achieve an increase in sensitivity. The scatter fraction for whole-body 3D PET studies increases from 10–20% in 2D PET to 40–60% in 3D PET.
(Sanchez-Crespo and Larsson 2006)

108. B – The high F-18 FDG uptake in normal brain tissue

Tumors with low metabolic activity, such as low-grade gliomas (LGG) in gray matter, may be obscured or even invisible, since F-18FDG accumulates physiologically in normal brain tissue, particularly in the gray matter, producing a high-metabolic background on PET scan.
(Lin and Alavi 2009)

109. A – Correcting for attenuation of gamma rays

At the present time the use of PET-MRI is mostly confined to brain disorders, where attenuation correction is a minor issue.
(Kaplan 2011)

110. B – the energy of positron and number of electrons in the immediate area of decay

In the annihilation event the identical mass of two particles (511 MeV each) is converted into energy according to $E=mc^2$ Einstein's equation.
(Lin and Alavi 2009)

111. C – Glucose metabolism

FDG uptake is associated with metabolic activity of the tumor itself, and as a result, F-18 FDG may detect metastases before bony destruction or osteoblastic healing.
(Brenner et al. 2012)

112. D – Anaplastic

Anaplastic thyroid carcinoma (ATC), with a median survival of 3 months, is the most aggressive solid cancer in man. ATC is characterized by the rapid onset and relentless progression of the disease and its dismal prognosis. Although 2% of all thyroid carcinomas are ATC, it accounts for 14–39% of thyroid carcinoma deaths.
(Kebebew et al. 2005)

113. A – Fat

−50, 30–45, >40 and >400 are CT numbers (Hounsfield units) assigned to fat, blood, muscle, and bone accordingly.
(Prokop and Galanski 2003)

114. A – Peak hyperemic and rest myocardial blood flow

Myocardial blood flow (MBF) and coronary vasodilator reserve (CVR) are inversely related to stenosis severity. A quantitative estimate of MBF by PET allows evaluation of relative perfusion in balanced ischemia.
(Zaret and Beller 2005)

115. B – Respiratory motion

Respiratory motion is not a problem with positron emission mammography (PEM) imaging since the breast is immobilized.
(Schilling et al. 2008)

116. B – Oral fatty acids loading

In ischemia, with limited delivery of oxygen, exogenous glucose becomes the preferred substrate. Increased insulin levels activate glucose transporters onto the cell membrane, resulting with increased exogenous glucose transport and utilization.
(Zaret and Beller 2005)

117. A – Deformable registration technique

Deformable registration methods compute the transformations on a pixel-by-pixel basis, which is computationally time consuming, and most of the time deformable registration methods cannot be clinically implemented in real time.
(Hajnal et al. 2001)

Answers

118. C – Deformable coregistration

Deformable registration methods employ techniques such as elastic transformation to correct deformations that rigid methods are not sufficient to correct.
(Zaidi and Thompson 2009)

119. B – 50%

Approximately 50% of the injected dose of 18 F-18 sodium fluoride is taken up by bone, comparable to 99 m-Tc-diphosphonates. Almost all causes of increased new bone formation result in increased localization of F-18 sodium fluoride.
(Grant et al. 2008)

120. D – 85 min

To solve this problem, utilize given times as an elapse time and decay 13 mCi of F-18 FDG.
For example, $13 \text{ mCi} \times e^{-(0.693)(85 \text{ min}/110 \text{ min})}$ will give you the desired answer of 7.6 mCi, which is under 8 mCi.
(Formula 16A)

121. A – hypoxia and perfusion

Hypoxia and perfusion are important parameters in tumor physiology and can have major implications in diagnosis, prognosis, treatment planning, and response to therapy. A Zn-62/Cu-62 microgenerator and rapid synthesis kits now provide a practical means of producing 62Cu-PTSM and 62Cu-ATSM on-site.
(Wong and Lacy 2008)

122. A – two planar detectors capable of detecting the 511-keV annihilation photons in a conventional mammography unit

High-resolution two flat detector heads are mounted to compression paddles that can be rotated to optimize breast views. The PET-FDG image can be acquired in positions that are analogous to those used in mammography, which allows for image coregistration and comparison. Another design consists of a boxlike detector arrangement that surrounds the breast, which allows a more comprehensive reconstruction of the activity within the breast.
(Zaidi and Thompson 2009)

123. C – C-11 acetate

Once taken up by the heart, acetate, a two-carbon chain free fatty acid, is rapidly converted to acetyl-CoA. Acetyl-CoA is metabolized through the tricarboxylic acid cycle, tightly coupled with oxidative phosphorylation.
(Bashir and Gropler 2009)

124. A – V shaped

    In general, physiologic uptake of FDG in the thymus disappears in adolescence in conjunction with involution of the thymus, but it has been reported in patients up to 54 years old.
    (Lin and Alavi 2009)

125. A – lower in tumors and higher background activity in the liver and bone marrow

    FLT-PET is considered a potentially powerful addition to staging by FDG-PET, providing additional diagnostic specificity for proliferating tissues.
    (Salskov et al. 2007)

126. C – Mesothelioma

    The disease manifests clinically 30–40 years after exposure to asbestos fibers. Other causes and/or cofactors for malignant pleural mesothelioma (MPM) include exposure to nonasbestos mineral fibers and therapeutic radiation.
    (Gerbaudo et al. 2011)

127. C – Use of collimator

    Image resolution is inferior to that of PET because emission of single photon requires the use of a collimator to acquire image data.
    (Christian et al. 2004)

128. C – The limbic system

    Limbic system structures—the hippocampus, amygdala, anterior thalamic nuclei, septum, limbic cortex, and fornix—are involved in many of our emotions and motivations related to survival (fear, anger) and to sexual behavior.
    (Christian et al. 2004)

129. D – Angiogenesis

    The expression of integrin receptor on sprouting capillary cells and its interaction have been shown to play a key role in angiogenesis and metastasis. Several radiolabeled ligands of the integrin receptor have been developed on the basis of the integrin's recognition of the tripeptide ArgGlyAsp (RGD) amino acid sequence.
    (Vallabhajosula et al. 2011)

130. C – Sagittal slice of the brain

    The sagittal plane divides the right and left side of the brain into parts. The midsagittal plane would divide the right and left sides of the brain into two equal parts.
    (Madden 2007)

131. C – 1.8 and 2 mm

    The contribution from non-collinearity worsens with a larger diameter ring, and it extends to 1.8–2 mm for 80–90-cm PET scanners.
    (Saha 2010)

132. C – C-11 epinephrine

    C-11 epinephrine is used for sympathetic neuronal catecholamine storage imaging. C-11 palmitate and C-11 acetate are used to trace uptake of fatty acids in the myocardium and Krebs cycle flux, oxidative metabolism accordingly.
    (Bengel et al. 2009)

133. B – Scatter correction

    The sensitivity to scattered coincidences is greater in 3D mode (the scatter fraction >40%) than in 2D mode (the scatter fraction ~15%). 3D mode the amount of scatter in the signal can become extremely large and accurate scatter correction methods are required.
    (Saha 2010)

134. A – Direct molecular imaging

    Examples of direct molecular imaging include: fluorodeoxyglucose (FDG) PET-FDG interacts directly with Glut-1 glucose transporters, and Tc-99 m methoxyisobutylisonitrile (MIBI) interacts directly with a p-glycoprotein (pgp)-scintigraphy.
    (Miles et al. 2007)

135. B – Resolution

    A longer crystal delivers a bigger chance of interaction and, for that reason, increased sensitivity.

    Since a longer crystal accepts a larger number of peripheral photons striking along its full vertical dimension, the spatial resolution is diminished. This drawback can be solved by detecting the depth of interaction (DOI) within the crystal, either by arranging two layers of crystals packed on each other or mathematically.
    (Mittra and Quon 2009)

136. C – Pattern of radiopharmaceutical distribution can be affected by auditory stimuli

    The gray matter–to–white matter flow proportion is circa 4:1. To reduce disparities modifying general pattern of radiopharmaceutical distribution, e.g., the visual, auditory, and somatosensory stimuli that the patient experiences, well-defined clinical practices should be used to control environmental influences.
    (Morano and Seibyl 2003)

137. A – A high-resolution gamma camera and Tc-99 m Sestamibi

    Latest innovations in technology have resulted in the improvement of high-resolution gamma cameras specifically designed to image the breast.
    (Brem and Petrovitch 2007)

138. B – Greater in magnitude and greater in extent

    In early-onset AD, the parietal, frontal, posterior cingulate cortices, and subcortical area are mostly affected; the limbic system and medial frontal lobe involvement is typical for late-onset AD.
    (Lin and Alavi 2009)

139. B – More precise localization of the source

    The key limitation to TOF is in the intrinsic scintillator decay time and the net time resolution of the detectors and electronics. If the time resolution could be cut to 15 picoseconds, the site of the original photon could be reduced to a few millimeters, and image reconstruction would be avoided.
    (Mittra and Quon 2009)

140. C – Indirect molecular imaging

    In indirect molecular imaging cellular work is modified so that the target gene induces a molecular change that can be evaluated with a matching imaging probe.
    (Miles et al. 2007)

141. C – 890 mRem (8.9 mSv)

    The radiation dose to the patient is 68% greater when 10 mCi (370 MBq) of F-18 sodium fluoride is used, compared with 25 mCi (925 MBq) of Tc-99 m MDP (5.3 mSv).
    (Segall et al. 2010)

142. C – Carbon-13

    A cyclotron-produced nitrogen-13 (N-13) has a half-life of 9.96 min, so it must be made at the PET site. Nitrogen-13 is used to tag ammonia molecules for PET imaging.
    (Early and Sodee 1995)

143. A – light detectors

    The main advantages of compact, solid-state APDs over PMTs rest in their small size, inexpensive production, and insensitivity to magnetic fields.
    (Mittra and Quon 2009)

Answers

144. D – Prevent tachyarrhythmias

    Intravenous procainamide, lidocaine, amiodarone, and beta blockers (metoprolol, esmolol, and propranolol) are used to suppress acute ventricular tachycardias.
    (Ferri 2007)

145. C – False-positive fraction

    ROC displays sensitivity and specificity as function of minimum image score needed to call image positive ROC analysis is considered to be the ultimate test of an imaging system and is used to compare one imaging system against another or one imaging technique against another.
    (Christian et al. 2004)

146. C – The data for the slice across all projection angles

    Notice that each projection image in SPECT represents the data acquired at projection angle across all slices.
    (Fahey 2002)

147. D – Scan provides resolution ~5 mm

    Resolution of PEM ~1.5 mm is higher than that of PET ~5 mm (PET). Breast immobilization used in PEM also limits the motion artifacts that can be a significant factor limiting the PET image quality.
    (Schilling et al. 2008)

148. B – Obese and women

    Attenuation artifacts are more frequent in obese populations and women. PET reduces the number of false-positive scans (specificity is increased) in this group of patients.
    (Zaret and Beller 2005)

149. B – N-13 ammonia

    The N-13 target produces N-13 ammonia in the target, which requires no additional synthesis, and minimal in-line purification.
    (Siemens 2012)

150. B – A scatter event

    A scatter event occurs when at least one of the two detected photons has undergone at least one Compton interaction prior to detection.
    (Christian et al. 2004)

151. B – Viable myocytes are metabolically active, whereas scarred or fibrotic tissue is metabolically inactive

    In the presence of reduced regional blood flow and function, techniques that assess metabolic processes provide unique insight into the presence or absence of myocardial viability.
    (Zaret and Beller 2005)

152. C – FDG uptake is proportional to iodine uptake

    Increased glucose metabolism is a sign of higher malignancy—FDG uptake is inversely proportional to iodine uptake and to tumor differentiation.
    (Mosci and Iagaru 2011)

153. B – Cell proliferation

    [F-18]-fluoromisonidazole is a marker of tumor hypoxia; F-18 Galacto-RGD and F-18AH111 (Fluciclatide) are radiotracers for imaging of angiogenesis.
    (Vallabhajosula et al. 2011)

154. D – Neurotransmitters imaging

    The capability to image tumor receptors is principally significant to breast cancer treatment, and includes the expression of estrogen receptors.
    (Mankoff and Lee 2009)

155. A – 1%

    Only 1% of energy is converted to X-rays that exit the tube usually perpendicular to the path of the electron beam as X-rays—the remaining 99% of energy creates heat. Tubes can be encircled by oil bath to remove heat and cooled air applied so that tubes do not require long cool down periods.
    (Prokop and Galanski 2003)

156. C – Aggrenox

    Aggrenox combines two different antiplatelet agents, aspirin and dipyridamole, which are used together for secondary stroke prevention. Dipyridamole coronary vasodilatory action involves an accumulation of the endogenous adenosine, a potent coronary vasodilator and inhibitor of platelet aggregation.
    (Aggrenox 2012)

157. B – Percentage change in the "hottest" lesion

    According to the PET Response Criteria in Solid Tumors (PERCIST) criteria, the hottest lesions per scan are not necessarily identical over time.
    (Boellaard 2011)

Answers

158. A – The basal ganglia

    The basal ganglia work with the cerebellum to coordinate fine motions, such as fingertip movements.
    (Christian et al. 2004)

159. B – Depolarization

    The return of heart muscle cells to their resting state after stimulation (depolarization) is called repolarization.
    (Goldberger 2006)

160. A – Acute

    Indolent or low-grade lymphomas—marginal zone lymphoma, chronic lymphocytic leukemia/small lymphocytic lymphoma; highly aggressive lymphomas include Burkitt lymphoma or lymphoblastic lymphoma; diffuse large B-cell lymphoma (DLBCL), peripheral T-cell lymphoma, and most forms of mantle cell lymphoma are classified as aggressive lymphomas.
    (Kumar and Abbas 2010)

161. C – Normalization

    Data are acquired in the absence of any object in the FOV. A standard phantom containing a low activity, to avoid the dead-time loss of positron emitters, is placed at the center of the scanner to expose all detectors uniformly. The multiplication factor for each detector is estimated by dividing the average of counts of all detector pairs by each individual detector pair count.
    (Saha 2010)

162. C – Oxygen and glucose

    The uptake of glucose is directly proportional to the functional requirements from the neurons-oxidation of glucose is responsible for providing energy to the brain. However, research has suggested that lactate may be a major source in cerebral energy metabolism.
    (Korf 2006)

163. B – SUV should be corrected for serum glucose levels

    Glucose corrections have been unpredictably useful, and errors in glucometer measurements are well known and may add errors in SUVs estimations.
    (Wahl 2009)

164. B – At rest and during peak stress

    In normal subjects, LVEF increases during peak vasodilator stress. In the presence of CAD, however, changes in LVEF (from baseline to peak stress)

are inversely related to the presence of myocardium at risk. Post-stress LVEF measurements are obtained with gated SPECT.
(Dorbala et al. 2007)

165. B – SUV × tumor volume

    TGV is a combination measure of both metabolic activity and tumor volume, and reflects the metabolically active tumor mass.
    (Gerbaudo et al. 2011)

166. C – Ranges from moderate to high

    Malignant mesothelioma is a rare type of cancer that occurs in the thin layer of cells lining the body's internal organs, known as the mesothelium. Pleural mesothelioma is the most common form of the disease, accounting for roughly 70% of cases. FDG uptake depends on the mesothelioma cell type, e.g., epithelial subtypes tend to be less metabolically active than mixed and sarcomatoid subtypes.
    (Gerbaudo et al. 2011)

167. C – Normal myocardial blood and decreased myocardial glucose metabolism

    Reverse mismatch pattern (normal perfusion, reduced metabolism relative to perfusion) can be detected in numerous patients with left bundle branch block (LBBB), in repetitive stunning, and in patients who have diabetes; its significance is still uncertain.
    (Thompson et al. 2006)

168. B – Amelanotic melanomas

    Amelanotic melanomas may be pink, red, or have light brown, tan, or gray at the edges and are usually detectable only on close examination of the skin.
    (Karakousis and Czerniecki 2011)

169. B – Fatty acid oxidation stops and anaerobic metabolism turns up

    This metabolic adjustment is essential for continued energy production and cell survival.
    (Bashir and Gropler 2009)

170. B – Quality factor

    The distribution factor considers the volume of irradiated tissue; the dose rate factor accounts for the differences in response to different dose rates.
    (Lombardi 1999)

171. C – is increased by 20 to 25%

    PET/CT is more accurate for tumor localization and assessing tumor extent for staging non-small cell lung cancer and other solid tumors, especially in the abdomen and pelvis; in the head and neck, PET/CT images can easily distinguish between abnormalities and physiological structures such as muscle and brown fat.
    (Saha 2010)

172. A – Decreased uptake in the caudate nucleus and putamen

    Huntington's disease (HD) results from genetically programmed loss and atrophy of neurons in the caudate nucleus and putamen. Neuronal degeneration causes uncontrolled movements, loss of intellectual faculties, and emotional disturbance.
    (Wahl 2009)

173. D – Recurrent disease

    The RECIST categories also include progressive disease categories when there is at least a 20% increase in the sum of all tumor diameters from the lowest tumor size is observed.
    (Wahl and Jacene 2009)

174. C – The lesion color homogeneity

    Presented clinical characteristics of a lesion are frequently referred as a "ABCDE": Asymmetry —the shape of one-half does not match the other, Border—the edges are ragged, blurred, or irregular, Color—the color in uneven and may include shades of black, brown, and tan, Diameter—there is a change in size, usually an increase, and Evolution—lesions with changing shapes, size, or color.
    (Karakousis and Czerniecki 2011)

175. C – Deformable registration techniques should be performed before rigid registration

    Given that rigid registration methods are less convoluted than deformable ones, rigidly aligning two images before performing nonrigid transformation reduces the time needed to nonrigidly align these images. Deformable registration methods apply techniques such as elastic transformations to register images that rigid methods are not sufficient to register.
    (Hajnal et al. 2001)

176. D – Ketoacidosis

    Diabetic ketoacidosis is an acute complication and it happens in patients with type I (insulin-dependent diabetes mellitus –IDDM) diabetes, and most frequently, when an incurrent sickness develops, e.g., infection. Symptoms include: dehydration, acidosis, electrolyte depletion.
    (Andreoli et al. 2001)

177. A – Random correction

    The number of coincidences in the standard window includes both the randoms plus trues; there will be no true coincidences in the delayed coincidence channel. Correction for randoms is made by subtracting delay channel counts from the typical window cts.
    (Brasse et al. 2005)

178. A – Ictal events

    Seizures or ictal events are caused by an imbalance in excitatory and inhibitory mechanisms leading to hypersynchrony and hyperexcitability. Rapid eye movement (REM) and non-rapid eye movement (NREM or non-REM) sleep are two types of sleep in mammals.
    (Dimitris et al. 2009)

179. C – 12.4 mm
    $2 mR/hr = 16 mR/hr \times e^{-.693(x/4.1\ HLVs)}$ (divide 2 mr/hr by 16mR/hr)
    $0.125 = e^{-.693(x/4.1\ HLVs)}$ (to move x out of exponent take the natural log (ln) of each side of equation)
    $\ln(0.125) = e^{-.693(x/4.1\ HLVs)}$ (remember inverse of is natural log (ln) of e)
    $-2.1 = e^{-.693(x/4.1\ HLVs)}$
    -2.1×4.1 mm HVL$/-.693 = 12.4$ mm
    *If the answer is needed in HVLs, then divide the thickness of the lead (answer) by 4.1 mm(HVL of F-18 FDG). For example, the above answer in HVL's is 12.4 mm/4.1 mm or 3.0 HVLs.
    Formula 13

180. B – Riedel's lobe

    Riedel's lobe is described as a downward tonguelike projection of the anterior edge of the right liver lobe to the right of the gallbladder, seen most frequently in women. Riedel's lobe appears to be a common variant of normal anatomy, its prevalence being dependent on age-related changes in liver size and skeletal shape.
    (Gillard et al. 1998)

181. B – Osteoblastic activity

    F-18 sodium fluoride bone uptake is similar to 99 m-Tc-diphosphonates, substitution for hydroxyl groups in hydroxyapatite, and is also dependent on new bone formation, covalently binding to the surface of new bone.
    (Brenner et al. 2012)

182. C – Endothelial function assessment

    Cold pressor testing increases myocardial blood flow (MBF) indirectly by sympathetic activation by the release of norepinephrine from cardiac sympathetic-nerve terminals, which causes vasodilation via an endothelium-dependent mechanism mediated by nitric oxide (NO).
    (Prior et al. 2005)

183. B – 20%

    According to the Response Evaluation Criteria in Solid Tumors, stable disease is described as neither partial response nor progressive disease.
    (Wahl and Jacene 2009)

184. B – Unpredictable

    The PET scan is reimbursable if used following a SPECT that was found to be inconclusive, and the PET scan must have been considered necessary in order to determine what medical or surgical intervention is required to treat the patient. A PET scan is not reimbursable if performed in addition to a emission SPECT.
    (National Coverage Determination 2012)

185. B – Calibration

    The CT system calibration is performed with a special manufacturer provided calibration phantom of known CT numbers after installation or major repair, and on an annual basis. The CT calibration is then checked daily with a water-filled cylinder to make sure that the error is not greater than 5 HU from the anticipated value of 0 HU.
    (Dilsizian et al. 2009)

186. A – Physiologic high uptake of FDG

    The glandular uptake of FDG in the breast can mask breast cancer in the postpartum woman undergoing PET scanning.
    (Kumar et al. 2009)

187. A – Deformable registration technique

    Registration techniques are divided into rigid registration methods, which only allow transformations such as translation, rotation, etc., and deformable

registration methods which register images that rigid methods are not sufficient to record.
(Hajnal et al. 2001)

188. B – Patient age 20–29 years

    PET SUV<2.5, lower lobe location, and no previous malignancy support diagnosis of benign lung disease.
    (Houseni et al. 2011)

189. A – 1.5–2 mm FWHM

    The closeness of the detectors and limited angle tomographic reconstruction results in an in-plane spatial resolution of 1.5 mm full-width-at-half-maximum (FWHM), compared with the 4.2–6.5-mm axial resolution available in commercial WB PET scanners.
    (Zaidi and Thompson 2009)

190. C – 0.3 ml

    Decay 15 mCi of F-18 60 min using formula 16A, which will give you 10.3 mCi. Obtain the concentration of 200 mCi in 4 ml using formula 17, which is 50 mCi/ml. Decay 50 mCi/ml to 3 h, which will be 16.1 mCi/ml at 1300 hours. The required dose amount is 15 mCi, and you only have 10.3 mCi at 1300 hours; therefore, 4.7 mCi is needed, which need to be obtained from the 16.1 mCi/ml concentration. To obtain the volume needed, use formula 18 and divide 4.7 mCi by 16.1 mCi/ml, which gives you 0.3 ml.
    (Formula16A, 17A and 18)

191. D – C-11 acetate

    C-11 acetate enters the tricarboxylic-acid (TCA) cycle, and because the TCA cycle activity is directly paired to myocardial oxygen consumption, clearance rates of C-11 acetate are used to evaluate regional myocardial consumption of oxygen.
    (Bengel et al. 2009)

192. A – Ionic agents cause fewer adverse reactions than nonionic medias

    An ionic compound dissolves into charged particles when it enters, e.g., blood and breaks down into cations (+) and anions (−). For every three iodine molecules present in an ionic media, one cation and one anion are produced when it enters a solution (3:2 compounds). Nonionic contrast media do not dissolve into charged particles when it enters, e.g., blood. For every three iodine molecules in a nonionic solution, one neutral molecule is produced (3:1compounds).
    (Antioch and Bockish 2009)

Answers 221

193. C – Neutropenia after cancer chemotherapy or radiotherapy

G-CSF and its analog, produced by recombinant DNA technology filgrastim, (Neupogen,Neugraf , Grastin, Religrast), is a growth factor that stimulates the production, maturation, and activation of white blood cells. In patients receiving chemotherapy, filgrastim can accelerate the recovery of neutrophils (a type of white blood cell), reducing the neutropenic phase (the time in which people are susceptible to infections).
(Mandell et al. 2010)

194. A – The basal ganglia

The basal ganglia is a core part of the brain, deep inside your skull, that helps control movement. This role in initiating and regulating motor commands becomes clearly apparent in people whose basal ganglia have been damaged, such as patients with Parkinson's disease. The largest component of the basal ganglia, the striatum, is composed of caudate and putamen.
(Christian et al. 2004)

195. B – Pleurodesis

Talc pleurodesis—talc induces an intense inflammatory reaction in pleura, resulting in chronic fibrosis that is evident on FDG-PET imaging, and may persist for years—is frequently performed in patients with malignant pleural mesothelioma to reduce pleural effusions.
(Gerbaudo et al. 2011)

196. D – Granulocyte colony-stimulating factor (G-CSF)

Erythropoietin stimulates red blood cell production and is widely employed clinically for the treatment of anemia. Thrombopoietin plays a key regulatory role in the growth and differentiation of megakaryocytes—large cells in bone marrow that fragments to produce blood platelets.
(Mandell et al. 2010)

197. A – Morphological evaluation

With increasing use of metabolic imaging with PET and PET/CT, there is a need to revise these criteria and include not only tumor size, as measured by anatomical imaging modalities like CT and MRI, but also tumor metabolism parameters, e.g., standardized uptake value (SUV).
(Wahl and Jacene 2009)

198. D – Increased membrane synthesis

The uptake of radiolabeled choline reflects the proliferative activity of membrane lipid synthesis. Tumor cells with high proliferation rate will have high uptake of choline to keep pace with increased demands for the synthesis of phospholipids (phosphatidylcholine is a major phospholipid of all membranes). (Wahl 2009)

199. B – An exercise-induced stress MPI study

N-13 NH3 is a cyclotron-produced radioisotope and has a physical half-life of 9.9 min, as opposed to Rb-82 with a very short physical half-life of 75 sec. The longer half-life of N-13 provides a larger imaging window opportunity. (Takalkar et al. 2011)

200. C – 2.9 mCi/ml

The concentration of 13 mCi/2.5 ml at 1300 hours is 5.2 mCi/ml. Decay the concentration of 5.2 mCi/ml 90 min, which will give you the final answer of 2.9 mCi/ml at 1430 hours.
(Formula 16A and 17A)

References and Suggested Readings

Abeloff DM, Armitage OJ. Abeloff's clinical oncology. 4th ed. Philadelphia, PA: Churchill Livingstone Elsevier; 2008.
ACC/AHA/SNM policy statement. Standardization of cardiac tomographic imaging. The Journal of Nuclear Medicine. 1992;33:1434–5.
Aggrenox. http://www.drugs.com/aggrenox.html. Accessed 22 Jan 2012
Al-Mallah HM, Sitek A, Moore CS, et al. Assessment of myocardial perfusion and function with PET and PET/CT. J Nucl Cardiol. 2010;17:498–513.
Andreoli TE, Bennett JC, et al. Cecil essentials of medicine. 5th ed. Philadelphia, PA: WB Saunders Company; 2001.
Antioch G, Bockish A. How to optimize CT/for PET/CT. In: Wahl R, editor. Principles and practice of PET and PET/CT. 2nd ed. Lippincott and Williams, a Walter Kluwer business: Philadelphia, PA; 2009. p. 131–8.
Bashir A, Gropler JR. Translation of myocardial metabolic imaging concepts into the clinics. Cardiol Clin. 2009;27:291–310.
Becherer A, Szabo M, Karanikas G, et al. Imaging of advanced neuroendocrine tumors with [18] F-FDOPA PET. J Nucl Med. 2004;45:1161–7.
Bengel MF, Higuchi T, Javadi SM, et al. Cardiac positron emission tomography. J Am Coll Cardiol. 2009;54:1–15.
Boellaard R. Need for standardization of F-18 FDG PET/CT for treatment response assessments. Journal of Nuclear Medicine. 2011;52:93S.
Brasse D, Kinahan EP, Lartizien C, et al. Correction methods for random coincidences in fully 3D whole-body PET: impact on data and image quality. J Nucl Med. 2005;46:859–67.
Brem FR, Petrovitch I. BSGI versus MRI for the detection of breast cancer. The Breast Journal. 2007;13(5):465–9.
Brenner IA, Koshy J, Morey J, et al. The bone scan. Semin Nucl Med. 2012;42:11–26.
Calhoun SP, Kuszyk SB, et al. Three-dimensional volume rendering of spiral CT data: theory and method. RadioGraphics. 1999;19:745–64.
Cannon B, Nedegaard J. Brown adipose tissue: function and physiological significance. Physiological Reviews. 2004;84(1):277–359.

Castellucci P, Valentina Ambrosini V, et al. PET/CT in Neuroendocrine tumors. PET Clin. Vol. 3, No. 2, April 2008.

Christian PE, Bernier DR, Langan JK. Nuclear medicine and PET: technology and techniques. 5th ed. St. Louis, MO: Mosby; 2004.

Di Carli MF, Lipton MJ, editors. Cardiac PET and PET/CT imaging. New York, NY: Springer; 2007.

Dilsizian V, Bacharach LS, Beanlands SR, et al. ASNC Imaging guidelines for nuclear cardiology procedures PET myocardial perfusion and metabolism clinical imaging. Journal of Nuclear Cardiology. 2009;16:651.

Dimitris G, Placantonakis GD, Schwartz HT. Localization in epilepsy. Neurol Clin. 2009;27:1015–30.

Dorbala S, Vangala D, Sampson U, et al. Value of vasodilator left ventricular ejection fraction reserve in evaluating the magnitude of myocardium at risk and the extent of angiographic coronary artery disease: A 82Rb PET/ CT study. J Nucl Med. 2007;48:349–58.

Early PJ, Sodee BD. Principles and practice of nuclear medicine. 2nd ed. St. Louis, MO: Mosby; 1995.

Fahey HF. Data Acquisition in PET Imaging. Journal of Nuclear Medicine Technology. 2002;30:2.

Ferri FF. Practical guide to the care of the medical patient. 7th ed. St. Louis, MO: Mosby; 2007.

Fletcher JW, Djulbegovic B, Soares HP, et al. Recommendations on the use of (18 F) FDG PET in oncology. J Nucl Med. 2008;49:480–508.

Fong Y, Saldinger PF, Akhurst T, et al. Utility of F-18 FDG positron emission tomography on selection of patients for resection of hepatic colorectal metastases. Am J Surg. 1999;178:282–7.

Gerbaudo HV, Katz IS, Nowak KA, et al. Multimodality imaging review of malignant pleural mesothelioma diagnosis and staging. PET Clin. 2011;6:275–97.

Gillard JH, Patel MC, Abrahams PH. et al Riedel's lobe of the liver: fact or fiction? Clin Anat. 1998;11(1):47–9.

Goldberger LA. Clinical electrocardiography: a simplified approach. 7th ed. St. Louis, MO: Mosby Elsevier; 2006.

Graham MM. The clinical trials network of the society of nuclear medicine. Semin Nucl Med. 2010;40:327–31.

Grant FD, Fahey FH, Packard AB, et al. Skeletal PET with 18 F-fluoride: applying new technology to an old tracer. J Nucl Med. 2008;49:68–78.

Hajnal GV, Hill LGD, Hawkes JD. Medical image registration (biomedical Engineering). Boca Raton, FL: CRC; 2001.

Hansell DM, Bankier AA, MacMahon H, et al. Fleischner society: glossary of terms for thoracic imaging. Radiology. 2008;246(3):697–722.

Hickeson M, Abikhzer G. Review of physiologic and pathophysiologic sources of fluorodeoxyglucose uptake in the chest wall on PET. PET Clin. 2011;6:339–64.

Houseni M, Chamroonrat W, Zhuang J, et al. Multimodality imaging assessment of pulmonary nodules. PET Clin. 2011;6:231–50.

Hutchings M. PET imaging in lymphoma. Expert Rev Hematol. 2009;2(3):261–76.

Inoue K, Okada K, et al. Diffuse bone marrow uptake on F-18 FDG PET in patients with myelodysplastic syndromes. Clin Nucl Med. 2006;31:721–3.

Jensen RT. Endocrine tumors of the gastrointestinaltract and pancreas. In: Kasper DL, Fauci AS, Longo DL, editors. Harrison's principles of internal medicine. 16th ed. New York: McGraw-Hill; 2005.

Jhanwar SY, Straus JD. The role of PET in Lymphoma. J Nucl Med. 2006;47:1326–34.

Kaplan AD. Advances in PET scanning. http://www.diagnosticimaging.com/pet-mr/content/article/113619/1877446.

Karakousis CG, Czerniecki JB. Diagnosis of melanoma. PET Clin. 2011;6:1–8.

Kebebew E, Greenspan FS, et al. Anaplastic thyroid carcinoma. Treatment outcome and prognostic factors. Cancer. 2005;103:1330–5.

Klein M, Cohen-Cymberknoh M, Armoni S, et al. F-18 Fluorodeoxyglucose-PET/CT Imaging of lungs in patients with cystic fibrosis. Chest. 2009;136:1220–8.

Korf J. Is brain lactate metabolized immediately after neuronal activity through the oxidative pathway? Journal of Cerebral Blood Flow & Metabolism. 2006;26:1584–6.

Kumar R, Rani N, et al. False-negative and false-positive results in FDG-PET and PET/CT in breast cancer. PET Clin. 2009;4:289–98.

Kumar V, Abbas KA. Robbins and Cotran pathologic basis of disease. 8th ed. Philadelphia, PA: Saunders Elsevier; 2010.

Lin CE, Alavi A. PET and PET/CT: a clinical guide, 2nd ed. New York, NY: Thieme; 2009.

Lombardi MH. Radiation safety in nuclear medicine. Boca Raton, FL: CRC Press; 1999.

Mach HR, Schwarz SW. Challenges for developing PET tracers: isotopes, chemistry, and regulatory aspects. PET Clin. 2010;5:131–53.

Machac J. Cardiac positron emission tomography imaging. Semin Nucl Med. 2005;35:17–36.

Madden EM. Introduction to sectional anatomy workbook and board review guide (Point). 2nd ed. Philadelphia, PA: Lippincott Williams & Wilkins; 2007.

Mandell LG, Bennett EJ, Dolin R. Mandell, Douglas, and Bennett's principles and practice of infectious diseases. 7th ed. Philadelphia, PA: Churchill Livingstone Elsevier; 2010.

Mankoff AD, Lee JH. Breast Cancer Imaging with Novel PET Tracers. PET Clin. 2009;4:371–80.

Miles AK, Blomley JKM, et al. Functional and physiological imaging in Grainger & Allison´s diagnostic radiology. Philadelphia, PA: Churchill Livingstone; 2007.

Mittra E, Quon A. Positron emission tomography/computed tomography: the current technology and applications. Radiol Clin North Am. 2009;47:147–60.

Moore LK, Dalley FA, Agur RMA. Clinically oriented anatomy. 6th ed. Philadelphia, PA: Lippincott Williams & Wilkins; 2010.

Morano NG, Seibyl JP. Technical overview of brain SPECT imaging: improving acquisition and processing of data. J Nucl Med Technol. 2003;31:191–6.

Mosci C, Iagaru A. PET/CT imaging of thyroid cancer. Clin Nucl Med. 2011;36(12):180–5.

National Coverage Determination (NCD) for PET Scans (220.6) https://www.cms.gov/medicare-coverage-database/details/ncd-details.aspx?NCDId=211&ver=2. Accessed 14 Jan 2012

National Electrical Manufacturers Association. NEMA standards publication NU 2–2007: performance measurements of positron emission tomographs. Rosslyn, VA: National Electrical Manufacturers Association; 2007.

Patton JA, Townsend WD, Brian F, Hutton FB. Hybrid imaging technology: from dreams and vision to clinical devices. Semin Nucl Med. 2009;39:247–63.

Placantonakis GD, Schwartz HT. Localization in epilepsy. Neurol Clin. 2009;27:1015–30.

Prior JO, Quinones MJ, Hernandez-Pampaloni M, et al. Coronary circulatory dysfunction in insulin resistance, impaired glucose tolerance, and type 2 diabetes mellitus. Circulation. 2005;111:2291–8.

Prokop M, Galanski M. Spiral and multislice computed tomography of the body. New York, NY: Thieme; 2003.

Rohren EM, Turkington TG, Coleman RE. Clinical application of PET in oncology. Radiology. 2004;231:305–32.

Roivainen A, Forsback S, Grönroos T, et al. Blood metabolism of [methyl-11 C]choline; implications for in vivo imaging with positron emission tomography. Eur J Nucl Med. 2000;27:25–32.

Saha GB. Basics of PET Imaging. New York, NY: Springer; 2010.

Salskov A, Tammisetti SV, et al. FLT: measuring tumor cell proliferation in vivo with positron emission tomography and 3'-Deoxy-3'-[18 F]Fluorothymidine. Semin Nucl Med. 2007;37:429–39.

Sanchez-Crespo A, Larsson SA. The influence of photon depth of interaction and non-collinear spread of annihilation photons on PET image spatial resolution. Eur J Nucl Med Mol Imaging. 2006;33:940–7.

Schilling K, Conti P, Adler L, et al. The role of positron emission mammography in breast cancer imaging and management. Applied Radiology. 2008;37:26–36.

Segall G, Delbeke D, Stabin MG, et al. SNM practice guideline for sodium 18 F-fluoride PET/CT bone scans 10. J Nucl Med. 2010;51:1813–20.

Siemens. Cyclotron solutions synthesizing the science of PET. www.siemens.com/healthcare. Accessed 13 Feb 2012

Soret M, Bacharach SL, Buvat I. Partial-volume effect in PET tumor imaging. Journal of Nuclear Medicine. 2007;48:932–45.

Sureshbabu W, Mawlawi O. PET/CT imaging artifacts. Journal of Nuclear Medicine Technology. 2005;33:156–61.

Takalkar A, Agarwal A, Adams S, et al. Cardiac assessment with PET. PET Clin. 2011;6:313–26.

Thompson K, Saab G, Birnie D, et al. Is septal glucose metabolism altered in patients with left bundle branch block and ischemic cardiomyopathy? J Nucl Med. 2006;47:1763–8.

Valk PE, Bailey DL, Townsend DW, Maisey MN, editors. Positron emission tomography: basic science and clinical practice. London: Springer; 2003.

Vallabhajosula S, Solnesn L, Vallabhajosula B. Broad overview of positron emission tomography radiopharmaceuticals and clinical applications: what is new? Semin Nucl Med. 2011;41:246–64.

Wahl RL, Buchanan JW, editors. Principles and practice of positron emission tomography. Philadelphia, PA: Lippincott Williams & Wilkins; 2002.

Wahl LR, Jacene H. From RECIST to PERCIST: evolving considerations for PET response criteria in solid tumors. The Journal of Nuclear Medicine. 2009;50(5):122s–50s.

Wahl RL. Principles and practice of PET and PET/CT. 2nd ed. Philadelphia, PA: Lippincott and Wilkins; 2009.

Wong TZ, Lacy LJ. PET of hypoxia and perfusion with 62Cu-ATSM and 62Cu-PTSM using a 62Zn/62Cu generator. AJR Am J Roentgenol. 2008;190:427–32.

Yoshinaga K, Chow BJ, Williams K, et al. What is the prognostic value of myocardial perfusion imaging using rubidium-82 positron emission tomography? J Am Coll Cardiol. 2006;48:1029.

Zaidi H, Thompson C. Evolution and developments in instrumentation for positron emission mammography. PET Clin. 2009;4:317–27.

Zaret BL, Beller GA. Clinical nuclear cardiology: state of the art and future directions. 3rd ed. Philadelphia, PA: Mosby; 2005.

Zielinski M, Hauer J, Hauer L, et al. Staging algorithm for diffuse malignant pleural mesothelioma. Interact Cardiovasc Thorac Surg. 2010;10(2):185–9.

Chapter 5
Practice Test # 4: Bonus Questions

Questions

1. What enzyme traps FDG inside the cell?
   (A) Glucoso-6-phosphatase
   (B) Hexokinase
   (C) Isomerase
   (D) GLUT-1

2. The standard uptake value (SUV) is:
   (A) The measured activity divided by the body mass
   (B) The amount of tracer needed for a particular body weight
   (C) The measured activity normalized for body weight/surface area and injected dose
   (D) The measured activity within a particular organ divided by the sampled volume

3. What should have been done to avoid the artifact illustrated in Fig. 5.1?
   (A) Administer insulin
   (B) Administer glucose
   (C) Keeping the patient warm during the uptake phase after the FDG injection
   (D) Keeping the patient cool during the uptake phase after the FDG injection

---

Answers to Test #4 begin on page 240.

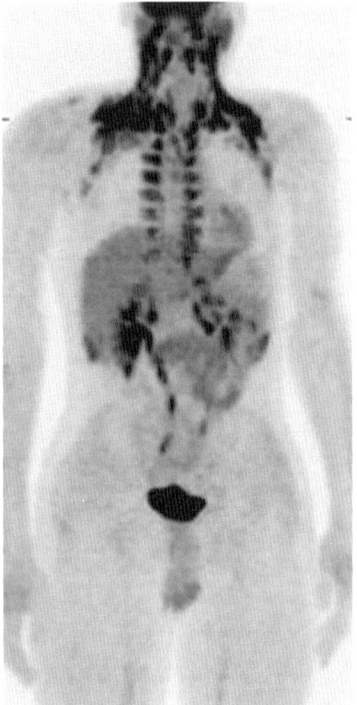

Fig. 5.1 PET/CT MIP image

4. The most common site of distant metastases in non-small cell lung cancer the most common distant metastasis is:
   (A) The liver
   (B) The spleen
   (C) The adrenal glands
   (D) The kidneys

5. The radiation absorbed dose (rad) of 350 is equal to how many grays (Gy)?
   (A) 350,000 Gy
   (B) 35,000 Gy
   (C) 3.5 Gy
   (D) 0.350 Gy

6. How can a patient's radiation exposure be minimized during FDG-PET imaging?
   (A) Shorter imaging time
   (B) Collimation
   (C) Using lead shields
   (D) Decreasing the administered FDG dose

7. The most common gastric cancer worldwide is:
   (A) Adenocarcinoma
   (B) Lymphoma
   (C) Leiomyosarcoma
   (D) Squamous cell carcinoma

8. The presented PET MIP image in Fig. 5.2 was obtained in routine PET/CT examination. Which of the following expressions can be found in the body of the radiologist's report describing the exam's findings?
   (A) Hypermetabolic activity in the infracarinal region…increased activity in both adrenal glands…
   (B) Mass at the right lung base with rim of increased activity…increased activity in the left adrenal…
   (C) The chest demonstrates several punctate hypermetabolic foci….liver metastases
   (D) The chest demonstrates several punctate hypermetabolic foci…physiologic uptake in the abdomen and pelvis

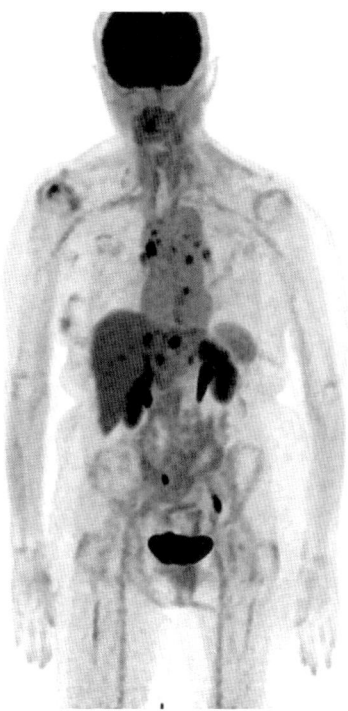

Fig. 5.2 PET/CT MIP image

9. The principal criteria by computed tomography (CT) for defining the presence of nodal metastases is:
   (A) Size
   (B) Shape
   (C) Metabolic activity
   (D) Presence of calcifications

10. An unshielded F-18 fluorodeoxyglucose dose is producing an exposure rate of 25 mR/h. How many HVLs of lead must be used to reduce the exposure rate to 1.5 mR/h? The half value layer of F-18 is 4.1 mm of lea(D)
    (A) 16.6 mm
    (B) 4 HVLs
    (C) 16.6 HVLs
    (D) 4 mm

11. FDG-PET imaging is not indicated for initial staging in what type of malignancy?
    (A) Breast cancer
    (B) Hodgkin's lymphoma
    (C) Prostate cancer
    (D) Lung cancer

12. The presented PET MIP image in Fig. 5.3 was obtained in routine PET/CT examination. Which of the following expressions can be found in the body of the radiologist's report describing the exam's findings?
    (A) Hypermetabolic activity in the infracarinal region…increased activity in both adrenal glands…
    (B) Mass at the right lung base with rim of increased activity…physiologic uptake in the bladder...
    (C) The chest demonstrates several punctate hypermetabolic foci….liver metastases
    (D) The chest demonstrates several punctate hypermetabolic foci…physiologic uptake in the abdomen and pelvis

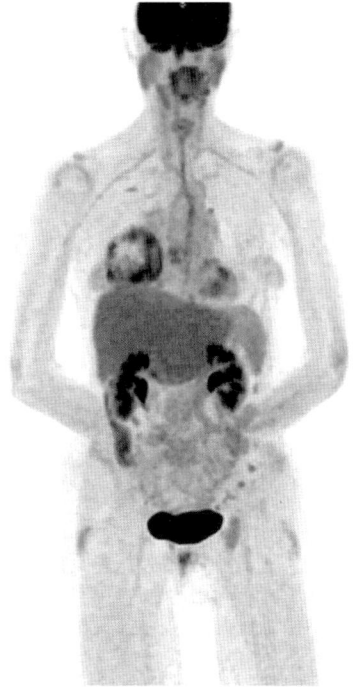

Fig. 5.3 PET/CT MIP image

13. The best FDG-PET results in epilepsy diagnosis have been obtained in what kind of condition?
    (A) Epilepsy occurring secondary to brain tumor
    (B) Epilepsy occurring secondary to arrest of neuronal migration
    (C) Epilepsy occurring secondary to mesial temporal sclerosis
    (D) Epilepsy occurring secondary to generalized brain atrophy

14. Convert 13,920 microcuries (μCi) to Curies (Ci).
    (A) 0.001392 Ci
    (B) 0.01392 Ci
    (C) 1392 Ci
    (D) 13920 Ci

15. What is the 5-year survival rate for a lung cancer patient with a Stage I disease?
    (A) 71%
    (B) 61%
    (C) 51%
    (D) 41%

16. The most common esophageal cancer worldwide is:
    (A) Squamous cell carcinoma
    (B) Adenocarcinoma
    (C) Sarcoma
    (D) Oat cell carcinoma

17. A PET imaging agent for Alzheimer's disease that gained FDA approval in 2012 is called:
    (A) Amiloride
    (B) Amyloid
    (C) Amyvid
    (D) Ambien

18. The pattern of myocardial blood flow combined with myocardial glucose metabolism in dysfunctional, but viable myocardium, is described as:
    (A) Decreased myocardial blood and decreased myocardial glucose metabolism
    (B) Decreased myocardial blood and retained myocardial glucose metabolism
    (C) Normal myocardial blood and decreased myocardial glucose metabolism
    (D) Normal myocardial blood and retained myocardial glucose metabolism

19. In the process of interpretation and analysis of PET/CT images, a study demonstrating a focal localized disease process, which could not be confirmed as being the cause of the fever of unknown origin (FUO) or malignancy, is called:
    (A) False positive
    (B) False negative
    (C) True negative
    (D) True positive

20. The pattern of FDG uptake/glucose metabolism in patients with Alzheimer disease (AD) is characterized by the presence of:
    (A) Frontal hypometabolism
    (B) Scattered foci of hypometabolism
    (C) Occipital hypometabolism
    (D) Parietotemporal hypometabolism

21. Excessive F-18 FDG metabolic activity in the thoracic expiratory musculature in patients with chronic obstructive pulmonary disease (COPD) is observed in:
    (A) The deltoid muscles
    (B) The sternocleidomastoid muscles
    (C) The trapezius muscles
    (D) The intercostal muscles

22. A Cancer facility has a protocol that implements a 14 mCi dose as the maximum activity limit of F-18 FDG that could be injected into patients. A dose of F-18 FDG is calibrated to have 14 mCi/2 ml at 16:00 h. If the patient shows up an hour early at 15:00 h for their appointment, what activity should be subtracted to make it 14 mCi at 15:00 h?
    (A) 0.6 ml
    (B) 1.4 ml
    (C) 6.4 mCi
    (D) 9.6 mCi

23. A rise in which of the following markers is suggestive of thyroid cancer recurrence in patients that have had a total thyroidectomy?
    (A) TSH (thyroid-stimulating hormone)
    (B) Tg (thyroglobulin)
    (C) T4 (thyroxin)
    (D) TRH (thyrotropin-releasing hormone)

24. Esophageal malignancy associated with Barrett's esophagus is:
    (A) Squamous Cell Carcinoma
    (B) Adenocarcinoma
    (C) Sarcoma
    (D) Oat cell carcinoma

25. What is the reason for the uptake pattern illustrated in Fig. 5.4?
    (A) Starvation
    (B) Hypoglycemia
    (C) Non-fasting state
    (D) High injected FDG dose

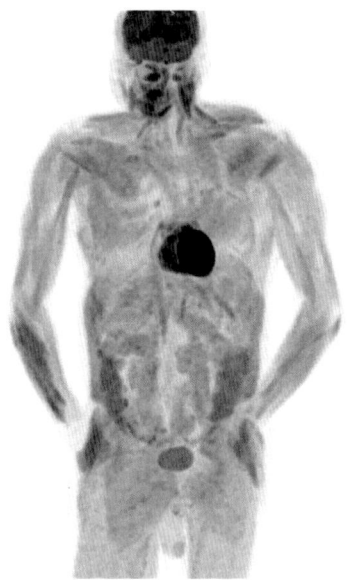

Fig. 5.4 PET MIP image

26. How many microcuries (μCi) is 5.7 megabecquerels (MBq)?
    (A) 153,900 μCi
    (B) 153.9 μCi
    (C) 21.09 μCi
    (D) 2.10900 μCi

27. Which statement describing an epileptogenic region is true?
    (A) The characteristic appearance of an epileptogenic region is a relative zonal hyperperfusion on ictal SPECT.
    (B) The characteristic appearance of an epileptogenic region is a relative zonal hypoperfusion on ictal SPECT.
    (C) The characteristic appearance of an epileptogenic region is a relative zonal hyperperfusion on interictal SPECT.
    (D) A PET brain perfusion examination is never useful in the detection of an epileptogenic region.

28. Luxury perfusion is characterized by:
    (A) Low cerebral blood flow, low oxygen extraction, and low cerebral oxidative metabolism
    (B) High cerebral blood flow, low oxygen extraction, and low cerebral oxidative metabolism
    (C) Low cerebral blood flow, high oxygen extraction, and low to normal cerebral oxidative metabolism
    (D) Low cerebral blood flow, high oxygen extraction, and high cerebral oxidative metabolism

29. Staging of a lung cancer depends on all of the following EXCEPT:
    (A) Histologic tumor grade
    (B) Size of the primary lesion
    (C) Nodal metastases
    (D) Distant metastases

30. Diaschisis is referred to as:
    (A) The dilation of lateral ventricles secondary to a lesion obstructing CSF flow
    (B) The focal increased uptake in an epileptogenic focus with hypermetabolic areas of seizure propagation
    (C) The coupled reduction in both the cortical perfusion and metabolism in an area of the brain due to a remote brain lesion
    (D) The focal decreased uptake in an epileptogenic focus in interictal SPECT imaging

31. If a lung cancer tumor size is 2 cm, without invasion of the pleura or main stem bronchus, includes a hypermetabolic lymph node in the contralateral mediastinum, and there are no distant metastases, what is the stage of the disease?
    (A) Stage II
    (B) Stage IIIA
    (C) Stage IIIB
    (D) Stage IV

32. Which thyroid cancer may produce calcitonin?
    (A) Papillary
    (B) Follicular
    (C) Medullary
    (D) Anaplastic

33. The exposure rate of an unshielded dose of F-18 FDG is 19 mR/h. If the dose is shielded with 6.0 mm of lead, what is the new exposure rate? The half value layer (HVL) of F-18 is 4.1 mm of lead (Pb).
    (A) 11.8 mR/h
    (B) 9.5 mR/h
    (C) 6.9 mR/h
    (D) 4.8 mR/h

34. Stroke penumbra is characterized by:
    (A) Low cerebral blood flow, low oxygen extraction, and low cerebral oxidative metabolism
    (B) High cerebral blood flow, low oxygen extraction, and low cerebral oxidative metabolism
    (C) Low cerebral blood flow, high oxygen extraction, and low to normal cerebral oxidative metabolism
    (D) Low cerebral blood flow, high oxygen extraction, and high cerebral oxidative metabolism

35. Focal thyroid uptake of F-18 FDG can occur with:
    (A) Graves' disease
    (B) Hashimoto thyroiditis
    (C) Endemic goiter
    (D) Autonomously functioning thyroid nodule

36. The event illustrated in the diagram in Fig. 5.5 is called:
    (A) A random event
    (B) A scatter event
    (C) A true event
    (D) An attenuated event

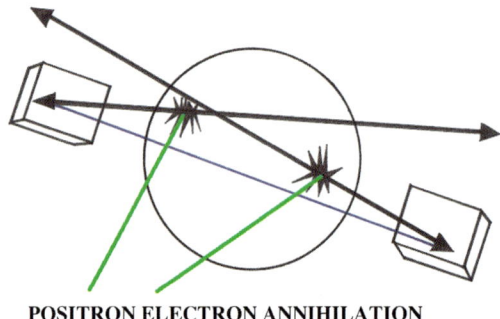

POSITRON ELECTRON ANNIHILATION

Fig. 5.5 Principle of positron emission tomography. *Illustration by Sabina Moniuszko*

37. The design of FDG molecule is based on labeling:
    (A) Carbon-2 atom in deoxyglucose with F-18
    (B) Carbon-4 atom in deoxyglucose with F-18
    (C) Carbon-2 atom in glucose with F-18
    (D) Carbon-4 atom in glucose with F-18

38. According to the PERCIST criteria for treatment response evaluation, the following requirements of PET scans performance have to be met EXCEPT:
    (A) Patients should have been fasting for at least 4–6 h
    (B) The measured serum glucose level must be less than 200 mg/dL
    (C) A baseline PET scan should be obtained at 50–70 min after tracer injection
    (D) The follow-up scan should be obtained within 30 min of the baseline scan

39. All of the following are examples of thyroid cancer EXCEPT:
    (A) Papillary
    (B) Hurthle cell
    (C) Anaplastic
    (D) Adenocarcinoma

40. A seizure can be classified as:
    (A) Generalized
    (B) Atrophic
    (C) Post-hemorrhagic
    (D) Spontaneous

41. Figure 5.6 presents the schematic drawing of the cardiac conduction system. The label B represents the:
    (A) Left bundle branch
    (B) Right bundle branch
    (C) Sinoatrial node
    (D) Atrioventricular node

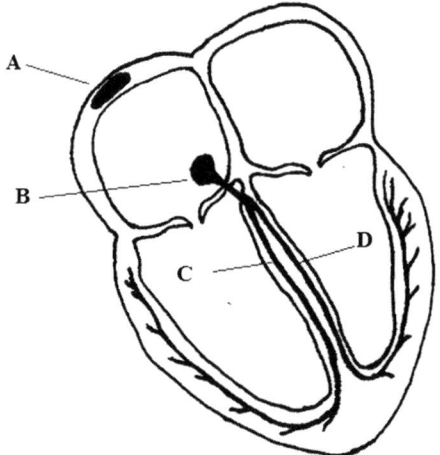

Fig. 5.6 Cardiac conduction system. *Illustration by Sabina Moniuszko*

42. The most common cancer in men is:
    (A) Lung cancer
    (B) Skin cancer
    (C) Lymphoma
    (D) Prostate cancer

43. A 13 mCi dose of F-18 FDG is calibrated for 11:00 A.M. If the patient is 15 min late, how many milicuries of F-18 FDG will be remaining at 11:15 A.M?
    (A) 14 mCi
    (B) 12 mCi
    (C) 6.5 mCi
    (D) 5.7 mCi

44. The average range of positrons in human tissue for the US Food and Drug Administration (FDA)-approved radiopharmaceuticals is about:
    (A) 0.6–4 mm
    (B) 4–5 mm
    (C) 5–10 mm
    (D) 1 cm

45. Estimates of absorbed organ doses as well as effective doses from nuclear medicine procedures are available from all of the following sources EXCEPT:
    (A) Patient information booklets
    (B) Nuclear medicine textbooks
    (C) Food and Drug Administration-required inserts
    (D) (D)SNM procedure guidelines

46. The biological tests establish the radiopharmaceutical:
    (A) Apyrogenicity
    (B) Purity
    (C) Chemistry
    (D) Osmolality

47. To verify that the survey meter has not been contaminated during the preceding operation the technologist should check the:
    (A) Background counting rate
    (B) Survey meter battery
    (C) Survey meter constancy of response
    (D) Survey meter accuracy of response

48. The tricuspid valve separates the:
    (A) Left atrium from the left ventricle
    (B) Right atrium from the right ventricle
    (C) Left ventricle from the aorta
    (D) Right ventricle from the pulmonary artery

49. An unshielded package containing F-18 FDG is reading 22 mR/h at its surface. If the package is shielded with 9.0 mm of lead, what will be the new exposure rate? Half value layer of F-18 is 4.1 mm of lead (Pb).
    (A) 4.8 mR/h
    (B) 5.5 mR/h
    (C) 11 mR/h
    (D) 16 mR/h

50. Figure 5.7 presents diagrammatic representation of end-systolic (dashed line) and end-diastolic (solid line) shape of left ventricle cineangiogram. The drawing A represents normal left ventricle wall motion. What left ventricle abnormality corresponds to the drawing B?
    (A) Hypokinetic left ventricle
    (B) Hyperkinetic left ventricle
    (C) Akinetic left ventricle
    (D) Dyskinetic left ventricle

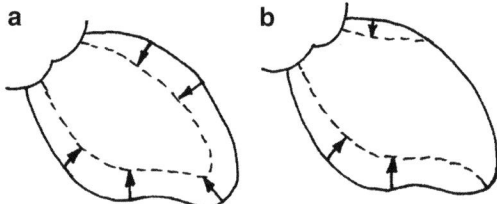

Fig. 5.7 Left ventricle cineangiogram. *Illustration by Sabina Moniuszko*

Answers

1. B – Hexokinase

   Hexokinase phosphorylates FDG, which results in intracellular trapping.
   (Lin and Alavi 2009)

2. C – The measured activity normalized for body weight/surface area and injected dose

   SUV is a simple way of determining activity in PET imaging, most commonly used in Flourodeoxyglucose (FDG) imaging. It is also known as the dose uptake ratio (DUR).
   (Lin and Alavi 2009)

3. C – Keeping the patient warm during the uptake phase after the FDG injection

   The MIP image demonstrates intense FDG uptake in brown fat, and excessive metabolism in the neck and paraspinal area. Keeping the patient warm and comfortable prior to injection can reduce such activity.
   (Lin and Alavi 2009)

4. C – The adrenal glands

   The most common types of NSCLC are squamous cell carcinoma, large cell carcinoma, and adenocarcinoma, but there are several other types that occur less frequently.
   (Jadver and Parker 2005)

5. C – 3.5 Gy
   (Formula 7 C)

6. D – Decreasing the administered FDG dose

   Decreasing the administered FDG dose decreases the patient's radiation exposure.
   (Jadver and Parker 2005)

7. A – Adenocarcinoma

   Adenocarcinoma of the stomach is a common cancer of the digestive tract worldwide, although it is uncommon in the USA.
   (Jadver and Parker 2005)

Answers 241

8. C – The chest demonstrates several punctate hypermetabolic foci....liver metastases

   Images obtained through the chest demonstrate several punctuate focal areas of hypermetabolic activity...images obtained of the abdomen show several punctate hypermetabolic foci within the liver ...are consistent with liver metastases...mildly increased activity in the right shoulder likely due to arthritic changes.
   (Radiology report frag)

9. A – Size

   Lymph nodes bigger than 1 cm are considered malignant, smaller lymph nodes that harbor cancer can be possibly unnoticed, and larger nodes can be a source of false positives. In large nodes, irregular borders may also suggest malignant spread.
   (Mittra and Quon 2009)

10. B – 4 HVLs $1.5 mR/h = 25 mR/h \times e^{-0.693(X/4.1HVLs)}$ (divide 1.5 mR/h by 25 mR/h) $0.06 = e^{-0.693(X/4.1HVLs)}$ (to move x out of exponent take natural log (ln) of each side of equation).
    $\ln(0.06) = e^{-0.693(X/4.1HVLs)}$ (remember inverse ofis natural log (ln) of e) -2.8×4.1 mm HVL/$-0.693 = 16.6$ mm.

    The answer is required in HVLs; therefore, 16.6 mm/4.1 mm(HVL of F-18FDG) = 4 HVLs.
    (Formula 13)

11. C – Prostate cancer

    FDG-PET imaging is not indicated for initial staging of prostate cancer.
    (Wahl 2009)

12. B – Mass at the right lung base with rim of increased activity...physiologic uptake in the bladder....

    Physiologic uptake is noted in the neck with asymmetric increased activity in prevertebral muscles on the right...Mass is noted at the posterior right lung base with the rim of increased activity...
    (Radiology report frag)

13. C – Epilepsy occurring secondary to mesial temporal sclerosis

    The best results have been obtained in epilepsy of originating in the temporal lobe origin corresponding to mesial temporal sclerosis, with evident abnormalities evident in as many as 90% of the surgical candidates.
    (Jadver and Parker 2005)

14. B – 0.01392 Ci
    (Formula 7A)

15. B – 61%
    Stage 1 lung cancer life expectancy can vary considerably among different people and depends on lung cancer type and location, age, sex, general health, etc.
    (Jadver and Parker 2005)

16. A – Squamous cell carcinoma
    Squamous cell carcinoma is responsible for 95% of all esophageal cancers worldwide.
    In the USA the incidence of adenocarcinoma of the distal esophagus and gastroesophageal junction has progressively increased since 1970 and, currently, it accounts for more than 50% of all new cases of esophageal cancer.
    (Jadver and Parker 2005)

17. C – Amyvid (solanezumab) binds to amyloid plaques, which are a telltale sign of Alzheimer's disease, making them detectable using a PET scan.
    (Lilly 2012)

18. B – Decreased myocardial blood and retained myocardial glucose metabolism
    Increased glucose uptake in areas with reduced blood flow at rest (perfusion–metabolism mismatch) on PET has been used successfully for diagnosing hibernating myocardium in patients with left ventricular dysfunction. Although the risk of bypass surgery is increased in these individuals, the high mortality of these patients, given medical therapy, may warrant an aggressive attempt to revascularize the coronary arteries.
    (Zaret and Beller 2005)

19. A – False positive
    False negative (FN)—reported as normal PET study when a focal inflammation or malignancy was subsequently detected by other diagnostic/therapeutic means.
    (Munro 2005)

20. D – Parietotemporal hypometabolism
    Envelopment of the frontal lobe in advanced cases is noted but with relative sparing of the motor cortices.
    (Mittra 2009)

21. D – The intercostal muscles
    Consequences of the compounded workload of the expiratory muscles in the thoracic and abdominal expiratory musculature, including the intercostal, subscapular, rectus abdominis, and abdominal oblique muscles, large and quite symmetric areas of excessive metabolic activity, are observed on FDG-PET examination.
    (Hickeson and Abikhzer 2011)

22. C – 6.4 mCi

    Pre-calibrate the given 14 mCi of F-18 FDG to 1 h, which is 20.4 mCi at 15:00 h. 14 mCi of FDG needs to be subtracted from 20.4 mCi, which will provide an answer of 6.4 mCi. Given that, 14 mCi/2 ml should be left alone and not included in the problem. One can solve this problem by obtaining a concentration of 14 mCi/2 ml, and then following proper steps; however, it adds unnecessary calculations.
    (Formula 16B)

23. B – Tg (thyroglobulin)

    Thyroglobulin is a protein produced by and used entirely within the thyroid gland. Its levels in the blood can be used as a tumor marker for certain types of thyroid cancer.
    (Mazzaferri et al. 2003)

24. B – Adenocarcinoma

    Barrett's esophagus is a condition in which the cells of your lower esophagus become damaged, usually from repeated exposure to stomach acid.
    (Jadver and Parker 2005)

25. C – Non-fasting state

    In a non-fasting state, increased levels of insulin result in skeletal muscle uptake.
    (Wahl 2009)

26. B – 153.9 µCi

    Since 1 GBq=27 mCi, convert 5.7 MBq to 0.0057 GBq and multiply by 27 to obtain which will give you 0.1539 mCi. Multiply 0.1539 mCi by 1,000 to obtain 153.9 µCi.
    Another way: 5.7 MBq/37 mCi/MBq=0.154 mCi, then multiply by 1,000 to get 154 uCi.
    (Formula 7B)

27. A – The characteristic appearance of the epileptogenic region is a relative zonal hyperperfusion on ictal SPECT.
    (Jadver and Parker 2005)

28. B – High cerebral blood flow, low oxygen extraction, and low cerebral oxidative metabolism

    In the luxury perfusion area, the cerebral blood flow is increased, but the tissue oxygen extraction ability and cerebral oxidative metabolism are decreased.
    (Jadver and Parker 2005)

29. A – Histologic tumor grade

    Staging of lung cancer depends on the size of the primary lesion, and nodal and distal metastasis.
    (Jadver and Parker 2005)

30. C – The coupled reduction in both the cortical perfusion and metabolism in an area of the brain due to a remote brain lesion

    Diaschisis is referred to as the reduction in both the cortical perfusion and metabolism in an area of the brain due to a remote brain lesion.
    (Jadver and Parker 2005)

31. C – Stage IIIB

    Stage 3A lung cancer is considered a "locally advanced" cancer, meaning the tumor has not spread to distant regions of the body but has spread to lymph nodes on the same side of the body as the tumor.
    (Jadver and Parker 2005)

32. C – Medullary

    Medullary thyroid cancer is a form of thyroid cancer which originates from the parafollicular cells, which produce the hormone calcitonin. Calcitonin regulates calcium levels and is involved in the process of bone building.
    (Hu et al. 2008)

33. C – 6.9 mR/h

    The Half value layer (HVL) of lead (PB) for F-18 FDG is 4.1 mm. This means that the exposure rate of F-18 FDG is reduced to half of its original intensity by placing 4.1 mm of lead (Pb) in front of it.
    (Formula 13)

34. C – Low cerebral blood flow, high oxygen extraction, and low to normal cerebral oxidative metabolism

    In stroke penumbra, the cerebral blood flow is decreased, but the tissue oxygen extraction capability is increased. This tissue is still viable, with low to normal cerebral oxidative metabolism.
    (Jadver and Parker 2005)

35. D – Autonomously functioning thyroid nodule

    Focal thyroid uptake can occur with autonomously functioning thyroid nodules and thyroid malignancies. A focal area of F-18 FDG uptake has a 30–50% chance of being cancer, most likely due to primary cancer of the thyroid, and patients with focal uptake should be further evaluated due to a higher risk of the result being associated with malignancy.
    (Chen et al. 2007)

Answers   245

36. A – A random event

    A random event occurs when two photons, which are not arising from the same annihilation event, are recorded by two opposite detectors within the coincidence time-window.
    (Wahl 2009)

37. A – Carbon-2 atom in deoxyglucose with F-18

    As a glucose analog, FDG enters the cell membrane using the same transporters as glucose.

    FDG is phosphorylated by hexokinase to FDG-6-phosphate, but in contrast to glucose, FDG-6-phosphate is not metabolized further and is essentially trapped in cells.
    (Vallabhajosula et al. 2011)

38. D – The follow-up scan should be obtained within 30 min of the baseline scan

    The follow-up scan performed on the same PET scanner with the same injected dose +/− 20% of radioactivity should be obtained within 15 min (but always 50 min or later after tracer injection) of the baseline scan.
    (Wahl and Jacene 2009)

39. D – Adenocarcinoma

    Thyroid cancers can be calcified according to their histopathologic characteristics. The following variants can be distinguished: papillary, follicular, medullary, and anaplastic thyroid cancer.
    (Thyroid cancer 2012)

40. A – Generalized

    A seizure is categorized according to whether the course of the seizure within the brain is localized (partial- or focal-onset seizures) or distributed (generalized seizure). Partial seizures are further divided on by the extent to which consciousness is affected.
    (Wahl 2009)

41. D – Atrioventricular node

    AV node is a small mass of specialized cardiac muscle fibers, located in the wall of the right atrium of the heart that receives heartbeat impulses from the sinoatrial node and directs them to the walls of the ventricles.
    (Goldberger 2006)

42. D – Prostate cancer

    Prostate cancer is more common among African-American men than men of other racial and ethnic groups, but medical experts do not know why. More men die from lung cancer than any other type of cancer.
    (CDC 2012)

43. B – 12 mCi
    (Formula 16A)

44. A – 0.6–4 mm

    In a PET camera of diameter 1 m and active transaxial FOV of 0.6 m, this results in a positional inaccuracy of 2–3 mm.
    (Alessi et al. 2010)

45. A – Patient information booklets

    For PET/CT it is important to include effective dose and organ dose estimates for both the radiopharmaceutical and the CT component of the examination.
    (Christian et al. 2004)

46. A – Apyrogenicity

    The physicochemical tests are used to determine the chemistry, purity, and the integrity of a formulation, while the biological tests ascertain the sterility and apyrogenicity of the radiopharmaceutical.
    (Vallabhajosula et al. 2010)

47. A – Background counting rate

    The background exposure should be measured daily in an area out-of-the-way from radioactive sources within the nuclear medicine facility.
    (Zanzonico 2008)

48. B – Right atrium from the right ventricle

    The tricuspid valve—a valve of three flaps—separates the right lower heart chamber (the right ventricle) from the right upper heart chamber (right atrium) and prevents reflux of blood from the right ventricle to the right atrium.
    (Andreoli et al. 2001)

49. A – 4.8 mR/h
    (Formula 13)

50. C – Akinetic left ventricle

    Segmental akinesis—seen there on the anteroapical surfaces—refers to absent contractile function of the left ventricle, e.g., after a heart attack. The heart muscle in the distribution of the involved vessels is often akinetic due to the lack or diminished blood supply.
    (Andreoli et al. 2001)

References and Suggested Readings

Alessi A, Farrell MB, Grabher JB, et al. Nuclear cardiology study guide. Reston, VA: SNM; 2010.

Andreoli TE, Bennett JC, et al. Cecil essentials of medicine. 5th ed. Philadelphia, PA: WB Saunders Company; 2001.

CDC. http://www.cdc.gov/Features/dsMenTop10Cancers/. Accessed 20 Feb 2012

Chen W, Li G, Parsons M, et al. Clinical significance of incidental focal versus diffuse thyroid uptake on FDG-PET imaging. PET Clin. 2007;2:321–9.

Christian PE, Bernier DR, Langan JK. Nuclear medicine and PET: technology and techniques. 5th ed. St. Louis, MO: Mosby; 2004.

Goldberger LA. Clinical electrocardiography: a simplified approach. 7th ed. St. Louis, MO: Mosby Elsevier; 2006.

Hickeson M, Abikhzer G. Review of physiologic and pathophysiologic sources of fluorodeoxyglucose uptake in the chest wall on PET. PET Clin. 2011;6(3):339–64.

Hu MI, Vassilopoulou-Sellin R, Lustig R, Lamont JP. Thyroid and parathyroid cancers. In: Pazdur R, Wagman LD, Camphausen KA, Hoskins WJ, editors. Cancer management: a multidisciplinary approach. 11th ed. Manhasset, NY: CMP Medica; 2008.

Jadver H, Parker JA. Clinical PET and PET/CT. London: Springer; 2005.

Lilly.http.newsroom.lilly.com. Accessed 9 April 2012

Lin CE, Alavi A. PET and PET/CT. A clinical guide. 2nd ed. New York, NY: Thieme; 2009.

Mazzaferri EL, Robbins RJ, Spencer CA, et al. A consensus report of the role of serum thyroglobulin as a monitoring method for low-risk patients with papillary thyroid carcinoma. J Clin Endocrinol Metab. 2003;88(4):1433–41.

Mittra E, Quon A. Positron emission tomography/computed tomography: the current technology and applications. Radiol Clin North Am. 2009;47:147–60.

Munro HB. Statistical methods for health care research. 5th ed. Philadelphia, PA: Lippincott Williams & Wilkins; 2005.

Thyroid cancer. http://en.wikipedia.org/wiki/Thyroid_cancer. Accessed 15 Feb 2012

Vallabhajosula S, Killeen R, Osborne J. Altered biodistribution of radiopharmaceuticals: role of radiochemical/pharmaceutical purity, physiological, and pharmacologic factors. Semin Nucl Med. 2010;40:220–41.

Vallabhajosula S, Solnesn L, Vallabhajosula B. Broad overview of positron emission tomography radiopharmaceuticals and clinical applications: what is new? Semin Nucl Med. 2011;41:246–64.

Wahl LR, Jacene H. From RECIST to PERCIST: evolving considerations for PET response criteria in solid tumors. J Nucl Med. 2009;50 Suppl 1:122s–50s.

Wahl RL. Principles and practice of PET and PET/CT. 2nd ed. Philadelphia, PA: Lippincott Williams & Wilkins; 2009.

Zanzonico P. Routine quality control of clinical nuclear medicine instrumentation: a brief review. J Nucl Med. 2008;49:1114–31.

Zaret BL, Beller GA. Clinical nuclear cardiology: state of the art and future directions. 3rd ed. Philadelphia, PA: Mosby; 2005.

Appendix A
Numbers and Formulas

Radiation Safety

The table below describes common radiation exposure limits for occupational and general public.

Occupational exposure limits	
Rem (Roentgen equivalent man) Sv (Sievert)	
Whole body	5 rem/year (0.05 Sv)
Skin or any extremity	50 rem/year (0.5 Sv)
Any organ or tissue	50 rem/year (0.5 Sv)
Lens of eye	15 rem/year (0.15 Sv)
Fetus of radiation worker	0.5 rem/year (0.005 Sv)
General public exposure limits	
Whole body	0.1 rem/year (0.001 Sv)

(Steves and Wells 2004)

Department of Transportation (DOT) Labels

Department of Transportation regulates the shipment of the radioactive materials; therefore, appropriate labels must be affixed to radioactive shipment packages.

Class	Exposure rate at the package surface cannot exceed (mR/h)	Exposure rate at 1 meter from the package cannot exceed (mR/h) Transportation Index (TI)
Radioactive I (white)	0.5	No detectable radiation
Radioactive II (yellow)	0.5–50	1 mR/hr
Radioactive III (yellow)	50–200	10 mR/hr

(Steves and Wells 2004)

Radiation Signs

- Caution: Radioactive Materials:
    - Posted in area where radioactive materials are stored and exceed the limit of 2 millirem within any given hour or 0.02 millisievert within any given hour.
- Caution: Radiation Area:
    - Posted where one can receive more than 5 mR/hr (0.05 millisievert) at 30 centimeters (cm)
- Caution: High Radiation Area:
    - Posted where one can receive more than 100 millirem per hour (1 millisievert) at 30 cm
    - Grave Danger: Very High Radiation Area:
    - Posted in area where one can receive more than 500 rads (5grays) in 1 hour at 1 meter from radiation source

(Steves and Wells 2004)

Physical Properties of Commonly Used Biological PET Radioisotopes

Isotope	Half-life (minutes)	Maximum energy (MeV)*	Range (mm) in H_2O*	Decay product
Fluorine-18	110	0.635	2.4	Oxygen-18
Carbon-11	20	0.96	4.1	Boron-11
Oxygen-15	2	1.72	8.2	Nitrogen-15
Nitrogen-13	10	1.19	5.4	Carbon-13
Rubidium-82	1.25	3.36	16.5	Krypton-82

*Theoretical maximum. Actual measured activities of above isotopes are about 5,000 times lower because of unavoidable dilution with the stable element
*Maximum linear range
(Wahl 2009)

Characteristics of the Scintillation Detectors for PET

Scintillation detector Material	Effective density or stopping power	Energy resolution or light output	Decay time or dead time
BGO Bismuth germinate Favored by GE	Highest	Lowest	Long
GSO Gadolinium orthosilicate Favored by Philips	Lower then LSO	Very High	Very Short
LSO or LYSO Lutetium orthosilicate or lutetium yttrium orthosilicate	High	High	Very Short

(continued)

Scintillation detector Material	Effective density or stopping power	Energy resolution or light output	Decay time or dead time
NaI (Tl)* Thallium-doped sodium iodide	Lowest	Highest	Long

Effective density—detector's ability to stop annihilation photon. Shorter the distance traveled by annihilation photon prior to deposition of the energy within the detector, the more preferable it is. Effective density determines scanner sensitivity; therefore, high effective density is more suitable.

Energy resolution—number of photon yield by each incident photon interaction with the detector. Higher energy resolution is preferable. Energy resolution determines energy and spatial resolution.

Decay time—the time required to process each scintillation event within the detector. Shorter decay time is desirable. Decay time determines dead time and random coincidences rate.

*Hygroscopic and no longer used in PET
(Lin and Alavi 2009)

Quality Control of Dose Calibrator

The quality control of dose calibrator, type of the test, and frequency and description of test are given in the following table.

Type of test	Rate of recurrence	Reason of the test
Constancy	Daily before use	To check consistency of the source of known activity from day to day
Linearity	Quarterly	To check ability of Dose calibrator to measure wide range of activity from millicurie (mCi) to microcurie (uCi) amounts
Accuracy	Annually	To check ability of Dose Calibrator to measure different level gamma energy (100–500 keV)
Geometry	At installation	Test for measurement of activity as the volume of radioactive source changes

*All test should be performed after installation of the new equipment, after adjustment and after repair
(Steves and Wells 2004)

Unit Conversions

A. Conversion between Ci (curie) to mCi (millicurie) to uCi (microcurie), and GBq (gigabecquerel) to MBq (megabecquerel) to kBq (kilobecquerel)
   - 1 Ci = 1,000 mCi = 1,000,000 uCi
   - 1 GBq = 1,000 MBq = 1,000,000 kBq

B. Conversion between Ci to GBq
   - 1 Ci = 37 GBq = 37,000 MBq = 37,000000 kBq
   - 1 GBq = 0.027 Ci or 27 mCi or 27,000 uCi
   - 1 Bq = 2.7×10^{-11} Ci

C. Conversion between rad (radiation absorbed dose) and gray (Gy)
   - 1 Gy = 100 rad = 100,000 mrad
   - 1 rad = 0.01 Gy = 10 mGy

D. Conversion of Sievert and rem (roentgen equivalent man)
   - 1 Sv = 100 rem
   - 1 rem = 0.01 Sv

E. Conversion between pound and kilogram
   - 1 lb = 0.45 kg
   - Kg = 2.2 lb

F. Conversion of length
   - 1 ft = 12 in. = 30.5 cm

(Wells and Martha 1999)

Calculation of Percent Error or Percent Difference

A. Percentage error or percentage difference
   - Percent error or percent difference = $\left| \dfrac{\text{Expected} - \text{Actual}}{\text{Expected}} \right| \times 100\%$

B. Correction factor
   - Correction factor = $\dfrac{\text{Expected activity}}{\text{Actual activity}}$

(Wells and Martha 1999)

Net Counts

Net counts = Gross counts − Background counts

(Wells and Martha 1999)

Standard Deviation of Series of Values

- $SD = \sqrt{\dfrac{\sum(n - \bar{n})^2}{N - 1}}$
    - Σ = symbol of sum, meaning value following this needs to be summed
    - $Mean = \dfrac{Sum\ of\ all\ values}{Total\ number\ of\ values}$
    - $\bar{n}$ = mean of value
    - n = individual value
    - N = total number of values
    - N–1 = degree of freedom

(Wells and Martha 1999)

How to Convert Counts Per Minute (cpm) to Disintegration Per Minute (dpm) Using Well Counter Efficiency

- $dpm = \dfrac{Gross\ cpm - Background\ cpm}{Efficiency\ expressed\ as\ decimal}$
    - divide given efficiency in % by 100 to obtain decimal

(Wells and Martha 1999)

Inverse Square Law

- $(I_1)(D_1)^2 = (I_2)(D_2)^2$
    - I_1 = Intensity at original distance D_1
    - I_2 = Intensity at newer distance D_2

(Wells and Martha 1999)

How to Calculate Change in Exposure Rate Due to Shielding

- $I = I_O \times e^{-(0.693)(x/HVL)}$
    - I = exposure rate being calculated
    - I_O = Original exposure rate
    - e = 2.718 constant know as Euler's number
    - x = thickness of the shielding material
    - HVL = half value layer for given shielding material

(Wells and Martha 1999)

Effective Half-life

- $T_e = \dfrac{T_P \times T_b}{T_P + T_b}$
  - T_e = effective half-life
  - T_P = physical half-life
  - T_b = biological half-life

(Wells and Martha 1999)

Well Counter Efficiency

- $\%\text{Efficiency} = \dfrac{\text{Counts per unit of time (cpm or cps)}}{(\text{Disintegration per unit time})(\text{Mean number per disintegration})} \times 100\%$

(Wells and Martha 1999)

Decay Calculation Using Half-life

A. $A_t = A_0 \times e^{-0.693 \times (t/t_{1/2})}$
  - A_t = activity at specific time
  - A_0 = original activity
  - e = Euler's number (2.718….) which remains constant in equation
  - t = elapsed time
  - $t_{1/2}$ = half-life

B. Use same formula as above for pre-calibration
- $A_t = A_0 \times e^{-0.693 \times (t/t_{1/2})}$
  - A_t = activity at time t (calibration time)
  - A_0 = activity at time 0 (pre-calibration time)

(Wells and Martha 1999)

How to Obtain Concentration and Specific Activity

A. Specific concentration
  - Specific concentration = $\dfrac{Activity}{Volume}$

B. Specific activity
  - Specific activity = Concentration × Volume

(Wells and Martha 1999)

How to Calculate Specific Volume

$$\text{Volume} = \frac{\text{Activity desired}}{\text{Specific concentration}} \quad or \quad \frac{\text{What you want}}{\text{What you have}}$$

(Wells and Martha 1999)

Pediatric Dose Calculation

A. Clark's formula (weight)
- $\text{Clark's formula} = \dfrac{(\text{Child's weight in lb})(\text{Adult dose})}{150 lb}$

B. Webster's formula (age)
- $\text{Webster's formula} = \dfrac{\text{Age}(\text{Years}) + 1}{\text{Age} + 7} \times \text{Adult dosage}$

C. Young's formula (age)
- $\text{Young's formula} = \dfrac{\text{Age}(\text{Years})}{\text{Age} + 12} \times \text{Adult dosage}$

(Steves and Wells 2004)

Cancers and Indications Eligible for Entry in the National Oncologic PET Registry (NOPR)

Cancer and indication covered for initial and subsequent treatment strategy	Cancer and indication that are covered for initial treatment but subsequent treatment is only covered with entry in the NOPR	Cancer and indication that are only covered upon certain condition (otherwise not covered) for initial treatment and subsequent treatment is covered (not eligible for entry in NOPR)
Lip, oral cavity, and pharynx	Stomach, Small intestine, Anus, Liver and intrahepatic bile ducts, Pancreas, Retroperitoneum and peritoneum	Melanoma of skin (B)
Esophagus		Female breast (B,C)
Colon		Male breast (B,C)
Nasal cavity, eat, and sinuses	Lung, small cell, Pleura, Thymus, heart, mediastinum, Bone/cartilage, Connective/other soft tissue,	Cervix
Larynx		
Lung, non-small cell	Non-melanoma of skin, Kaposi's sarcoma	
Ovary	Uterus, unspecified, Placenta, Uterus, body, Uterine adnexa, Other and unspecified female genitalia, Testis	
Lymphoma		
Myeloma	Penis and other male genitalia, Bladder	
	Kidney and other urinary tract, Eye, Primary brain, Other endocrine glands and related structures, Metastatic cancer/unknown primary, Other and unspecified nervous system, Neuroendocrine tumors and All other solid tumors	
Cancer that is not covered under initial treatment, but subsequent treatment is covered with entry in NOPR		
Prostate		
Cancer and indication that are covered for initial treatment but subsequent treatment is either covered or covered by submission to NOPR (see footnote D)		
Thyroid cancer (D)		

Cancers and Indications Eligible for Entry in the NOPR

Cancer and indication that are not eligible for submission in NOPR for neither initial nor subsequent treatment

Leukemia

All other cancers not listed in here

A. Some Medicare contractors include anal cancer in their local coverage of "colorectal cancer"; for PET facilities served by those carriers, PET for subsequent treatment evaluation of anal cancer would be a covered indication.

B. PET is non-covered for initial staging for auxiliary lymph nodes in patients with breast cancer and of regional lymph nodes in patients with melanoma, but is covered for detection of distant metastatic disease in high-risk patients with breast cancer or melanoma.

C. PET is non-covered for "diagnosis" of breast cancer to evaluate a suspicious breast mass. However, PET is covered for initial treatment strategy evaluation of a patient with axillary nodal metastasis of unknown primary origin or in a patient with a paraneoplastic syndrome potentially caused by an occult breast cancer.

D. PET is non-covered for "diagnosis" of cervical cancer. However, PET is covered for initial staging of cervical cancer.

E. To qualify as a covered indication for subsequent treatment strategy evaluation, thyroid cancer must be of follicular cell origin and been previously treated by thyroidectomy and radioiodine ablation and the patient must have a serum thyroglobulin > 10ng/ml and negative whole-body I-131 scan. Patients who do not qualify for this covered indication (e.g., because tumor is of other than follicular cell origin, the thyroglobulin is not elevated, or I-131 whole-body imaging was not performed or is positive) can be entered on NOPR

(http://www.cancerpetregistry.org)

Radiation Exposure of the Commonly Performed Radiological Procedures

Radiological Procedure	Effective dose in millisievert (mSv)
Chest X-Ray	0.1
Chest CT (standard)	7.0
Chest CT (R/O PE)	15
Bone scan	5.3
Lung scan (VQ)	2.2
PET/CT Low-dose protocol	
Topogram	0.2
Low-dose CT	1.3
PET with 10mCi F-18 FDG	7.0
Total exposure	8.5
PET/CT High-quality protocol	
Topogram	0.2
Diagnostic CT with contrast	17.6
PET with 10mCi F-18 FDG	7.0
Total exposure	24.8

Above radiation exposure were derived from set protocol and may very as scan parameters change.
(Brix et al. 2005)

Appendix B
Commonly used Abbreviations and Symbols in Nuclear Medicine

AAA	Abdominal aortic aneurysm
ABC	Airway, breathing, circulation
ABG	Arterial blood gases
ABW	Adjusted body weight
AC	Attenuation corrected
A/C	Assist control ventilation
ACD	Acid-citrate-dextrose
ACE	Angiotensin-converting enzyme
ACLS	Advance cardiac life support
ACS	Acute coronary syndrome
ACTH	Adrenocorticotropic hormone
AD	Alzheimer's disease
ADC	Analog-to-digital converter
ADL	Activities of daily living
AED	Automated external defibrillator
AF	Atrial fibrillation
AFB	Acid fast bacilli
AFL	Atrial flutter
AIPES	Association of imaging producers and equipment Suppliers
AICD	Automatic Implantable Cardiac defibrillator
AKA	Above knee amputation
AKA	Also known as
ALDN	Axillary lymph nodes dissection
ALS	Advance life support
ALI	Annual limit on intake
AMA	Against medical advice
AMI	Acute myocardial infarction

AMV	Assisted mechanical ventilation
ANDA	Abbreviated new drug application
ANL	Argonne national laboratory
Angio.	Angiogram; angiography
ANSI	American national standards institute
AO	Aorta
APC	Atrial premature contraction
Approx.	Approximately; approximated
APUD	Amine precursor uptake and decarboxylation
AR	Androgen receptor
ARF	Acute renal failure
ARS	Acute radiation syndrome
ASA	Acetylsalicylic Acid (Aspirin)
ASAP	As soon as possible
ASNC	American society of nuclear cardiology
ASTM	American standards for testing and materials
ATR	Advanced test reactor
AV	Arteriovenous
A-V	Arterioventricular
AVM	Arteriovenous malformation
AVN	Avascular necrosis
AVR	Aortic valve replacement
Ax	Axilla, axillary
BASIC	Beginner's all-purpose symbolic instruction code
BaF2	Barium fluoride
BBB	Bundle branch block
BBB	Blood–brain barrier
BE	Barium enema
BERT	Background equivalent radiation time
BG	Blood glucose
BGO	Bismuth germinate, $Bi_4Ge_3O_{12}$
BGSI	Breast-specific gamma Imaging
BID	Twice daily
Bil	Bilateral
BLS	Basic life support
BM	Bowel movement
BMI	Body mass index
BP	Blood pressure
BPH	Benign prostatic hypertrophy
Bpm	Beats per minute
BRADY	Bradycardia
BRH	Bureau of radiological health
BSA	Body surface area
BUN	Blood urea nitrogen
Bx	Biopsy

Appendix B: Commonly used Abbreviations and Symbols in Nuclear Medicine

CA	Cancer, carcinoma
CABG	Coronary artery bypass graft
CACS	Coronary artery calcium score
CAD	Coronary artery disease
CAP	Community acquired pneumonia
CAT	Computed axial tomography
Cath	Catheterization
CBC	Complete blood count
CBF	Cerebral blood flow
CCT	Cardiac computed tomography
CCTA	Cardiac computed tomographic angiography
CDE	Committed dose equivalent
CDRH	Center for devices and radiological health
CE	Cardiac enzymes
CE	Cardiac events
CEA	Carcinoembryonic antigen
CF	Calibration factor
CFR	Coronary flow reserve
CFR	Code of federal regulations
CGS	Centimetre–gram–second system
CHF	Congestive heart failure
CHIPES	Chloral hydrate, heavy metals, iodides, phenothiazines, enteric-coated, solvents
Chol	Cholesterol
Chr	Chronic
CK-MB	Creatine kinase-myocardial band
cm	Centimeter
CMR	Cardiac magnetic resonance
CMS	Centers for medicare and medicaid services
CNA	Certified nursing assistant
CO	Cardiac output
COD	critical organ dose
CO_2	Carbon dioxide
COPD	Chronic obstructive pulmonary disease
COR	Center of rotation
CORAR	Council on radionuclides and radiopharmaceuticals
CP	Chest pain
CPR	Cardiopulmonary resuscitation
CPT	Current procedural terminology
CPU	Central processing unit
CRADA	Cooperative research and development agreement
CRF	Chronic renal failure
CRP	C-reactive protein
CRP	Coordinated research project
CRT	Cathode ray tube

CPT	Current procedural terminology
CSF	Cerebrospinal Fluid
CSF	Colony-stimulating factor
CT	Computed tomography
CTA	Computed tomography angiogram
CTDI	CT dose index
CVA	Cerebrovascular accident
CVD	Cardiovascular disease
DAC	Digital-to-analog converter
DAC	Derived air concentration
DARLing	Diagnostic acceptable reference level
DCE	Dynamic contrast-enhanced
D/C	Discharge
DDE	Deep dose equivalent
DEXA	Dual-energy X-ray absorptiometry
DICOM	Digital Imaging and Communications in Medicine
DIF	Dedicated Isotope Facilities
DLB	Dementia with lewy bodies
DLBCL	Diffuse large B-cell lymphoma
DLP	Dose length product
DM	Diabetes mellitus
DMA	Direct memory access
DMF	Drug master file
DNA	Deoxyribonucleic acid
DNR	Do not resuscitate
D. O.	Doctor of osteopathy
DOA	Dead on arrival
DOB	Date of birth
DOE	Dyspnea on exertion
DOE	U.S. department of energy
DOE-NNSA	U.S. department of energy, national nuclear security Adm
DOPA	DihydrOxyPhenylAlanine
DOTA	Dodecanetetraacetic acid-chelated somatostatin analogue
TOC	Tyr^3 octreotide
TATE	Tyr^3, Thr^8 octreotide
NOC	1-Nal^3 octreotide
dpm	Disintegrations per minute
DR	Digital radiography
DRE	Digital Rectal Examination
DTC	Differentiated thyroid cancer
DTPI	Dual time-point imaging
DVT	Deep venous thrombosis
Dx	Diagnosis
e.g.	For example
E. S.R.D.	End-stage renal disease

Appendix B: Commonly used Abbreviations and Symbols in Nuclear Medicine

Ea.	Each
EBL	Estimated blood loss
ECG	Electrocardiogram
EENT	Eye, ear, nose, and throat
ED	End diastole
ED	Effective dose
EDE	Effective dose equivalent
EF	Ejection fraction
EGD	EsophagoGastroDuodenoscopy
EMG	ElectroMyography
EMR	Electronic medical records
EOB	End of bombardment
EP	Electrophysiology
Eq	Equal
ERNA	Equilibrium radionuclide angiography
ES	End Systole
ESR	Erythrocyte sedimentation rate
et	and
ET	Emory toolbox
Etc	Et cetera
ETT	Endotracheal tube
ETT	Exercise tolerance test
Eval	Evaluation
Excl.	Exclude
Exp.	Expired
Extr.	Extremities
FAD	Fetal absorbed dose
FBP	Filtered back projection
FBS	Fasting blood sugar
FDA	Food and drug administration
FDG	FluoroDeoxyGlucose
FDHT	Fluoro-dihydrotestosterone
FISS	Fissile solution storage
Fluoro	Fluoroscopy
FLT	Fluorothymidine
F-MISO	Fluoromisonidazole
FN	False negative
FNA	Fine needle aspiration
FNAC	Fine needle aspiration cytology
FNAB	Fine needle aspiration biopsy
Ft	Feet (Length)
FORE	Fourier rebinning
FOV	Field of view
FP	False positive
f/u	Follow-up

FUO	Fever of unknown origin
Fx	Fracture
GCS	Glasgow coma scale
G-CSF	Granulocyte colony-stimulating factor
GERD	GastroEsophageal reflux disease
GFR	Glomerular filtration rate
GI	GastroIntestinal
GIST	Gastrointestinal stromal tumor
GLU	Glucose
Gm	Gram
GM-CSF	Granulocyte-macrophage colony-stimulating factor
GRAE	Generally regarded as effective.
GRAS	Generally regarded as safe
GSO	Gadolinium silicate, $GaSiO_5$
GSW	Gunshot wound.
G-tube	Gastrostomy tube
GTRI	Global threat reduction initiative
HAMA	Human anti-mouse antibodies
HAP	Hospital-acquired pneumonia
Hb	Hemoglobin
HbA1c	Glycosylated hemoglobin
HCFA	Health care financing administration
HCG	Human chorionic gonadotropin
Hct	Hematocrit
HCTZ	Hydrochlorothiazide
HD	High definition
HDL	High-density lipoprotein
HDP	Hydroxyethylene diphosphonate
HEENT	Head, eyes, ears, nose, throat
HELLP	Hemolysis, elevated liver enzymes, low platelets
HEU	Highly enriched uranium
HFR	High flux reactor
H/H	Hemoglobin/Hematocrit
HIV	Human immuodeficiency virus
HLTx	Heart and lung transplant
HLW	High-level waste
HMO	Health maintenance organization
HMPAO	Hexamethylpropyleneamine Oxime
H/O	History of
H&P	History and physical
HR	Heart rate
HRCT	High-resolution CT
HRES	High resolution
HRT	Hormone replacement therapy
HTN	Hypertension

Appendix B: Commonly used Abbreviations and Symbols in Nuclear Medicine 265

HV	High voltage
IBS	Irritable bowel syndrome
IBW	Ideal body weight
ICCU	Intensive coronary care unit
ICD-9	International classification of diseases (9th revision)
ICU	Intensive care unit
IDDM	Insulin-dependent diabetes mellitus
IAEA	International atomic energy agency
Ig	Immunoglobin
IHD	Ischemic heart disease
IMACS	Image (management) archiving and communications system
IMP	IodoaMPhetamine
inc	Incontinent
INF	Inferior
Inj	Injection
Insuff	Insufficiency
INT	Interior
I/O	Intake and output
ISO	International standards organization
ITLC	Instant thin layer chromatography
IV	Intravenous(ly)
IVC	Inferior vena cava
JCAHO	Joint commission on accreditation of healthcare organizations
JPEG	Joint photographic experts group
k	Kilo
K	Thousand
Kcal	Kilocalories
KCl	Potassium chloride
keV	Kiloelectronvolts
Kg	Kilogram
KUB	Kidneys, ureters, and bladder X-ray
L	Liter
LA	Left atrium
LAD	Left anterior descending
LAN	Local area network
LBBB	Left bundle branch block
LCA	Left coronary artery
LCX	Left circumflex artery
LDE	Lens dose equivalent
LDL	Lower density lipoprotein
LE	Lower extremity
LEAP	Low energy, all purpose
LEHR	Low energy, high resolution
LEHS	Low energy, high sensitivity
LET	Linear energy transfer

LFOV	Large field of view
LFT	Liver function tests
LIMA	Left internal mammary artery
LLAT	Left lateral
LLL	Left lower lobe
LLQ	Left lower quadrant
LMA	Left main artery
LMP	Last menstrual period
LOR	Line of response
LPN	Licensed practical nurse
LPO	Left posterior Oblique
L-S	Lumbo-sacral
LUE	Left upper extremity
LUL	Left upper lobe
LUQ	Left upper quadrant
LUT	Lookup table
LYSO	Cerium-doped lutetium yttrium ORthosilicate
LV	Left ventricle
LVEF	Left ventricle ejection fraction
LVG	Left ventriculography
LVH	Left ventricular hypertrophy
m	Meter
MAA	Macroaggregated Albumin
MAG 3	MercaptuAcetyltriGlycine
MBF	myocardial blood flow
MBq	MegaBecquerel
MCA	Middle cerebral artery
MCHC	Mean corpuscular hemoglobin concentrate
mCi	Millicurie
MCL	Medial collateral ligament
MS-CSF	Macrophage colony-stimulating factor
MCV	Mean Corpuscular Volume
MDCT	Muti-row detector CT scanner
MEAP	Medium Energy, All Purpose
MEN	Multiple endocrine neoplasia
mEq	milliequivalent
MET	Metabolic equivalent of task
mg	Milligram
MHR	Multiple head registration
MI	Myocardial infarction
MIBG	MetaIodoBenzylGuanidine
MIRD	Medical internal radiation dose
MIP	Maximum-intensity projection
µCi	Microcurie
µg	Microgram

Appendix B: Commonly used Abbreviations and Symbols in Nuclear Medicine 267

MIP	Maximum-intensity projection
ml	Milliliter
MLEM	Maximum likelihood expectation maximization
M&M	Morbidity and mortality
MMAD	Mass median aerodynamic diameter
MoAb	Monoclonal antibody
MOD	Magnetic optical disc
MPD	Maximum permissible dose
MPI	Myocardial perfusion imaging
MPM	Malignant pleural mesothelioma
MPR	Multiplanar reconstruction
MR	Mitral regurgitation
MRI	Magnetic resonance imaging
MRSA	Methicillin-resistant staphylococcus aureus
MSAD	Multiple slice average dose
msec	Millisecond(s)
MTF	Modulation transfer function
MTV	Metabolic tumor volume
MUGA	Multigated acquisition scan
MV	Mitral valve
MVO_2	Myocardial oxygen consumption
MVP	Mitral valve prolapse
MVR	Mitral valve replacement.
N/A	Non applicable
NaCl	Sodium chloride
NAC	Non-attenuation corrected
NC	Nasal Cannula
NDA	New drug application
NECR	Noise equivalent count rate
NEMA	National electrical manufacturers association
NET	Neuroendocrine tumor
ng	Nanogram(s)
NGT	NasoGastric tube
NHL	Non-Hodgkin's lymphoma
NIDDM	Non-insulin-dependent diabetes mellitus
NIH	National Institutes of Health
NIST	National Institute of Standards and Technology
NKA	No known allergies
NOPR	National Oncologic PET Registry
NPH	Normal pressure hydrocephalus
NPO	Nothing per oral
NRC	Nuclear regulatory commission
NREM	Non-rapid eye movement
NSLC	Non-small cell lung cancer
NSTEMI	NON-ST-segment elevation myocardial infarction

NSR	Normal sinus rhythm
N&T	Nose and throat
NTG	Nitroglycerine
N/V/D	Nausea/vomiting/diarrhea
ODS	One day surgery
OOB	Out of bed
OSEM	Ordered subsets expectation maximization
OP-OSEM	Ordinary Poisson OSEM
AW-OSEM	Attenuation-weighted OSEM
OSHA	Occupational safety and health administration
OT	Occupational therapy
OTC	Over the counter
p	After
P	P wave
PA	Pulmonary artery
PAC	Premature atrial contraction
PACS	Picture archiving and communication systems
PAPR	Powered air-purifying respirator
PCN	Penicillin
PE	Pulmonary embolism
PEG	Percutaneous endoscopic gastrostomy
PEM	Positron emission mammography
PERCIST	PET response criteria in solid tumors
PET	Positron emission tomography
PET/CT	Positron emission tomography/computed tomography
PFT	Pulmonary function tests
PH	Pulmonary hypertension
PHA	Pulse height analyzer
pH	Degree of acidity or alkalinity
PICC	Peripherally inserted central catheter
PIOPED	Prospective investigation of pulmonary embolism diagnosis
PMH	Past medical history
PMTs	Photomultiplier tubes
PN	Parenteral nutrition
PNS	Peripheral nervous system
PO	Per Os
PPE	Personal protective equipment
PRN	Pro re nata: as necessary, as needed
Prox	Proximal
PSA	Prostate-specific antigen
PSRF	Point source response function
PT	Physical therapy
PTCA	Percutaneous transluminal coronary angioplasty
PVC	Premature ventricular contractions
PVD	Peripheral vascular disease

Appendix B: Commonly used Abbreviations and Symbols in Nuclear Medicine

PVE	Partial-volume effect
PYP	Pyrophosphate
q	Every
QC	Quality control
QF	Quality factor
q.h.	Every hour
q.i.d.	Four times daily
QPS-QGS	Quantitative perfusion SPECT/quantitative gated SPECT
QRS	QRS complex
QS	QS complex
QT	Q to T interval
RA	Right atrium
RAIU	Radioactive iodine uptake
RAM	Random access memory
ROC	Receiver-operator characteristic
RAO	Right anterior oblique
RBBB	Right bundle branch block
RBC	Red Blood Cells
RBE	Relative biologic effectiveness
RCA	Right coronary artery
RCC	Renal cell carcinoma
RECIST	Response evaluation criteria in solid tumors
REM	Rapid eye movement
RES	ReticuloEndothelial system
RF	Renal failure
Rh	Rhesus blood factor
RIS	Radioimmunoscintigraphy
RISA	Radioactive iodine serum albumin
RLAT	Right lateral
RLE	Right lower extremity
RLL	Right lower lobe
RLQ	Right lower quadrant
RLS	Restless leg syndrome
R/O	Rule out
ROM	Read only memory
RN	Registered nurse
RNA	Radionuclide angiography
RNA	Ribonucleic acid
R/O	Rule out
ROM	Range of motion
RP	RadioPharmaceutical
RR	Respiratory rate
RSC	Radiation safety committee
RSO	Radiation safety officer
RT	Radiation therapy

RUE	Right upper extremity
RUL	Right upper lobe
RUQ	Right upper quadrant
RV	Right ventricle
Rx	Prescription
S1, S2, S3 etc	First sacral, second sacral, third sacral vertebra, etc.
SA	SinoAtrial
SAD	Surface absorbed dose
SC	Sulfur colloid
SB	Sinus bradycardia
SCA	Sudden cardiac arrest
SCLC	Small cell lung carcinoma
SDS	Same day surgery
SDS	Summed difference (stress-rest perfusion) Score
SICU	Surgical intensive care unit
SN	Sentinel node
SNB	Sentinel node biopsy
SNM	Society of nuclear medicine
SNR	Signal-to-noise ratio
SOAP	A standardized method for recording patient progress notes: S—subjective patient complaint; O—objective findings; A—assessment of the program; P—plan of action
SOB	Short of breath
S/P	Status post
SPECT	Single-photon emission computed tomography
SRS	Summed rest score
S and S	Signs and symptoms
SSKI	Saturated solution of potassium iodide
SSN	SupraSternal notch
SSS	Summed stress score
SSS	Sick sinus syndrome
SSTR	Somatostatin receptor
ST	Sinus tachycardia
ST	ST segment
Stat	Immediately
STD	Sexually transmitted disease
STEMI	ST-segment elevation myocardial infarction
Strep	Streptococcus
SUL	SUV normalized to lean body mass
Sup	Supine
SUV	Standardized uptake value
SVC	Superior vena cava
SVT	Supraventricular tachycardia
T	T wave
T3	Triodothyronine

T4	Thyroxine
TB	Tuberculosis
t_b	Biological half-life
TBG	Thyroxine binding globulin
TCP/IP	Transmission control protocol / internet protocol
TDD	Telecommunications device for the deaf
t_e	Effective half-life
TED	Thrombo embolic deterrent (Ted stockings)
TEDE	Total effective dose equivalent
TEE	Transesophageal echocardiogram
TF	Tube feeding
TGV	Tumor's glycolytic volume
THR	Target heart rate
TIA	Transient ischemic attack
TID	Transient ischemic dilation
t.i.d.	Three times a day
TIE	Total imparted energy
TIFF	Tagged Image File Format
TLD	ThermoLuminescent Dosimeter
TLG	Total lesion glycolysis
TMJ	Temporal mandibular joint
TN	True negative
TNM	Tumor nodes metastasis
TOD	Tail on detector
TP	True positive
TPN	Total parenteral nutrition
TPR	Temperature, pulse, respiration
TRH	Thyrotropin-releasing hormone
TSH	Thyroid-stimulating hormone
TTE	TransThoracic echocardiography
TURP	Trans-urethral resection of prostate
U/A	Urinalysis
UE	Upper extremity
UGI	Upper gastrointestinal
UTI	Urinary tract infection
VF SCA	Ventricular fibrillation sudden cardiac arrest
via	By way of
VMA	Vanillymandelic acid
VOI	Volume of interest
V-P shunt	Ventriculo-peritoneal shunt
VRE	Vancomycin resistant enterococcus
VRT	Volume rendered techniques
VS	Vital signs
V-tach	Ventricular tachycardia
WAN	Wide area network

WBC	White blood cell
W/C	Wheelchair
WHO	World health organization
WLCQ	Wackers–Liu circumferential quantification
WPW	Wolff–Parkinson–White syndrome
XRT	Radiation therapy treatment
YTD	Year to date

Symbols

&	And
@	At
√	Check
↓	Decrease
=	Equal
♀	Female
←	From
>	Greater than
↑	High
↑	Increased
+++	Large amount
<	Less than
↓	Low
↓	Decreased
♂	Male
++	Moderate amount
+	More or less
-	Negative
o	No; null; none; nothing
#	Number
o	Objective findings
+	Positive
1°	Primary
(?)	Questionable
2nd	Secondary; SECOND
2°	Secondary to
2°	Second degree
c̄	With
s̄	Without

Appendix C
Glossary

Absorbed dose The energy imparted by ionizing radiation per unit mass of irradiated material. The units of absorbed dose are the rad and the gray (Gy). 1 rad is equivalent to 0.01 Gy.

Actinide Any of a series of radioactive elements with atomic numbers 89 (actinium) to 103 (lawrencium). All of these elements are radioactive, and two of the elements, uranium and plutonium, are used to generate nuclear energy.

Activity The rate of disintegration (transformation) or decay of radioactive material. The units of activity are the curie (Ci) and the becquerel (Bq).

Aerobic respiration A form of cellular respiration that requires oxygen in order to generate energy

Agreement State A State that has signed an agreement with the NRC authorizing the State to regulate certain uses of radioactive materials within the State

Airborne radioactive material Radioactive material dispersed in the air in the form of dusts, fumes, particulates, mists, vapors, or gases.

Air-purifying respirator A respirator with an air-purifying filter, cartridge, or canister that removes specific air contaminants by passing ambient air through the air-purifying element

Algorithm A mathematical process applied to raw data for the purposes of reconstruction and filtering

Alpha particle A particle emitted from the nucleus of an atom, which contains two protons and two neutrons. It is identical to the nucleus of a Helium atom, without the electrons.

Analog signal Analog signals are a representation of time varying quantities as voltage, light or x-rays in a continuous signal using small fluctuations in the signal itself to pass information.

Anaerobic respiration A form of cellular respiration that occurs when oxygen is absent or insufficient

Annihilation Reaction in which a particle and its antiparticle collide and disappear, releasing energy.

Annual limit on intake (ALI) The derived limit for the amount of radioactive material taken into the body of an adult worker by inhalation or ingestion in a year.

Anode The (+) terminal of the x-ray tube where the target material is deposited.

Antibody Immune system-related proteins called immunoglobulins, produced because of the introduction of an antigen into the body, and which possesses the remarkable ability to form a specific complex with the very antigen that initiated its production.

Antigen An antigen is any substance that causes the immune system to produce antibodies against it.

Aperture The donut-shaped opening in the gantry through the patient and patient table will pass during the scan.

Arthroplasty A generic term for any joint surgery designed to restore joint function.

Atelectasis Reduced inflation of all or part of the lung

Autograft A graft in which material is transferred from one part of a person's body to another part.

Average variance The square sum of the differences of the relative crystal efficiencies between the two scans weighted by the inverse variances of the differences, for example. The daily acquired blank sinogram is compared with a reference blank sinogram obtained during the last setup of the scanner.

Axial field-of-view The maximum length parallel to the long axis of a PET scanner along which the instrument generates transaxial tomographic images (NEMA definition).

Background radiation Radiation from cosmic sources; naturally occurring radioactive material, including radon (except as a decay product of source or special nuclear material); and global fallout as it exists in the environment from the testing of nuclear explosive devices or from past nuclear accidents.

Beam-hardening artifact A type of computed tomographic artifact that occurs because the x-ray beam in CT scanners is not monochromatic and becomes progressively "harder" (of shorter wavelength) as it passes through tissue.

Becquerel (Bq) The SI derived unit of radioactivity. One Becquerel is that quantity of a radioactive material that will have 1 transformation in one second. There are 3.7×10^{10} Bq in one curie.

Beta particle A high speed particle, identical to an electron which is emitted from the nucleus of an atom.

Bioassay (radiobioassay) The determination of kinds, quantities, or concentrations and, in some cases, the locations of radioactive material in the human body, whether by direct measurement (in vivo counting) or by analysis and evaluation of materials excreted or removed from the human body.

Biomaterial A material brought into contact with living tissue for the treatment of medical and dental conditions.

Bleb A small gas-containing space within the visceral pleura or in the subpleural lung, not larger than 1 cm in diameter.

Appendix C: Glossary

Bone stimulator An electronic device used for stimulating bone growth in cases of poor fracture healing and in cases of extensive spine surgery.

Brachytherapy A type of radiation therapy in which the source of the ionizing radiation is applied directly to or is only a short distance away from the body area being treated.

Bremsstrahlung "Braking radiation" and is retained from the original German to describe the radiation which is emitted when electrons are decelerated or "braked" when they are fired at a metal target. Braking radiation comprises 80% to 90% of the x-rays used in CT scanning.

Bronchiolitis Bronchiolar inflammation of various causes

Calandria A sealed drum-shaped vessel that contains the heavy-water moderator for the reactor. This vessel is penetrated by a series of horizontal fuel channels and vertical channels for control rods.

Casting The process of melting a metal and pouring into a mold.

Cathode The (-) terminal of x-ray tube where the negatively charged electrons flow into the tube from the HV generator

Chemical shift artifact A type of magnetic resonance imaging artifact commonly seen at the interface of fat and soft tissue

Chi-square test A statistical test commonly used to compare observed data with data we would expect to obtain according to a specific hypothesis

Cold testing Testing conducted without the use of radioactive material.

Collective dose The sum of the individual doses received in a given period of time by a specified population from exposure to a specified source of radiation.

Committed dose equivalent (HT,50) The dose equivalent to organs or tissues of reference (T) that will be received from an intake of radioactive material by an individual during the 50-year period following the intake.

Committed effective dose equivalent (HE,50) The sum of the products of the weighting factors applicable to each of the body organs or tissues that are irradiated and the committed dose equivalent to these organs or tissues (HE,50 = ΣWTHT.50).

Consolidation Refers to an exudate or other product of disease that replaces alveolar air, rendering the lung solid (as in infective pneumonia).

Constraint (dose constraint) A value above which specified licensee actions are required.

Contiguous Having no gaps between adjacent slices.

Controlled area An area, outside of a restricted area but inside the site boundary, access to which can be limited by the licensee for any reason

Critical organ The organ or physiological system that would first be subjected to radiation in excess of the maximum permissible amount as the dose of a radioactive material is increased.

Cross plane Geometric plane between two physical rings of detector crystals

CT dose index The cumulative dose along the patient's axis for a single tomographic image

Curie (Ci) A unit of radioactivity, defined as 1 Ci = 3.7×10^{10} decays per second. The relationship between becquerels and curies is: 3.7×10^{10} Bq in one curie.

Cyst Any round circumscribed space that is surrounded by an epithelial or fibrous wall of variable thickness.

Declared pregnant woman A woman who has voluntarily informed the licensee, in writing, of her pregnancy and the estimated date of conception. The declaration remains in effect until the declared pregnant woman withdraws the declaration in writing or is no longer pregnant.

Deep-dose equivalent (Hd) applies to external whole-body exposure: the dose equivalent at a tissue depth of 1 cm (1,000 mg/cm^2).

Digital signal A type of electrical signal that is in the form of binary code.

Direct-use material Material that is directly usable in nuclear weapons. Such materials include highly enriched uranium (HEU) and separated plutonium.

Discrete source A radionuclide that has been processed so that its concentration within a material has been purposely increased for use for commercial, medical, or research activities.

Distinguishable from background The detectable concentration of a radionuclide is statistically different from the background concentration of that radionuclide in the vicinity of the site or, in the case of structures, in similar materials using adequate measurement technology, survey, and statistical techniques.

Doppler phenomenon An eponymous term to describe the apparent change in frequency of a waveform, such as light or sound, whenever the wave source and an observer are in motion relative to each other.

Dose or radiation dose A generic term that means absorbed dose, dose equivalent, effective dose equivalent, committed dose equivalent, committed effective dose equivalent, or total effective dose equivalent.

Dose equivalent (HT) The product of the absorbed dose in tissue, quality factor, and all other necessary modifying factors at the location of interest. The units of dose equivalent are the rem and sievert (Sv).

Dosimetry processor An individual or organization that processes and evaluates individual monitoring equipment in order to determine the radiation dose delivered to the equipment.

Drug master file (DMF) A submission to the Food and Drug Administration (FDA) that may be used to provide confidential detailed information about facilities, processes, or articles used in the manufacturing, processing, packaging, and storing of one or more human drugs.

Effective dose equivalent (HE) The sum of the products of the dose equivalent to the organ or tissue (HT) and the weighting factors (WT) applicable to each of the body organs or tissues that are irradiated (HE = ΣWTHT).

Effective half-life The time in which the quantity in the body will decrease to half as a result of both radioactive decay and biological elimination

Electron capture Process that unstable atoms can use to become more stable. During electron capture, an electron in an atom's inner shell is drawn into the nucleus where it combines with a proton, forming a neutron and a neutrino. The neutrino is ejected from the atom's nucleus.

Embryo/fetus The developing human organism from conception until the time of birth.

Appendix C: Glossary

Enriched uranium Uranium With A Higher concentration of the U-235 isotope than found naturally.

Enrichment Process used to increase the concentration of the uranium-235 (U-235) isotope in a material relative to U-238.

Entrance or access point Any location through which an individual could gain access to radiation areas or to radioactive materials. This includes entry or exit portals of sufficient size to permit human entry, irrespective of their intended use.

Exposure Being exposed to ionizing radiation or to radioactive material.

External dose That portion of the dose equivalent received from radiation sources outside the body.

Extremity Hand, elbow, arm below the elbow, foot, knee, or leg below the knee.

Filament A structure on the cathode (-) terminal of the x-ray tube from which the electron beam is released

Filtering facepiece (dust mask) A negative pressure particulate respirator with a filter as an integral part of the facepiece or with the entire facepiece composed of the filtering medium, not equipped with elastomeric sealing surfaces and adjustable straps.

Fission Process whereby a large atomic nucleus (such as uranium) is split into two (and sometimes three) smaller nuclei.

Fission fragments Smaller atomic fragments resulting from fission of a large nucleus.

Fit factor A quantitative estimate of the fit of a particular respirator to a specific individual, and typically estimates the ratio of the concentration of a substance in ambient air to its concentration inside the respirator when worn.

Fit test The use of a protocol to qualitatively or quantitatively evaluate the fit of a respirator on an individual.

Fourier transform A mathematical process that converts matrix information into frequency domain

Frame mode A method of computer data collection where x and y positional signals are stored in a single matrix.

Frequency The number of occurrences of a repeating event per unit time (temporal frequency).

Full-Width Half-Maximum (FWHM) A measurement of curve peak characteristics by comparing the curve width at half the peak height with the value at which the peak occurs. It is commonly used to express energy or spatial resolution to describe a measurement of the width of an object in a picture, when that object does not have sharp edges.

Gamma rays Electromagnetic waves or photons emitted from the nucleus (center) of an atom.

Generally applicable environmental radiation standards Standards issued by the Environmental Protection Agency (EPA) under the authority of the Atomic Energy Act of 1954, as amended, that impose limits on radiation exposures or levels, or concentrations or quantities of radioactive material, in the general environment outside the boundaries of locations under the control of persons possessing or using radioactive material.

Genetic effects Effects from some agent that are seen in the offspring of the individual who received the agent. The agent must be encountered preconception.

Gibbs (truncation) artifact A frequency artifact produced by magnetic resonance imaging that is similar to chemical shift and magnetic artifacts.

Gray (Gy) The derived SI unit for the absorbed dose of ionizing radiation, equal to the absorption of 1 joule per kilogram, replaces the traditional cgs unit, the rad (equivalent to 0.01 Gy).

Gray scale A continuous spectrum of shades of the color gray used to differentiate structures on a digital image.

Greenfield filter A type of inferior vena cava filter for use in the prevention of clot propagation to the lungs.

Half-life The time required for a quantity of radioactive material to decay to half of its initial value.

Half-value layer The thickness of specified material which reduces the intensity of radiation entering the material by half.

Helical scan A study of cross-sectional images characterized by continuous table movement during x-ray tube rotation.

Heterograft A graft of tissue or an organ from one species to another species

High-level waste Highly radioactive materials containing fission products and transuranic elements produced as a by-product of the reactions that occur inside nuclear reactors.

Highly enriched uranium Uranium enriched to concentrations greater than or equal to 20 percent by weight of U-235.

High radiation area An area, accessible to individuals, in which radiation levels from radiation sources external to the body could result in an individual receiving a dose equivalent in excess of 0.1 rem (1 mSv) in 1 hour at 30 centimeters from the radiation source or 30 centimeters from any surface that the radiation penetrates.

Hilum A generic term that describes the indentation in the surface of an organ, where vessels and nerves connect with the organ.

Homograft A graft of tissue or an organ from a donor of the same species as the recipient

Hot cell Shielded workspace for working with highly radioactive materials.

Hot rolling Heating metal above its recrystalization temperature before rolling it to form sheets.

Hydroxyapatite A fundamental inorganic constituent of bone matrix and teeth.

Hyperemia The increase of blood flow to different tissues in the body.

Hyperplasia Increased cell production in a normal tissue or organ. Hyperplasia may be a sign of abnormal or precancerous changes.

Immobilization device Any device to immobilize a patient so that a procedure may be performed.

Implant Generic term used for materials or devices placed in vivo for the treatment of medical or dental conditions

Individual monitoring devices (individual monitoring equipment) Devices designed to be worn by a single individual for the assessment of dose equivalent such as film badges, thermoluminescence dosimeters (TLDs), pocket ionization chambers, and personal ("lapel") air sampling devices.

Injection artifact A type of nuclear medicine artifact that originates from the injection of radiotracer

Insulin A hormone, produced by the pancreas, which is central to regulating carbohydrate and fat metabolism in the body.

Internal conversion A transition of energy within a molecule or atom from a high energy state to a lower energy state without an accompanying photon.

Ionizing radiation Radiation with enough energy so that during an interaction with an atom, it can remove tightly bound electrons from their orbits, causing the atom to become charged or ionized, e.g., gamma rays and neutrons.

Internal dose That portion of the dose equivalent received from radioactive material taken into the body.

Intrathecal (drug) delivery pump A battery-operated pump placed in a subcutaneous pocket and connected to a catheter situated in the spinal subarachnoid space.

Isomeric transition Radioactive decay process in which the nucleus of a metastable isotope has an elevated energy state and releases this energy by emitting a gamma ray.

Lens dose equivalent (LDE) Applies to the external exposure of the lens of the eye and is taken as the dose equivalent at a tissue depth of 0.3 cm (300 mg/cm^2).

Licensed material Source material, special nuclear material, or by-product material received, possessed, used, transferred, or disposed of under a general or specific license issued by the Commission.

Ligand An ion or molecule that binds to a central metal atom to form a coordination complex.

Limits (dose limits) The permissible upper bounds of radiation doses.

Linear artifact A type of computed tomographic artifact seen at the edges of tissues with different attenuation.

List mode A method of computer data collection where x and y positional signals are stored sequentially in memory in the form of list.

Localizer scan A single projection scan obtained with a stationary x-ray tube and a moving patient table.

Lost or missing licensed material Licensed material whose location is unknown. It includes material that has been shipped but has not reached its destination and whose location cannot be readily traced in the transportation system

Low enriched uranium Uranium enriched to concentrations less than 20 percent by weight of U-235.

Lymphadenopathy Usually restricted to enlargement, due to any cause, of the lymph nodes. Synonyms include lymph node enlargement (preferred) and adenopathy.

Mammary prosthesis A breast augmentation-reconstruction implant.

Mass attenuation coefficient The quotient of the linear attenuation coefficient divided by the density of the matter through which it passes.

Mass defect The amount by which the mass of an atomic nucleus is less than the sum of the masses of its constituent particles; also called mass deficiency.

Mass pulmonary Any pulmonary, pleural, or mediastinal lesion seen on chest radiographs as an opacity greater than 3 cm in diameter (without regard to contour, border, or density characteristics).

Member of the public Any individual except when that individual is receiving an occupational dose.

Metastable state Excited state of an atom, nucleus, or other system that has a longer lifetime than the ordinary excited states and generally has a shorter lifetime than the ground state

Minor An individual less than 18 years of age.

Million instructions per second (MIPS) A general measure of computing performance and, by implication, the amount of work a larger computer can do.

Mirror imaging artifact A type of ultrasound artifact that may be created adjacent to a highly reflective acoustic interface.

Monitoring (radiation monitoring, radiation protection monitoring) The measurement of radiation levels, concentrations, surface area concentrations, or quantities of radioactive material and the use of the results of these measurements to evaluate potential exposures and doses.

Multiplanar reconstruction (MPR) The reformatting of images acquired in the original axial plane to produce images in either the coronal, sagittal, or oblique plane.

Myeloid Referring to bone marrow or to the spinal cord

Nasogastric tube A generic term for any rubber or plastic tube used for decompression of the stomach.

Neutron capture Process involving the capture of neutrons by an atomic nucleus to form a heavier nucleus.

Neutron flux Measure of the intensity of neutron radiation, defined as the number of neutrons crossing a unit area of a square centimeter in one second (neutrons/cm^2–s).

Neutrons Neutral particles that are normally contained in the nucleus of all atoms and may be removed by various interactions or processes like collision and fission

New drug application (NDA) A written application to the Food and Drug Administration seeking approval to sell a pharmaceutical in the USA.

Negative pressure respirator (tight fitting) A respirator in which the air pressure inside the facepiece is negative during inhalation with respect to the ambient air pressure outside the respirator.

Nephrostomy tube A tube placed into the pelvis of the kidney for the external drainage of urine.

Nodule The chest radiographic appearance of a nodule is a rounded opacity, well or poorly defined, measuring up to 3 cm in diameter.

Noise Extraneous interference in electronic circuit of statistical manipulation

Nonionizing radiation Radiation without enough energy to remove tightly bound electrons from their orbits around atoms. Examples are microwaves and visible light.

Nonstochastic effect Health effects, the severity of which varies with the dose and for which a threshold is believed to exist.

Normalize A term used in association with computer defined ROI to indicate that counts contained in the regions have been converted to the same size of region

Nyquist frequency The highest frequency that can be coded at a given sampling rate that can be represented in an image.

Occupational dose The dose received by an individual in the course of employment in which the individual's assigned duties involve exposure to radiation or to radioactive material from licensed and unlicensed sources of radiation, whether in the possession of the licensee or other person.

Opacity Refers to any area that preferentially attenuates the x-ray beam and therefore appears more opaque than the surrounding area.

Orogastric tube Any tube going into the stomach through the mouth rather than through the nose.

Orotracheal tube A tube inserted in the mouth to keep the mouth open and the teeth from biting the tongue.

Pair production Formation or materialization of two electrons, one negative and the other positive (positron), from a pulse of electromagnetic energy traveling through matter, usually in the vicinity of an atomic nucleus

Parenchyma Refers to the gas-exchanging part of the lung, consisting of the alveoli and their capillaries.

Particle accelerator Any machine capable of accelerating electrons, protons, deuterons, or other charged particles in a vacuum and of discharging the resultant particulate or other radiation into a medium at energies usually in excess of 1 megaelectron volt.

PEG tube A gastrostomy tube placed by means of percutaneous endoscopic technique

Peritoneal jugular (LeVeen) shunt A shunt designed to drain fluid from the peritoneal cavity to the central venous system.

Phantom Cylinder with fillable inserts, mimicking some of the body organs, which once filled with the radioactive material and scanned, offers the standard measurements for characterization of scanner performances

Photoelectric effect Process by electrons are emitted from matter (metals and nonmetallic solids, liquids, or gases) as a consequence of their absorption of energy from electromagnetic radiation of very short wavelength, such as visible or ultraviolet radiation

Pigtail Used to describe the appearance of the end of a drainage catheter or angiography catheter with a curvature similar to that of a pig's tail.

Pitch Defined as the table travel per rotation divided by the collimation of the x-ray beam

Poisson distribution A discrete frequency distribution that gives the probability of a number of independent events occurring in a fixed time

Porcine graft (valve) A biologic body part derived from a pig.

Port-A-Cath A type of vascular access port.

Positive pressure respirator A respirator in which the pressure inside the respiratory inlet covering exceeds the ambient air pressure outside the respirator.

Positron Also called positive electron, positively charged subatomic particle having the same mass and magnitude of charge as the electron and constituting the antiparticle of a negative electron.

Precision Also called reproducibility or repeatability, is the degree to which repeated measurements under unchanged conditions show the same results

Pressure demand respirator A positive pressure atmosphere-supplying respirator that admits breathing air to the facepiece when the positive pressure is reduced inside the facepiece by inhalation.

Prosthesis Artificial substitute for a missing body part.

Public dose The dose received by a member of the public from exposure to radiation or to radioactive material released by a licensee, or to any other source of radiation under the control of a licensee. Public dose does not include occupational dose or doses received from background radiation, from any medical administration the individual has received, from exposure to individuals administered radioactive material and released under § 35.75, or from voluntary participation in medical research programs.

Quality Factor (Q) The modifying factor that is used to derive dose equivalent from absorbed dose.

Rad - r adiation a bsorbed d ose A unit of measurement of the absorbed dose of ionizing radiation, corresponding to an energy transfer of 100 ergs per gram of any absorbing material. The unit can be used for any type of radiation, but it does not describe the biological effects of the different radiations.

Radiation (ionizing radiation) Alpha particles, beta particles, gamma rays, x-rays, neutrons, high-speed electrons, high-speed protons, and other particles capable of producing ions.

Radiation area An area, accessible to individuals, in which radiation levels could result in an individual receiving a dose equivalent in excess of 0.005 rem (0.05 mSv) in 1 hour at 30 centimeters from the radiation source or from any surface that the radiation penetrates.

Radiopaque Used to describe the ability of a substance to absorb x-rays and appear opaque (white) on radiographs

Rate meter Device that measures the rate of activity of a radioisotope usually in units cts/min or cts/sec

Receptor A structure on the surface of a cell (or inside a cell) that selectively receives and binds a specific substance

Reference man A hypothetical aggregation of human physical and physiological characteristics arrived at by international consensus. These characteristics may be used by researchers and public health workers to standardize results of experiments and to relate biological insult to a common base.

Rem—Roentgen equivalent man A unit used to derive a quantity called equivalent dose and relates the absorbed dose in human tissue to the effective biological damage of the radiation. To determine equivalent dose (rem), you multiply absorbed dose (rad) by a quality factor (Q) that is unique to the type of incident radiation.

Residual radioactivity Radioactivity in structures, materials, soils, groundwater, and other media at a site resulting from activities under the licensee's control.

Respiratory protective device An apparatus, such as a respirator, used to reduce the individual's intake of airborne radioactive materials.

Restricted area An area, access to which is limited by the licensee for the purpose of protecting individuals against undue risks from exposure to radiation and radioactive materials

Retrospective reconstruction Image reconstruction after raw data have been saved, e.g., MPR and 3D volume rendering.

Ring artifact A type of computed tomographic artifact usually caused by a faulty detector producing rings or concentric circles on computed tomographic images.

ROC curve A plot of the true positive rate against the false-positive rate for the different possible cutpoints of a diagnostic test. The ROC curve is a fundamental tool for diagnostic test evaluation

Roentgen (R) A unit used to measure a quantity called exposure. The main advantage of this unit is that it is easy to measure directly, but it is limited because it is only for deposition in air, and only for gamma and x rays.

Scintillation A flash of light produced in certain materials when they absorb ionizing radiation

Sensitivity Measures the proportion of actual positives which are correctly identified as such (e.g., the percentage of sick people who are correctly identified as having the condition)

Shallow-dose equivalent (Hs) Applies to the external exposure of the skin of the whole body or the skin of an extremity and is taken as the dose equivalent at a tissue depth of 0.007 centimeter (7 mg/cm^2).

Sievert A unit used to derive a quantity called equivalent dose. One sievert is equivalent to 100 rem.

Significant quantity Approximate quantity of material from which the possibility of manufacturing a nuclear explosive device (i.e., a device that can achieve a prompt critical mass) cannot be excluded

Sinogram A two-dimensional projection space representation of a transaxial image where one dimension refers to radial distance from the center and the second dimension refers to projection angle

Site boundary That line beyond which the land or property is not owned, leased, or otherwise controlled by the licensee.

Slip ring An electromechanical device that allows the transmission of power and electrical signals from a stationary to a rotating structure and which eliminates the need for power and data cables

Spinal column stimulator An electronic device with leads implanted in the epidural space, the dura, or the subarachnoid space to provide an electrical signal for the relief of pain or muscle spasticity.

Specificity Measures the proportion of negatives which are correctly identified (e.g., the percentage of healthy people who are correctly identified as not having the condition).

Standard deviation The square root of the variance where variance is the average of the squared differences from the Mean

Stochastic effects Health effects that occur randomly and for which the probability of the effect occurring, rather than its severity, is assumed to be a linear function of dose without threshold.

Student's *t*-testAssesses whether the means of two groups are statistically different from each other

Supplemental new drug application (sNDA) Additional written documentation submitted for approval by the FDA when a producer makes major changes to the process or raw materials it uses to make a pharmaceutical.

Survey An evaluation of the radiological conditions and potential hazards incident to the production, use, transfer, release, disposal, or presence of radioactive material or other sources of radiation.

Table increment The advancement, in mm, of the patient table between consecutive conventional slices. It describes the overlap or gap between neighboring slices.

Target Material containing U-235 that is designed to be irradiated in a nuclear reactor

Target organ An organ intended to receive a therapeutic dose of irradiation and/or to receive the greatest concentration of a diagnostic radioactive tracer

Technetium generator Device used to store Mo-99 and extract its decay product Tc-99m.

Total Effective Dose Equivalent (TEDE) The sum of the effective dose equivalent (for external exposures) and the committed effective dose equivalent (for internal exposures).

Teratogenic effects Effects from some agent that are seen in the offspring of the individual who received the agent. The agent must be encountered during the gestation period.

Thoracostomy tube Is used to drain pleural fluid collections or reexpand the lung in cases of a pneumothorax (chest tube).

Thorotrast Thorium dioxide, formerly used as a radiologic contrast agent. It was discontinued because of its carcinogenic properties.

Tissue weighting factor (w_T)The values of w_T take into account the numbers of (1) fatal cancers and (2) risk of hereditary disease above normal incidence per unit of ionizing radiation for each organ system for which such effects are known to occur.

Total-body or Whole-body dose The total energy deposited in the body divided by the mass of the body. This approach assumes a uniform whole-body exposure to radiation.

Tracheostomy tube A tube directly inserted into the trachea through the anterior tracheal cartilage.

Transaxial field-of-view The maximum diameter circular region perpendicular to the long axis of a PET scanner within which objects might be imaged

Tube current (mA) Determines the number of x-ray photons produced by the CT x-ray tube

T-tube drain A type of traditional gravity drain configured in a T shape. T-tubes are most often used for common bile duct drainage.

Tube voltage (kV) Determines the energy level of x-ray photons produced by the CT x-ray tube

Unrestricted area An area, access to which is neither limited nor controlled by the licensee

Uranium fuel cycle The operations of milling of uranium ore, chemical conversion of uranium, isotopic enrichment of uranium, fabrication of uranium fuel, generation of electricity by a light-water-cooled nuclear power plant using uranium fuel, and reprocessing of spent uranium fuel to the extent that these activities directly support the production of electrical power for public use.

Urinary stent A generic term used for any stent employed in the urinary system to traverse benign and malignant strictures and bypass areas of dehiscence or obstructing calculi.

Variance Degree of change

Vascular Referring to the vessels

Ventricular assist device (VAD) A device used to assist the heart in its blood pumping function (univentricular or biventricular)

Ventriculoperitoneal shunt A shunt system designed to reduce intracranial pressure and prevent the development of hydrocephalus

Very high radiation area An area, accessible to individuals, in which radiation levels from radiation sources external to the body could result in an individual receiving an absorbed dose in excess of 500 rads (5 grays) in 1 hour at 1 meter from a radiation source or 1 meter from any surface that the radiation penetrates.

Vertebroplasty Percutaneous injection of methylmethacrylate or similar material into a vertebral body to provide pain relief from a vertebral lesion.

Viscosity The thickness of the substance. Describes the thickness of contrast media in CT

Waste Low-level radioactive wastes containing source, special nuclear, or by-product material that are acceptable for disposal in a land disposal facility.

Whole body For purposes of external exposure means head, trunk (including male gonads), arms above the elbow, or legs above the knee.

Windowing The process of selecting some segment of the total pixel value range and then displaying the pixel values within that segment over the full brightness (shades of gray) range from white to black

X rays Electromagnetic waves or photons not emitted from the nucleus, but normally emitted by energy changes in electrons. These energy changes are either in electron orbital shells that surround an atom or in the process of slowing down such as in an X-ray machine.

Xenograft Same as a heterograft.

Zipper artifact A type of computed radiographic artifact caused by missing information being reflected in the image as a lucent vertical band.

Z-stent A generic term for a variety of metallic stents used to overcome areas of narrowing in such tubular structures as vessels, bile ducts, ureters, and the urethra.

References

Austin JH, Müller NL, Friedman PJ, et al. Glossary of terms for CT of the lungs: recommendations of the Nomenclature Committee of the Fleischner Society. Radiology. 1996;200:327–31.

Brix G, Lechel U, Glatting G, et al. Radiation exposure of patients undergoing whole-body dual-modality 18 FDG PET/CT examinations. The Jurnal of Nuclear Medicine. 2005;46(4):608–13.

Christian PE, Bernier DR, Langan JK. Nuclear medicine and PET: technology and techniques. 5th ed. St. Louis, MO: Mosby; 2004.

Early PJ, Sodee BD. Principles and practice of nuclear medicine. 2nd ed. St. Louis, MO: Mosby; 1995.

Hamilton B, Guidos B. Medical acronyms, symbols, and abbreviations. 2nd ed. New York, NY: Neal-Schumann; 1988.

Health Physics Society. http://hps.org/publicinformation/radterms/. Accessed 20 January 2011

Hunter BT, Taljanovic SM. Glossary of medical devices and procedures: abbreviations, acronyms, and definitions. RadioGraphics. 2003;23:195–213.

Jablonski S. Dictionary of medical acronyms and abbreviations. Philadelphia, Pa: Hanley and Belfus; 1987.

Lin E, Alavi A. PET and PET/CT a clinical guide. 2nd ed. New York, NY: Thieme Medical Publishers; 2009.

Logan CM, Rice MK. Logan's medical and scientific abbreviations. Philadelphia, Pa: Lippincott; 1987.

Glanze WD, Anderson KN, Anderson LE. Mosby's medical, nursing, and allied health dictionary. 3rd ed. St Louis, Mo: Mosby, 1990

National Oncologic PET Registry. Cancers and indications eligible for entry in the NOPR. http://www.cancerpetregistry.org/pdf/FDG%20Indications.pdf. Accessed 2 March2012

REMM. Dictionary of Radiation Terms. http://www.remm.nlm.gov/dictionary.htm. Accessed December 20, 2011

Steves AM, Wells AM. Review of nuclear medicine technology: preparation for certification examinations. Reston, VA: Society of Nuclear Medicine; 2004.

U.S. NRC Glossary. http://www.nrc.gov/reading-rm/basic-ref/glossary.html. Accessed December 15, 2011

Wahl RL. Principles and practice of PET and PET/CT. 2nd ed. Philadelphia, PA: Lippincott Williams & Williams; 2009.

Webster JG, editor. Encyclopedia of medical devices and instrumentation, vol. 1–4. New York, NY: Wiley; 1988.

Webster's New World™ Medical Dictionary, 3rd edition, Medicinenet.com, 2008

Wells P, Martha P. Practical mathematics in nuclear medicine technology. Reston, VA: Society of Nuclear Medicine; 1999.

Appendix D
Useful Websites

ACR American College of Radiology:
http://www.acr.org/

AHA:
http://www.heart.org/

Amedeo. The Medical Literature Guide:
http://www.amedeo.com/

American AED/CPR Association:
http://www.aedcpr.com/

ANMS American Neurogastroenterology and Motility Society:
http://www.motilitysociety.org/

ARRT American Registry of Radiologic Technologists:
https://www.arrt.org/index.html

ASRT American Society of Radiologic Technologists:
https://www.asrt.org/

ASNC American Society of Nuclear Cardiology:
http://www.asnc.org/

AuntMinnie.com:
http://www.auntminnie.com/

Author Stream (slide sharing):
http://www.authorstream.com

Brain Atlas:
http://www.med.harvard.edu/AANLIB/home.html

CDC Centers for Disease Control:
http://www.cdc.gov/

Consultants in Nuclear Medicine:
http://www.nucmedconsultants.com/

Dose Estimates for Nuclear Medicine Scans:
http://ehs.columbia.edu/Dosimetry%20Help/NMDoseEstimates.html

DOT Department of Transportation:
http://www.dot.gov/

Drugs.com:
http://www.drugs.com/

Emedicine:
http://emedicine.medscape.com

EPA Environmental Protection Agency:
http://www.epa.gov/

Family Health Guide. Harvard Medical School:
http://www.health.harvard.edu/fhg/

FDA Food and Drug Administration:
http://www.fda.gov/

HFAP Healthcare Facilities Accreditation Program:
http://www.hfap.org/

HPS. Health Physics Society:
http://www.hps.org/

GE (General Electric) Healthcare:
https://hls.gehealthcare.com/gehc/

HealthImaging.com:
http://www.healthimaging.com/

ICANL Intersocietal Commission for the Accreditation of Nuclear Medicine Laboratories:
http://www.icanl.org/icanl/index.htm

ICRP International Commission on Radiological Protection:
http://www.icrp.org/

ICRU International Commission on Radiation Units:
http://www.icru.org/

IAEA International Atomic Energy Agency:
http://www.iaea.org/

IMAIOSE E-anatomy.
http://www.imaios.com/en/e-Anatomy/

Internet Journal of Nuclear Medicine
http://www.ispub.com/ostia/index.php?xmlFilePath=journals/ijnuc/vol3n1/scan.xml

Jefferson Lab.
http://www.jlab.org/div_dept/train/rad_guide/effects.html

JCAHO Joint Commission on Accreditation of Healthcare Organizations:
http://www.jointcommission.org/

Appendix D: Useful Websites

Mallinckrodt Inst of Radiology WU in St Louis Teaching file:
http://gamma.wustl.edu/

Mallinckrodt Institute of Radiology cases:
http://www.radquiz.com/Nucs-Teaching.htm

MDConsult:
http://www.mdconsult.com

MDS Nordion:
http://www.mds.nordion.com/

Medical Physics Dep:
http://www.nuclearmedicine.org.uk/ Pilgrim Hosp, Boston

Medscape:
http://www.medscape.com/

Molecular Imaging:
http://www.molecularimaging.net/

NCI National Cancer Institute:
http://www.cancer.gov/

NCRP National Council on Radiation Protection & Measurements:
http://www.ncrponline.org/

NEMA National Electrical Manufacturer's Association:
http://www.nema.org/

North American Center for Continuing Medical Education:
http://www.naccme.com/

Nuclear Medicine. Radiochemistry Society:
http://www.radiochemistry.org/nuclearmedicine/

Nuclear Medicine Technology Certification Board:
http://www.nmtcb.org/root/default.php

Oxford Journals. Radiation Protection Dosimetry:
http://rpd.oxfordjournals.org/content/

Philips: http://www.healthcare.philips.com/

RadiologyInfo.org:
http://www.radiologyinfo.org/

NCBI. PubMed.gov National Center for Biotechnology Information:
http://www.ncbi.nlm.nih.gov/pubmed/

Radiological Society of North America (USA):
http://www.rsna.org

NMTCB Nuclear Medicine Technology Certification Board:
http://www.nmtcb.org/root/default.php

Radiopharmacy, Inc.:
http://www.radiopharmacy.com/Newsletters.htm

REMM Radiation Emergency Medical Management:
http://www.remm.nlm.gov/dictionary.htm

RSNA Radiological Society of North America:
http://www.rsna.org/

Scintigraphy of the Paediatric Skeleton:
http://www.medical-atlas.org/

Siemens:
http://www.medical.siemens.com/

SNM Society of Nuclear Medicine:
http://www.snm.org/

Societies of Nuclear Medicine of Latin America:
http://www.alasbimnjournal.cl/

Society of Nuclear Medicine:
http://www.snm.org/

UpToDate:
http://www.uptodate.com/home/

U.S. NRC Nuclear Regulatory Commission:
http://www.nrc.gov/

WIKIPEDIA:
http://www.wikipedia.org/

Author Index

A
Abbas, K.A., 55, 58–62, 64, 69, 199, 201, 215
Abeloff, D.M., 71, 132, 197
Abikhzer, G., 55, 142, 144, 202, 242
Alavi, A., 47, 51–58, 61, 62, 65–69, 72, 123, 124, 128–131, 133–137, 144, 145, 147, 148, 195, 196, 200–204, 206, 207, 210, 212, 240, 251
Albert, R.H., 145
Alessi, A., 246
Al-Mallah, H.M., 59, 204
Andreoli, T.E., 57, 64, 69, 72, 138, 142, 147, 206, 218, 246
Antioch, G., 122, 220
Armitage, O.J., 71, 132, 197
Austin, J.H., 286

B
Balink, H., 69
Barger, R.L., 57
Bashir, A., 205, 209, 216
Becherer, A., 206
Beller, G.A., 57–59, 67, 70, 121, 123, 125, 208, 213, 214, 242
Bengel, M.F., 60, 196, 197, 211, 220
Bernier, D.R., 56
Blake, G.M., 49
Bockish, A., 122, 220
Boellaard, R., 53, 130, 214
Brant, E.W., 60
Brasse, D., 218
Brem, F.R., 212
Brenner, I.A., 207, 219
Brix, G., 60, 147, 258
Buchanan, J.W., 137, 200
Burrell, S., 67

C
Calhoun, S.P., 191
Cannon, B., 47, 122, 193
Castellucci, P., 132, 142, 144, 199, 201, 203
Chen, W., 244
Cheson, D.B., 142
Christian, P.E., 49–52, 56, 58, 59, 64, 66, 125–130, 135, 137–140, 191, 197–200, 204, 205, 210, 213, 215, 221, 246
Collins, J., 69
Cotran, R.S., 46
Czerniecki, J.B., 48, 53, 121, 216, 217

D
Delbeke, D., 137
Dementia, 62
Di Carli, M.F., 59, 191, 193
Dilsizian, V., 219
Dimitris, G., 218
Dorbala, S., 216

E
Early, P.J., 46, 48, 50, 126, 132, 204, 212
Einstein, A.J., 120
Erwin, W.D.J., 68, 148

F
Fahey, H.F., 68, 139–141, 146, 213
Ferri, F.F., 213
Ferrif, F., 133, 139, 146
Fletcher, J.W., 203
Fong, Y., 198
Frohlich, E.D., 52, 64

G

Galanski, M., 49, 60, 70, 72, 126, 127, 133, 138, 145, 146, 198, 199, 208, 214
Gerbaudo, H.V., 60, 138, 142, 200, 210, 216, 221
Gillard, J.H., 218
Goldberger, L.A., 46, 68, 71, 121, 124, 201, 206, 215, 245
Graham, M.M., 192
Grant, F.D., 209
Groch, M.W., 68
Groch, W.M., 148
Gropler, J.R., 205, 209, 216

H

Hajnal, G.V., 54, 208, 217, 220
Hallett, W.A., 63
Hamblen, M.S., 63, 68, 136
Hamilton, B., 286
Hanaoka, K., 134
Hansell, D.M., 61, 71, 195
Harvey, R.A., 65–67, 69, 125, 130, 140, 143, 147
Heller, G.V., 145
Hickeson, M., 55, 136, 142, 144, 202, 242
Hicks, J.R., 64
Houseni, M., 58, 59, 69, 196, 220
Hu, M.I., 244
Hunter, B.T., 286
Hutchings, M., 129, 198

I

Iagaru, A., 56, 130, 135, 205, 214
Inoue, K., 197
Isasi, C.R., 141

J

Jablonski, S., 286
Jacene, H., 130, 131, 134, 217, 219, 221, 245
Jadver, H., 240–244
Jensen, R.T., 204
Jhanwar, S.Y., 56, 128, 137, 197, 198

K

Kaplan, A.D., 207
Karakousis, C.G., 47, 48, 53, 121, 216, 217
Kazama, T., 143
Kebebew, E., 208

Kim, S.K., 71
Klein, M., 203
Korf, J., 215
Kumar, R., 56, 67, 70, 141, 142, 146, 206, 219
Kumar, U., 47
Kumar, V., 55, 58–62, 64, 69, 199, 201, 215

L

Lacy, L.J., 209
Larsson, S.A., 207
Lee, J.H., 214
Lin, C.E., 123, 124, 128–131, 133–137, 144, 147, 148, 195, 196, 200–204, 206, 207, 210, 212, 240
Lin, E.C., 47, 51–58, 61, 62, 65–69, 251
Lipton, M.J., 59, 191, 193
Logan, C.M., 286
Lombardi, M.H., 48, 67, 69, 127, 131, 136, 138, 202, 203, 216
Lowe, J.V., 63, 68, 136
Lucignani, G., 72, 122

M

MacDonald, A., 67
Mach, H.R., 125, 126, 194, 197, 199
Machac, J., 194
Madden, E.M., 63, 129, 134, 210
Maecke, H.R., 139
Mandell, L.G., 130, 131, 221
Mankoff, A.D., 214
Martha, P., 252–255
Mawlawi, O., 45, 122, 191, 193
Mazzaferri, E.L., 243
Miles, A.K., 66, 68, 139, 194, 211, 212
Miletich, S.R., 129, 143
Mittra, E., 71, 140, 146, 192, 211, 212, 241, 242
Moore, L.K., 62, 63, 129, 196
Morano, N.G., 211
Mosci, C., 130, 135, 205, 214
Munro, H.B., 70, 126, 242
Mycek, M.J., 65–67, 69, 125, 130, 140, 143, 147

N

Nair, A., 66
Nandular, R.K., 57
Nedegaard, J., 47, 122, 193
Newberg, B.A., 72, 145

Author Index

P
Parker, J.A., 240–244
Patton, J.A., 48, 53, 54, 57, 133, 140, 202
Perry, A.G., 71
Petrovitch, I., 212
Placantonakis, G.D., 52, 131, 142, 146, 194, 195, 198
Potter, P.A., 71
Prior, J.O., 219
Prokop, M., 49, 60, 70, 72, 126, 127, 133, 138, 145, 146, 198, 199, 208, 214

Q
Quon, A., 71, 140, 146, 192, 211, 212, 241

R
Rahmim, A., 62, 140
Reubi, J.C., 139
Rice, L.S., 148
Robbins, S.L., 46
Rohren, E.M., 144, 205
Roivainen, A., 50, 194
Russell, J.J., 145

S
Saha, G.B., 45, 48, 72, 120, 121, 127, 132, 135, 147, 193, 194, 201, 211, 215, 217
Salskov, A., 210
Sanchez-Crespo, A., 207
Sarji, A.S., 123, 145
Schilling, K., 208, 213
Schwartz, H.T., 52, 131, 142, 146, 194, 195, 198
Schwarz, S.W., 125, 126, 194, 197, 199
Segall, G., 212
Seibyl, J.P., 211
Shukla, A.K., 47
Sodee, B.D., 46, 48, 50, 126, 132, 204, 212
Soret, M., 45, 120, 191
Soyka, D.J., 125
Spaepen, K., 141

Steves, A.M., 249–251, 255
Straus, J.D., 56, 128, 137, 197, 198
Sureshbabu, W., 45, 122, 191, 193

T
Takalkar, A., 62, 131, 133, 222
Thompson, C., 61, 144, 209, 220
Thompson, K., 216
Turkington, G.T., 124

V
Valk, P.E., 205
Vallabhajosula, S., 45–47, 49, 121, 123–126, 143, 193, 195, 204, 210, 214, 245, 246
Vines, C.D., 58
Visvikis, D., 65, 120, 123, 126

W
Wahl, L.R., 130, 131, 134, 217, 219, 221, 245
Wahl, R.L., 48–57, 59, 62, 63, 66, 68, 70, 120, 121, 124, 127–129, 132, 137–139, 143, 145, 147, 148, 191, 192, 194, 196, 200–202, 215, 217, 222, 241, 243, 245, 250
Webster, J.G., 286
Wells, A.M., 249–251, 255
Wells, P., 252–255
Wong, T.Z., 209

Y
Yoshinaga, K., 202

Z
Zaidi, H., 61, 62, 140, 144, 209, 220
Zanzonico, P., 246
Zaret, B.L., 57–59, 67, 70, 121, 123, 125, 208, 213, 214, 242
Zhuang, H., 143
Zielinski, M., 196

Subject Index

A
Abbreviations and symbols, nuclear medicine, 259–272
Abdominal mass evaluation, 158, 195
Absorbed dose, 273
Absorbed organ doses, 238, 246
Accessory organs, digestive system, 87, 127
Accuracy testing, 88, 127
Acetate C-11, 169, 204
Actinide, 273
Active lesions, 166, 202
Activity, 273
Adenocarcinoma, 229, 233, 237, 240, 243, 245
Adrenal glands, 228, 240
Aerobic respiration, 273
Aggrenox, 182, 214
Agreement State, 273
Airborne radioactive material, 273
Airflow direction
  negative pressure rooms, 163, 198
Air-purifying respirator, 273
Akinetic left ventricle, 239, 246
Algorithm, 273
Alimentary canal, 15, 52
Allergic reaction, 6, 46
Alpha particle, 273
Alpha radiation, radioactivity, 161, 197
Altered metabolism (PET) and areas of structural change (CT), 17, 53
Alzheimer's disease, 82, 93, 111, 123, 131, 143
Amelanotic melanomas, 184, 216
Amino acids, 90, 128
  as building blocks, 8, 47
Aminophylline, 92, 130

Amyvid, 232, 242
Anaerobic glycolysis, 114, 145
Anaerobic respiration, 273
Analog signal, 273
Anaphylaxis, 6, 46
Anaplastic thyroid cancer scintigraphy, 170, 205
Anaplastic thyroid carcinomas (ATC), 93, 130, 174, 208
Anatomic diagnostic modality, 14, 52
Angiogenesis, 10, 49, 177, 210
Annihilation, 273
Annihilation event, photons, 7, 46
Annual allowable limit, radiation exposure, 164, 200
Annual limit on intake (ALI), 274
Anode, 274
Anterior mediastinum, 173, 207
Antibody, 274
Antigen, 274
Anxiolytic medication, 32, 65
Aorta, 91, 129
Aperture, 274
Apoptosis, 105, 139
Apyrogenicity, 238, 246
Arms position, malignant melanoma scanning, 13, 51
Arrangement of Ps, 8, 47
Arthroplasty, 274
Ascending aorta, 172, 206
ATC. *See* Anaplastic thyroid carcinomas (ATC)
Atelectasis, 274
Atoms measurement, 87, 127
Atrial fibrillation, 79, 121
Atrioventricular node, 237, 245

Attenuation-corrected and reconstructed positron emission tomography (PET-FDG), 155, 192
Attenuation-corrected (AC) PET images, 165, 200
Attenuation correction, 15, 52
Auditory information, temporal lobe, 31, 64
Autograft, 274
Auxillary lymph node metastasis, 172, 206
Average variance, 166, 201, 274
Axial field-of-view, 274

B

Background counting rate, 238, 246
Background radiation, 274
Back projection, 84, 125
Basal ganglia, 182, 189, 215, 221
Baseline PET-FDG scan, 39, 69
BAT. *See* Brown adipose tissue (BAT)
Bayesian analysis, 160, 196
Beam current and exposure time, 16, 53
Beam-hardening artifact, 274
Becquerel (Bq), 274
Benign nodules, 116, 145
Beta particle, 274
Bioassay (radiobioassay), 274
Biological PET radioisotopes, 250
Biomaterial, 274
Bismuth germinate (BGO), 8, 47
Blank scan, 11, 50
Bleb, 274
Blood perfusion radiopharmaceutical, brain, 178, 211
Blood vessels formation process, 10, 49
Bone marrow
 hyperplasia, 99, 135
 radiation effects, 160, 196
Bone stimulator, 275
Brachytherapy, 275
Brain metabolism and blood flow, 94, 116, 131, 146
Brain metabolism rate, 183, 215
Braking radiation, 84, 124
Breast benign lesions, 110, 142
Breast cancer, 109, 141
Breast-feeding patient referred for PET imaging, 28, 61
Breast-specific gamma imaging (BGSI), 179, 212
Breathing protocols, 80, 122
Bremsstrahlung, 275
Bremsstrahlung radiation, 86, 126
Bronchiolitis, 275

Bronchioloalveolar carcinoma, 117, 147
Brown adipose tissue (BAT), 157, 193
Brown fat localization, 8, 47

C

C-11 acetate, 171, 176, 188, 205, 209, 220
Calandria, 275
Calculation, percent error, 83, 124
Calibration, 154, 187, 191, 219
Calibration and constancy, 10, 49
Cancer tissue, molecular and functional alterations, 156, 189, 192, 221–222
Carbon-13, 179, 212
Carbon-2 atom, deoxyglucose with F-18, 236, 245
Carbon-11-labeled Pittsburgh Compound B (C-11 PiB), 20, 55
Carbon-11-methionine PET, 165, 201
Cardiac conduction system, 237, 245
Cardiac imaging studies
 lowest estimated effective radiation dose, 153, 191
Cardiac scanning processing, 156, 193
Cardiovascular compression rate, 40, 70
Casting, 275
Cathode, 275
Cathode filament, X-ray tube, 13, 51
Cecum, colon, and rectum, 92, 129
Cell proliferation, 181, 214
Cellular apoptosis, 105, 139
C-11 epinephrine, 178, 211
C-F-2, 156, 193
Chemical shift artifact, 275
Chest compressions, Airway, Breathing (C-A-B), 118, 148
Child's dose for PET scan, 81, 122
Chi-square test, 275
Cholesterol metabolic pathway, 104, 139
Choline, 11, 50, 168, 204
Chronic obstructive pulmonary disease, 19, 55
Circle of Willis, 10, 49
Circulatory system, 23, 58
Clinical follow-up excluding focal inflammation or malignancy, 40, 70
Clinical stress perfusion studies with Rb-82, 22, 57
Clinical utility, PET/CT-FDG imaging *vs.* PET-FDG imaging, 91, 129
C-11 L-leucine, 85, 125
C-11 L-methionine, 85, 125
C-11 L-tyrosine, 85, 125
Coincidence events, 34, 66, 84, 124
Cold pressor testing, PET MPI, 187, 219

Cold testing, 275
Collective dose, 275
Colon inflammation, 98, 134
Colonoscopy, 95, 132
Colony-stimulating factors (CSFs), 92, 130
Colorectal cancer, 41, 71, 96, 133, 161, 197
Combined whole-body effective dose, diagnostic PET/CT, 9, 48
Committed dose equivalent (HT,50), 275
Committed effective dose equivalent (HE,50), 275
Computed tomography (CT)
  assessment, pulmonary nodules, 27, 60
  nodal metastases, 230, 241
  X-ray tube, 40, 70
Concentration and specific activity, 254
Concept, clinical SPECT/CT system, 18, 54
Conscious sedation, 101, 136
Consolidation, 275
Constancy, dose calibrator quality control procedure testing, 11, 50
Constraint (dose constraint), 275
Contiguous, 275
Contrast agents, 114, 145
Contrast media, 43, 72
Controlled area, 275
Conversion, 14 mCi to megabecquerels (MBq), 35, 67
Convolution, 118, 148
Coronal maximum-intensity projection PET image, 169–170, 204
Coronal slice of the brain, 97, 134
Coronary artery disease (CAD), 97, 133
  mean sensitivity and specificity, 157, 194
Coronary flow reserve (CFR), 162, 197
Coronary vasodilator reserve (CVR), 174, 208
Correction for table speed, 33, 65
Cotswold system, 89, 128, 161, 197
  single lymph node region, 162, 198
Counts per minute (cpm) conversion, 253
Critical organ, 275
Cross plane, 275
CSFs. *See* Colony-stimulating factors (CSFs)
Cs-137 measurement, 167, 203
CT attenuation correction, 153, 191
CT dose index, 275
CT X-ray tube, 10, 49
Curie (Ci), 102, 136, 275
Cyclotron produced positron-emitting radionuclide, 9, 48
Cyst, 276
Cystic fibrosis (CF), 167, 203

D
3D acquisition *vs.* 2D, 105, 139
Daily quality control checks, PET scanner, 13, 51
Decay calculation, half-life, 254
Decay constant, 6, 45
Declared pregnant woman, 276
Decontamination, 99, 135
Deep-dose equivalent (Hd), 276
Deformable coregistration, 175, 209
Deformable registration techniques, 175, 185, 187, 208, 217, 219–220
Delay time, positron emission tomography scan, 13, 51
Dementia, 43, 72
Dementia with Lewy bodies (DLB), 160, 196
Dental fillings, hip prosthetics, chemotherapy port, 6, 45
Department of Transportation (DOT) labels, 249
Depolarization, 182, 215
Depth of interaction (DOI), 178, 211
Descending aorta, 110–111, 142
Diabetes, chronic complications, 185, 218
Diagnostic CT, 27, 60
Diaphragmatic crus F-18 FDG uptake, 98, 134
Diaschisis, 235, 244
DICOM. *See* Digital Imaging and Communications in Medicine (DICOM)
Dicumarol, 85, 125
Differentiated thyroid cancer (DTC), 28, 62
Diffuse large B-cell lymphoma, 20, 56
Diffusely increased marrow FDG uptake, 162, 197
Diffuse muscular and myocardial uptake, 19, 55
Diffuse, symmetric uptake, F-18 FDG, 36, 68
Digital Imaging and Communications in Medicine (DICOM), 107, 140
Digital signal, 276
Dipirydamole, 112, 143
Direct molecular imaging, 178, 211
Direct-use material, 276
Discrete source, 276
Distant metastasis, 228, 240
Distinguishable from background, 276
2D mode septa, 36, 68
DNA synthesis, cell proliferation, 10, 49
Dobutamine, 107, 140
Doppler phenomenon, 276
Dose calibrator and quality control, 251

Dose calibrator quality control procedure, 7, 46
Dose equivalent (HT), 276
Dose extravasation, antecubital injection site, 28, 62
Dose of F-18 FDG, 8, 47
Dose/radiation dose, 276
Dosimetry processor, 276
Drug master file (DMF), 276
3D surface rendering, 154, 191
DTC. See Differentiated thyroid cancer (DTC)
Dual time point FDG-PET imaging, 22, 57
Dynamic contrast-enhanced (DCE) CT, 160, 196

E

Earliest disposal, decay-in-storage waste material, 14, 52
ECG order, electrical currents, 166, 201
Effective dose equivalent (HE), 276
Effective half-life, 254, 276
  radiopharmaceutical, 20, 55, 79, 121
Eipe test, 112, 144
Electrocardiogram (ECG or EKG), 37, 68
Electroencephalography (EEG), 110, 142
Electron capture, 276
Electronic collimation, 104, 138
Electronic ventricular pacemaker, 41–42, 71,
Electrons, cathode filament, 153, 191
Embryo/fetus, 276
Emits electrons, 13, 51
Endometrial uptake F-18 FDG, 97, 133
Endothelial function assessment, 187, 219
Enriched uranium, 277
Enrichment, 277
Entrance/access point, 277
Epilepsy, mesial temporal sclerosis, 231, 241
Epileptic focus, 159, 195
Epileptogenic region, 234, 243
Epinephrine, 116, 146
ERC. See Exposure rate constant (ERC)
Esophageal cancer, 232, 242
Esophageal malignancy, Barrett's esophagus, 233, 243
Esophageal sphincter, 160, 196
Estimated effective radiation dose, 77, 120
Estrogen receptor, 87, 126
Evaluation of brain injuries, 107, 140
Excessive F-18 FDG metabolic activity, 233, 242

Exercise-induced stress MPI study, 189, 222
Exposure, 277
Exposure rate, 239, 246
  change calculation, shielding, 253
  at distance, F-18 FDG, 43, 72
  radiation source, 117, 147
  radioactive source, 44, 73
Exposure rate constant (ERC), 5, 45
External dose, 277
Extracellular β-amyloid plaques (Aβ), 82, 123
Extremity, 277

F

F-18, 7, 46
Falling CEA levels, 32, 64
False-negative PET scans in lung cancer imaging, 15, 53
False-positive fraction, 180, 213, 232, 242
False-positive uptake in FDG-PET images, 14, 51
Fat tissue, 174, 208
FDG injection, 227, 240
FDG molecule design, 236, 245
FDG-PET imaging
  malignant mesotheliomas, 103, 138
  malignant pleural mesothelioma (MPM), 164, 200
  prostate cancer, 230, 241
  radiation exposure minimization, 228, 240
  staging, Hodgkin's lymphoma (HL), 163, 198
FDG-PET over conventional scintigraphy, 39, 69
FDG-PET sensitivity and specificity, 171, 205
FDG uptake
  by cancer cells, 41, 70
  mesotheliomas, 183, 216
  period, 16, 53
F-18 DOPA, 165, 201
F-18 FDG, 14, 32, 51, 64
  dosage, 175, 188, 190, 209, 220, 222, 233, 238, 243, 246
  dose in brain, 114, 145
  time and dosage, 162, 198
F-18 FDG-PET imaging, 20, 56
  thyroid carcinoma, 181, 214
F-18 FDG unit, 161, 197
F-18 FDG uptake, 101, 105, 136, 139
  atherosclerotic lesions, 164, 200
  in fracture, 111, 143
  in gallbladder/biliary tract, 90, 129
F-18 fluoride bone uptake mechanism, 10, 49

Subject Index

F-18 fluorocholine, 157, 194
F-18 fluorodeoxyglucose (FDG), 28, 61, 173, 207
F-18 fluoro-dihydrotestosterone (FDHT), 110, 142
F-18 fluoroestradiol (FES), 87, 126
6-[F-18]fluoro-L-DOPA, 171, 206
F-18 fluorothymidine, 83, 124
Filament, 277
Filtering facepiece (dust mask), 277
Fission, 277
Fission fragments, 277
Fit factor, 277
Fit test, 277
Fluorine-18, 15, 52, 88, 128
Fluoromisonidazole (F-18 MISO), 159, 195
Focal colon activity, 98, 134
Focal FDG uptake, lungs, 18, 55
Focal thyroid uptake, F-18 FDG, 236, 244
Focal uptake, 28, 61
Focal ureteral activity, 159, 195
Fourier rebinning, 154, 192
Fourier transform, 37, 68, 277
Frame mode, 277
Free fatty acids and glucose, 27, 60
Frequency, 277
Frontal lobe of the brain, 14, 52
F-18 sodium fluoride
  radiation dose, 179, 212
  uptake
    bone, 175, 209
    mechanism, 186, 219
Full-width half-maximum (FWHM), 277
Fused coronal, 12, 50

G
Ga-68 DOTA-peptides, 96, 132
Gallbladder, 31, 63
Gamma and beta radiation
  radioactivity, 161, 197
Gamma rays, 277
Gastric cancer, 229, 240
Gastroesophageal junction, 23, 58
G-CSF. *See* Granulocyte-colony stimulating factor (G-CSF)
Geiger–Muller counter output, 87, 127
Generalized seizure, 237, 245
Generally applicable environmental radiation standards, 277
Genetic effects, 278
Geometric efficiency, PET scanner, 112, 143
Germanium-68, 21, 56
Gibbs (truncation) artifact, 278

Glucose, 170, 205
Glucose metabolism, 174, 207
Glucose metabolism, early-onset *versus* late-onset Alzheimer's disease, 179, 212
Glutamine synthetase pathway, 93, 131
Granulocyte-colony stimulating factor (G-CSF), 32, 65, 92, 94, 98, 130, 131, 134, 188, 189, 221
Granulocyte-macrophage colony-stimulating factor (GM-CSF), 92, 130
Gray (Gy), 278
Gray scale, 278
Greenfield filter, 278

H
Half-life, 278
Half value layer (HVL), 230, 235, 241, 244, 278
Helical scan, 278
Hemoptysis, 39, 69
Heterograft, 278
Hexokinase, 227, 240
Hiatal hernias, 21, 57
Hibernatic myocardium, 81, 123
HIF-1. *See* Hypoxia inducible factor-1 (HIF-1)
High-definition PET, 107, 140
Highest light output scintillators, 20, 56
High-level waste, 278
Highly enriched uranium, 278
High radiation area, 91, 129, 278
Hilum, 278
Histologic evaluation, diagnosis of melanoma, 9, 48
Hodgkin's disease, 163, 199
Homograft, 278
Hot cell, 278
Hot-for-cold substitution, 87, 126, 158, 194
Hot rolling, 278
Hounsfield unit scale, 88, 127
Housing info, 30, 63
Huntington's disease, 184, 217
Hybrid PET-CT scanners, 160, 196
Hydroxyapatite, 278
Hyperemia, 278
Hyperinsulinemic state, 19, 55
Hypermetabolic activity, 93–94, 112–113, 131, 144
  right hemithorax, 107–108, 140
Hyperplasia, 278
Hyperthermia, 104, 138
Hypoglycemia, 39, 69

Hypometabolic area, radiation therapy, 165, 201
Hypothalamus, 103, 137
Hypothyroidism, 82, 123
Hypoxia
  extent assessment, 159, 195
  growing tumor, 159, 195
  and perfusion, 175, 209
Hypoxia inducible factor-1 (HIF-1), 119, 148

I
I-124, 99, 135
Ictal events, 185, 218
Image-guided transthoracic needle aspiration/biopsy, 22, 58
Image registration, 17, 54, 88, 127
Immobilization device, 278
Implant, 278
Improved noise-to-signal ratios, 29, 62
Inconclusive CCTA, 82, 123
Inconclusive test, 29, 62, 187, 219
Increased membrane synthesis, 189, 221
Increased sensitivity, 96, 133
Indirect molecular imaging, 179, 212
Individual monitoring devices, 278–279
Infiltrated dose, 35, 67
Injected blood clot, 18, 55
Injection artifact, 279
In situ carcinoma, 171, 206
Insulin, 34, 66, 279
Intense F-18 FDG activity, 114, 144
Intercostal muscles, 233, 242
Interictal PET scans, 170, 205
Interictal state, 116, 146
Internal conversion, 279
Internal dose, 279
Intraictal state, 94, 131
Intraneuronal neurofibrillary tangles (NFTs), 82, 123
Intrathecal (drug) delivery pump, 279
Inverse square law, 253
Inverted C shape, 168, 203
Ionic agents, 188, 220
Ionizing radiation, 279
IR. *See* Iterative Reconstruction (IR)
Isomeric transition, 279
Iterative Reconstruction (IR), 78, 121

K
Kernel into raw data, 118, 148
Ketoacidosis, 185, 218

L
Laryngeal F-18 FDG uptake, 113, 144
Lateral brain localizer image, 26, 60
Lead shielding, 186, 218
Left ventricle, 29–30, 63
Left ventricular ejection fraction (LVEF), 183, 215–216
Lens dose equivalent (LDE), 279
Lesion color homogeneity, 185, 217
Licensed material, 279
Ligand, 163, 199, 279
Light detectors, 179, 212
Light output, 11, 50
Limbic system, 177, 210
Limitations of PET head and neck imaging, 21, 56
Limits (dose limits), 279
Linear artifact, 279
Linear attenuation coefficient, 79, 121
Linearity, 7, 46
Lipoma, 19, 55
Liposarcoma, 110, 142
List mode, 279
Liver, 87, 127
Liver metastasis, 168, 204
Lobe, 27, 61
Localizer scan, 279
Longest half-life, positron-emitting nuclides, 15, 52
Lost/missing licensed material, 279
Low-dose CT scan, 22, 57
Low enriched uranium, 279
Lower sensitivity, F-18 L-Thymidine (FLT) PET, 176, 210
Lowest radiation dose, PET/CT scanning protocols, 117, 147
LSO. *See* Lutetium oxyorthosilicate (LSO)
Luer-activated device, 42, 71
Lung activity observation, 16, 53
Lung cancer patient
  5-year survival rate, 232, 242
Lung disease, benign nature, 188, 220
Lutetium oxyorthosilicate (LSO), 90, 128
  detector, 156, 193
  radioactivity, 157, 194
Luxury perfusion, 234, 243
Lymphadenopathy, 279
Lymphatic system, 23, 58
Lymphocyte, 21, 56
Lymphoma, 21, 25, 28, 57, 59, 61, 109, 141
Lymphoma evaluation, 32, 64
LYSO, 80, 122

Subject Index

M
Macrophage colony-stimulating factor (M-CSF), 92, 130
Magnetic resonance imaging (MRI), 14, 52
Magnotherapy, 43, 72
Malignancy, 83, 123
Malignant lung nodules, 41, 71
Malignant neoplasm, skin, 8, 47
Mammary prosthesis, 279
Mass attenuation coefficient, 279
Mass defect, 280
Mass pulmonary, 280
Maximum-intensity projection, 23–24, 58
11 mCi, 8, 47
M-CSF. *See* Macrophage colony-stimulating factor (M-CSF)
Mediastinal soft tissues, 118, 148
Medicare coverage, 40, 70
Medicare reimbursement, 101, 136
Medicare reimbursement, PET-FDG Myocardial Viability imaging, 82, 123
Medullary thyroid cancer, 24, 235
Megabecquerels (MBq), 234, 243
Melanoma, 8, 47, 78, 121
Member of the public, 280
Membrane lipid synthesis measurement, 157, 194
Mesothelioma, 176, 210
Mesothelioma stage, treatment selection, 161, 196
Metabolic lesion characteristics, 27, 60
Metabolic tracers, viability evaluation, 181, 214
Metallic implants artifacts, 6, 45
Metastable state, 280
Metastases to regional lymph nodes, 96, 133
Metformin, 85, 125
Microcuries (mCi) to Curies (Ci), 231, 242
Mild to moderate myocardial ischemia, 184, 216
Million instructions per second (MIPS), 280
Mineralocorticoids, 167, 202
Minimization physiologic muscular uptake, 31, 63
Minor, 280
Mirror imaging artifact, 280
Misregistration artifacts, 80, 122
Mixed attenuation, 162, 198
Molecular imaging, 6, 45
Monitoring (radiation monitoring, radiation protection monitoring), 280
Motion artifacts, 15, 16, 53, 154, 191
Mucinous adenocarcinoma, 162, 198

Multi-infarct dementia
  FDG uptake, 158, 194
Multiplanar reconstruction (MPR), 280
Multiple-choice test
  elements, 1
  methods and strategies, 1–2
  physical strategy, 3–4
  study strategy, 3
Multiple focal cortical and subcortical defects, 17, 54
Multiple myeloma, 165, 201
Myeloid, 280
Myocardial blood flow (MBF), 162, 197
Myocardial glucose metabolism, 232, 242
Myocardial oxygen consumption (MVO_2), 176, 209
Myocardial viability, 79, 121

N
NaI (Tl) (thallium-doped sodium iodide), 20, 56
N-13 ammonia, 180, 189, 213, 222
Nasogastric tube, 280
The National Oncologic PET Registry (NOPR), 101, 136, 255–257
NECR. *See* Noise equivalent count rate (NECR)
Necrosis, 36, 67
Negative pressure respirator (tight fitting), 280
Nephrostomy tube, 280
Net counts, 252
Neuroendocrine tumors (NET), 164, 167, 199, 203
Neurotransmitters imaging, 181, 214
Neutron capture, 280
Neutron flux, 280
Neutrons, 280
Neutropenia, 31, 64, 188, 221
New drug application (NDA), 280
Nigral degeneration and striatal dopamine deficiency, 96, 132
Nitrogen-13 (N-13), 9, 48
  isotope, 179, 212
Nitrogen-13-ammonia, 99, 135
Nitroglycerine, 35, 67
Nodule, 280
Noise, 280
Noise equivalent count rate (NECR), 43, 72
Non-attenuation-corrected (NAC) images, 37–38, 69, 92, 100, 130, 135
Non-collinearity
  annihilation photons, 178, 211
  pair of annihilation photons, 28, 61

Non-contrast low radiation dose scan, 82, 123
Non-fasting state, 233, 234, 243
Non-Hodgkin lymphomas (NHLs), 182, 215
Noninvasive myocardial blood flow (MBF) quantitation, 169, 204
Nonionizing radiation, 280
Non-small cell lung carcinoma, 102, 137
Nonstochastic effect, 281
Nonviable myocardium, 86, 125
NOPR. See The National Oncologic PET Registry (NOPR)
Normalization, 86, 126, 183, 215, 281
Normal saline, 99, 135
Normal sinus rhythm (NSR), 7, 46
Normal thymic activity, 176, 210
NU 2-2007, 172, 206
Nuclear medicine study *vs.* PET-FDG study, 22, 57
Nyquist frequency, 281

O

O-18 (oxygen enriched water), 112, 143
Occupational dose, 281
One standard deviation, 86, 126
Opacity, 159, 195, 281
Oral fatty acids loading, 175, 208
Oral route, F-18 FDG administration, 34, 66
Orogastric tube, 281
Orotracheal tube, 281
Osmolality, 114, 145
Osteoblastic activity, 186, 219
Ovarian uptake of F-18 FDG, 83, 123
Overestimated standardized uptake value (SUV), 33, 65
Overestimation, attenuation coefficients, 77, 120
Oxygen-15, 11, 50
Oxygen and glucose consumption, 183, 215

P

Pair production, 281
Papillary and follicular, DTC, 28, 62
Parathyroid glands, F-18 FDG-PET scintigraphy, 101, 136
Parenchyma, 281
Parietotemporal hypometabolism, 232, 242
Parkinson's disease (PD), 96, 132
Partial simple seizures, 157, 194
Partial-volume effect (PVE), 5, 45, 77, 78, 120, 153, 191

Particle accelerator, 281
Path distance, positron, 174, 207
Patient age for SUV calculation, 43, 72
Patient's fluid intake, 30, 63
Pattern, F-18 FDG, 28, 33, 61, 65
PD. See Parkinson's disease (PD)
Pediatric dose calculation, 255
Pediatric F-18 FDG dose, 40, 70
PEG tube, 281
Percentage change, "hottest" lesion, 182, 214
Percent error/difference calculation, 252
Percent error, dose calibrator, 11, 50
PERCIST-criteria, 182, 183, 214, 215
    requirements, PET scans, 236, 245
Perfusion study, 36, 68
Peripheral and thoracic lymph nodes involvement, 102, 137
Peristalsis, 15, 52
Peritoneal jugular (LeVeen) shunt, 281
PET. See Positron emission tomography (PET)
PET/CT examination, 80–81, 122, 184, 217
    punctate hypermetabolic foci, 229, 241
    right lung base mass, 230, 231, 241
PET/CT imaging, 154, 191
PET/CT scans, 118, 148
PET-FDG imaging, RCC, 154, 192
PET-FDG scan, Barrett esophagus, 113, 144
PET-FDG studies, Huntington's disease, 184, 217
PET F-18 FDG, prominent right ventricle, 166, 202
PET imaging in colorectal cancer, 102–103, 137
PET/MR scanner, 173, 207
PET myocardial perfusion imaging, 159, 195
    incremental prognostic value, 167, 202
    obese and women, 180, 213
    Rb-82, 155, 192
PET radiotracer, physicochemical property, 161, 197
Phantom, 281
Pharmacist, clinical FDG-PET imaging work, 78, 121
Pharynx, 20, 56
Photoelectric effect (PE), 168, 204, 281
Photomultiplier tube, 116, 146
Photon collinearity, 173, 207
Photon non-collinearity, 118, 147
Physiological breast uptake, postmenopausal women, 173, 206
Physiologic high uptake, FDG, 187, 219

Subject Index

Pick's disease, 169, 204
Picturing, description and measurement of
    biological processes, 6, 45
Pigtail, 281
Pitch, 87, 126, 281
Pleurodesis, 189, 221
PN. *See* Pulmonary nodule (PN)
Point spread function, 168, 204
Poisson distribution, 281
Polarity of charge, 33, 66
Porcine graft (valve), 281
Port-A-Cath, 281
Positional inaccuracy, 13, 51
Positive pressure respirator, 281
Positron, 282
Positron–electron annihilation diagram, 33–34,
    66, 89, 128
Positron–electron annihilation process,
    21–22, 57
Positron emission mammography (PEM),
    176, 209
    detectors arrangement, 188, 220
    imaging, 180, 213
    vs. PET-FDG, 112, 143
Positron emission tomography (PET), 24, 58
    biological radioisotopes, 250
    cardiac tracers, 188, 220
    gating, 23, 58
    imaging, 173, 207
    myocardial perfusion imaging *vs.*
        single-photon emission computed
        tomography, 35, 67
    radiopharmaceutical, U.S. FDA approval,
        6, 46
    reduced sensitivity, 162, 198
    scanning process raw data, 9, 48
    scintillation detectors, 250–251
    system capacity, 6, 46
    tracers, 8, 47
Positron-emitting imaging agents, 181, 214
Positron-emitting radionuclides, 7, 46
Positron, mass, 9, 48
Positrons average range, human tissue,
    238, 246
Posterior association cortex hypometabolism,
    111, 143
Post-processing measures, 78, 120
Postsurgical F-18 FDG uptake, 166, 202
Posttraumatic breast hematoma, 117, 146
Precision, 282
Pressure demand respirator, 282
Pretest probability of disease, 17, 54, 101, 136
Primary symptom of dementia, 29, 62
Primary tumor mass proximity, 171, 205

Prominent right ventricle PET F-18 FDG,
    166, 202
Propranolol, 80, 122
Proprietary agents, 154, 192
Prostate cancer, 237, 245
Prosthesis, 282
Prosthetic mitral valve, 106, 139
Protein synthesis, 85, 125
Proton-rich isotopes, 95, 132
Proximal stomach uptake, 18, 54
Public dose, 282
Pulmonary infarction, 84, 124
Pulmonary mass, 42, 71
Pulmonary nodule (PN), 25, 59
Pulmonology, 8, 47
Pulse height analyzer, 9, 48
Pulse pileups, 103, 137

Q
Quality control testing for PET agents, 84, 125
Quality factor (Q), 184, 216, 282
Quantitative bias, 5, 45

R
Rad, 93, 131
Radiation
    area, 282
    breast-feeding infant, 32, 64
    dose equivalency, 166, 202
    exposure
        from FDG-PET, 109, 141
        radiological procedures, 258
    rate, 164, 200
    necrosis, 90, 129, 201
    safety, 249
    sensitivity of tissue, 35, 67
    signs, 250
Radiation (ionizing radiation), 282
Radiation absorbed dose (rad), 228, 240, 282
Radioactive spill, 89, 128
Radiodensity, distilled water, 10, 49
Radionuclidic identity, 84, 125
Radiopaque, 282
Radiopharmacy, vial of F-18 FDG, 108, 141
Radiotherapy planning, 103, 138
Random correction, 185, 218
Random events, 88, 127, 236, 239, 245
Rate meter, 282
Rate of cell proliferation, 104, 138
Rb-82, 114, 145
    myocardial perfusion imaging, 101, 136
    rest and stress, 77, 120

Receiver operating characteristic curve (ROC) analysis, 180, 213
Receptors, 282
Recommended compression depth, 82, 123
Reconstruction method, 78, 121
Reed-Sternberg cells, 163, 199
Reference man, 282
Reference worker, 98, 134
Region of interest, 33, 65
Regular insulin, 118, 147
Residual radioactivity, 283
Residual/recurrent gliomas, 173, 207
Resolution, scanner, 178, 211
Respiratory motion, 156, 174, 193, 208
Respiratory protective device, 283
Response Evaluation Criteria in Solid Tumors (RECIST), 94, 131, 185, 217
   morphological evaluation, 189, 221
   progressive disease, 187, 219
Restricted area, 283
Retrospective reconstruction, 283
Reverse mismatch pattern, 184, 216
Riedel's lobe, 186, 218
Ring artifact, 283
Ring dosimeters, 167, 203
ROC curve, 283
Roentgen (R), 283
Roentgen equivalent man (rem), 42, 71, 282
ROI and lesion size, 98, 134
Rubidium-82 (Rb-82), 6, 13, 23, 41, 46, 51, 58, 70

S
Sagittal slice, brain, 177, 210
Saline flush, 36, 68
Scanner sensitivity, 114, 145
Scanning order, PET/CT protocol, 13, 50
Scatter coincidences, 156, 193
Scatter correction, 178, 211
Scattered foci of hypometabolism, 41, 71
Scatter events, 173, 180–181, 207, 213
Scatter-to-true ratio, 100, 135
Scintillation, 283
Scintillation detectors, PET, 250–251
Scintillators used, PET imaging, 8, 47
Scout scan, 25, 59
Screening, 27, 60
Sealed sources inventory and leak test, 105, 139
Semiology, seizures, 163, 198
Sensitivity, 283
Sensitivity of PT scanner operation in 3D mode, 107, 140

"Sensory relay," 163, 199
Sentinel node biopsy, 16, 53
Sentinel node localization, 25, 59
Shallow-dose equivalent (Hs), 283
Short-axis slices, 18–19, 55
Short half-life, Rb-82, 22, 57
Sievert, 283
Signal-to-noise ratio (SNR), 92, 130, 171, 205
Signet-ring cell carcinoma, 89, 128
Significant quantity, 283
Sinoatrial node, 172, 206
Sinograms, 9, 48, 283
Site boundary, 283
Skeletal muscles, 25, 59
Skin cancer–related mortality, 8, 47
Slip ring, 283
Small intestine, 30, 63
SNR. *See* Signal-to-noise ratio (SNR)
Somatostatin, 111, 142
Somatostatin receptors, 113, 144
Specificity, 283
Specific volume calculation, 255
SPECT imaging, 108, 140
Spinal column stimulator, 283
Squamous cell carcinoma, 232, 242
Stage IIIB lung cancer, 235, 244
Stage III, lymphoma, 161, 197
Stage I, lymphoma, 162, 198
Stage IV of the Cotswold system, 102, 137
Staging, lung cancer, 235, 244
Standard deviation, 284
Standard deviation, series of values, 253
Standardized uptake value (SUV), 15, 30, 52, 63, 80, 86, 122, 126, 227, 240
Standard pressure and temperature (STP), 88, 127
Stochastic effects, 284
Stomach reflux disease, 23, 58
Stopping power, 78, 79, 120, 121
STP. *See* Standard pressure and temperature (STP)
Straton x-ray tube, 166, 202
Stroke penumbra, 235, 244
Student's *t*-test, 88, 127, 284
Stunned or hibernating myocardium, 29, 62
Superficial nodal lesions, 98, 134
Supplemental new drug application (sNDA), 284
Surrogate molecular imaging, 157, 194
Survey, 284
Survey meter, 238, 246
   proper functioning of, 10, 49
SUV. *See* Standardized uptake value (SUV)
SUV max, 17, 53

SUV min, 26, 60
SUV normalization, 92, 130

T
Table increment, 284
Tachyarrhythmias prevention, 180, 213
Tactile sensation, 86, 125
Target, 284
Target organ, 284
Tc-99 m methylenediphosphonate (MDP), 10, 49
Technetium generator, 284
Teratogenic effects, 284
Thalamus, 163, 199
Thallium Tl-201, 25, 59
Therapy monitoring, 95, 132
Thoracostomy tube, 284
Thorotrast, 284
Thymus, 39, 69
Thyroglobulin (Tg) levels, 168, 203, 233, 243
Thyroid, 27, 60
Thyroid cancer, 235, 244
Time delay, coincident annihilation photons detection, 179, 212
Time interval
  PET-FDG imaging after chemotherapy, 18, 54
  PET imaging after biopsy, 14, 52
Time-of-flight imaging, 96, 132
Tissue weighting factor (w_T), 284
Topogram, 114–115, 145
Total-body/whole-body dose, 284
Total effective dose equivalent (TEDE), 164, 200, 284
Tracheostomy tube, 284
Transaxial field-of-view, 284
Transverse colon, 29, 62
Tricuspid valve, 238, 246
True coincidences, 7, 46
True event, 95, 132
Truncation, 77, 120
Truncation artifacts, 5, 45, 82, 123
T-tube drain, 285
Tube current (mA), 153, 191, 284
Tube voltage (kV), 90, 129, 285
Tumor node metastasis (TNM) staging system, 25, 59
Tumors
  low/variable FDG uptake, 165, 200
  recurrence, 102, 111, 137, 143
  total glycolytic volume (TGV), 183, 216
Type II diabetes, 117, 147

U
Unit conversions, 252
Unrestricted area, 285
Uranium fuel cycle, 285
Urinary stent, 285
Use of collimator, 176, 210
Uterine carcinoma, 90, 129

V
Valium administration, 35, 67
Valium administration in dementia imaging, 29, 62
Variance, 285
Variations in count densities, 40, 70
Vascular, 285
  dementia, 17, 54
  system, 34, 66
Vasodilation, 39, 69
Ventricular assist device (VAD), 285
Ventricular bigeminy, 83, 124
Ventricular premature beats (VPBs), 83, 124
Ventriculoperitoneal shunt, 285
Vertebroplasty, 285
Vertical long axis slices, 99–100, 135
Very high radiation area, 285
Virtual colonography, 95, 132
Viscosity, 116, 146, 285
Visual information, 93, 130
Volume of interest (VOI) analysis, 84, 124
Volume-rendered techniques (VRT), 103, 138
VPBs. *See* Ventricular premature beats (VPBs)
VRT. *See* Volume-rendered techniques (VRT)

W
Wash-in study, 105, 139
Waste, 285
Water-15, 156, 193
Water-equivalent contrast agent, 80, 122
Water O-15, 25, 41, 59, 71
Websites, 287–290
Weighted equivalent doses, 9, 48
Well counter efficiency, 253, 254
Whole body, 285
Whole-body dosimeter, 38, 69
Windowing, 285
Wipe test records, 17, 54
Wipe tests, 34, 66, 110, 142

X

X-axis, data plotted on PET, 109, 141
Xenograft, 285
X-ray beam, 96, 133, 164, 199
X rays, 285
X-ray tube current (mA), 104, 138
X-ray tube kV, 117, 147
X-ray tube system energy, 182, 214

Y

Y-axis, data plotted on PET sinogram, 36, 68

Z

Zero Hounsfield units (HU), 10, 49
Zipper artifact, 285
Z-stent, 285

Made in the USA
San Bernardino, CA
16 July 2013